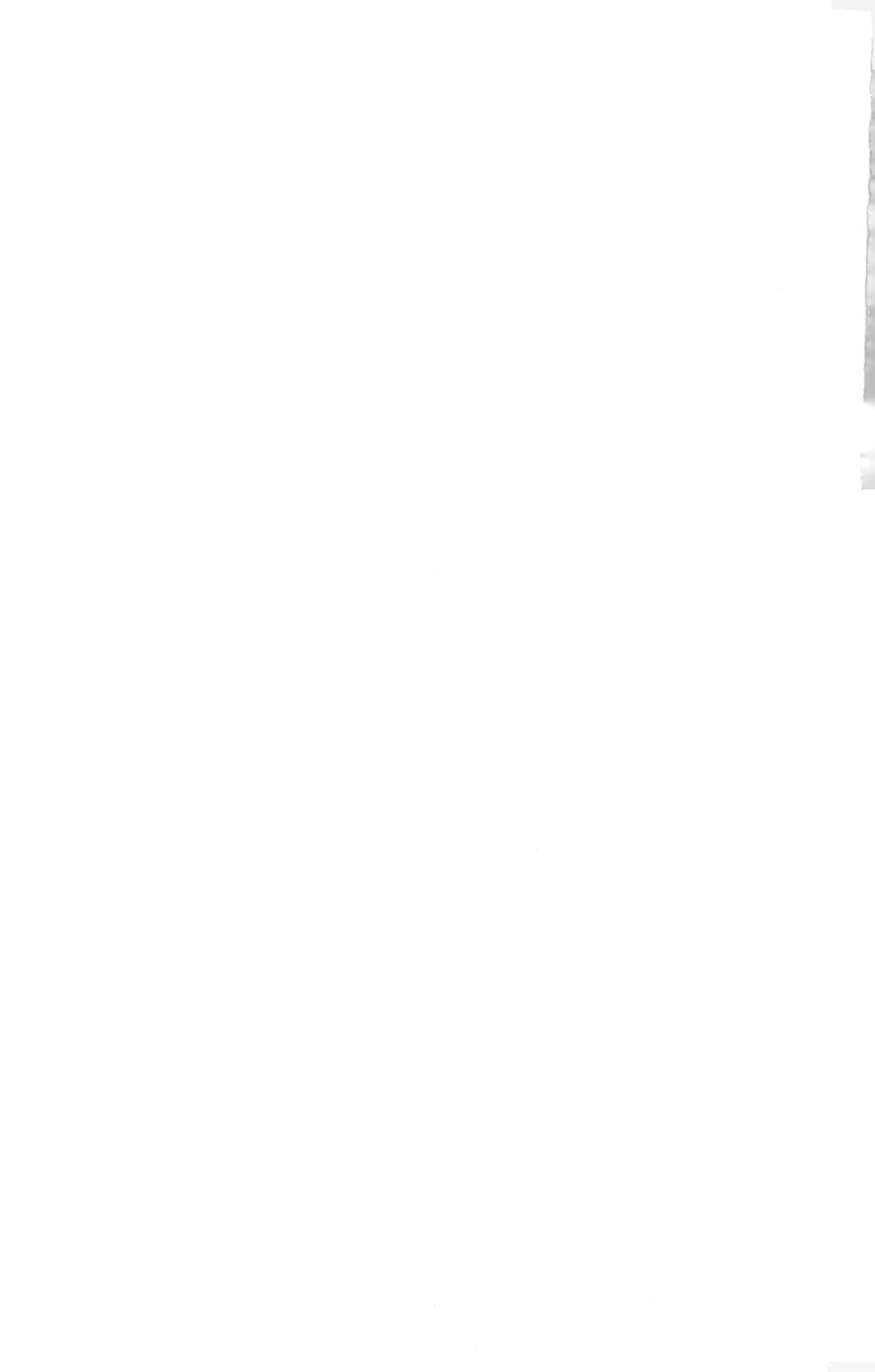

Essential Concepts of Prostate Cancer

Essential Concepts of Prostate Cancer

Edited by **Karl Meloni**

hayle
medical

New York

Published by Hayle Medical,
30 West, 37th Street, Suite 612,
New York, NY 10018, USA
www.haylemedical.com

Essential Concepts of Prostate Cancer
Edited by Karl Meloni

International Standard Book Number: 978-1-63241-215-7 (Hardback)

Printed in the United States of America.

Contents

Preface   VII

Part 1   Introduction   1

Chapter 1   **Prostate Cancer: Essential Diagnostic
and Therapeutic Considerations**   3
Paul Bradley and Philippe E. Spiess

Part 2   Methods in Cancer Biology   11

Chapter 2   **Prostate Cancer, the Long Search
for Etiologic and Therapeutic Factors:
Dietary Supplementation Avoiding Invasive Treatment**   13
Thomas Tallberg and Faik Atroshi

Chapter 3   **Effective Methodologies
for Statistical Inference on Microarray Studies**   33
Makoto Aoshima and Kazuyoshi Yata

Chapter 4   **Advanced Models for Target Validation
& Drug Discovery in Prostate Cancer**   53
Malin Åkerfelt, Ville Härmä and Matthias Nees

Part 3   Signaling Pathways   91

Chapter 5   **Signalling Pathways
and Gene Expression Profiles in Prostate Cancer**   93
Sophia Marsella-Hatziieremia, Pamela McCall and Joanne Edwards

Chapter 6   **Prostate Cancer Dephosphorylation Atlas**   115
Carmen Veríssima Ferreira, Renato Milani,
Willian Fernando Zambuzzi, Thomas Martin Halder,
Eduardo Galembeck and Hiroshi Aoyama

Chapter 7   **TRP-Channels and Human
             Prostate Carcinogenesis**   133
             V'yacheslav Lehen'kyi and Natalia Prevarskaya

Chapter 8   **Clinical Relevance of Circulating Nucleic Acids
             in Blood of Prostate Cancer Patients**   143
             Heidi Schwarzenbach

Chapter 9   **Epidermal Growth Factor Receptor (EGFR)
             Phosphorylation, Signaling and
             Trafficking in Prostate Cancer**   161
             Yao Huang and Yongchang Chang

Chapter 10 **Integrins as Determinants of Genetic Susceptibility,
             Tumour Behaviour and Their Potential
             as Therapeutic Targets**   191
             James R. Marthick, Adele F. Holloway and Joanne L. Dickinson

Chapter 11 **Cytotoxic Endonucleases:
             New Targets for Prostate Cancer Chemotherapy**   215
             Xiaoying Wang, Marina V. Mikhailova and Alexei G. Basnakian

Chapter 12 **Modulation of One-Carbon Metabolism by
             B Vitamins: Implications for Transformation
             and Progression of Prostate Cancer**   231
             Glenn Tisman

Chapter 13 **MAP Kinases and Prostate Cancer**   283
             Gonzalo Rodríguez-Berriguete, Benito Fraile, Laura Galvis,
             Ricardo Paniagua and Mar Royuela

            Permissions

            List of Contributors

Preface

This book throws light on a number of exciting discoveries made in the diagnosis and treatment of prostate cancer over the past decade. International experts have contributed to this book giving a descriptive and advanced review of essentials in diagnostics, methods in cancer biology and signaling pathways essential in prostate cancer. The book serves as a valuable resource for scientists and healthcare professionals related to this field. It is dedicated to the efforts and developments made by our scientific community, realizing we have a lot to learn in striving to cure this disease specifically among those with aggressive tumor biology.

This book is a comprehensive compilation of works of different researchers from varied parts of the world. It includes valuable experiences of the researchers with the sole objective of providing the readers (learners) with a proper knowledge of the concerned field. This book will be beneficial in evoking inspiration and enhancing the knowledge of the interested readers.

In the end, I would like to extend my heartiest thanks to the authors who worked with great determination on their chapters. I also appreciate the publisher's support in the course of the book. I would also like to deeply acknowledge my family who stood by me as a source of inspiration during the project.

Editor

Part 1

Introduction

Prostate Cancer: Essential Diagnostic and Therapeutic Considerations

Paul Bradley and Philippe E. Spiess

Department of Urologic Oncology, Moffitt Cancer Center, Tampa, FL
USA

1. Introduction

The potential impact imparted by prostate cancer on our society is immense. In this chapter, we provide a general overview of current concepts, diagnostic advances, and novel therapeutic approaches to the management of prostate cancer. It is widely reported that prostate cancer is the most common malignancy diagnosed in U.S. males. The current lifetime risk of developing prostate cancer is 17%, with an estimated lifetime cancer-specific mortality risk of 3%. The diagnosis of prostate cancer rapidly increased in the mid-1980s, with the advent of the serological biomarker prostate specific antigen (PSA) which has played a pivotal role in the screening and early detection of prostate cancer worldwide.

From what was almost uniformly a poor prognostic malignancy associated with highly morbid therapies, prostate cancer emerged as a potentially curable disease, with state of the art diagnostic and therapeutic approaches. Advancements in the last 30 years have redefined the surgical approach of localized prostate cancer with minimally invasive surgical approaches for the most part being our primary treatment approach. Additionally radiotherapy techniques have been refined increasing the efficacy and limiting the toxicity to adjacent organs. New systemic and vaccine therapies have most recently emerged as effective approaches to advanced disease.

2. Prostate cancer screening

Prostate cancer screening has evolved since the initial introduction of serum PSA in our screening armamentarium. The discovery of PSA in the 1980s along with an appreciation of its prognostic significance has greatly impacted patient education and surveillance recommendations. Over the last two decades, a stage migration has occurred in favor of small volume, localized disease which we believe is in large part as a direct consequence of the utilization of serum PSA screening. Between 1986 and 1999, there has been a dramatic reduction in the incidence of locally advanced, high volume disease for the similarly proposed reasons. The Prostate, Lung, Colorectal, and Ovary (PLCO) cancer trial of the National Cancer Institute (NCI) was designed to evaluate the effectiveness of prostate cancer screening. It began accruing patients between 1993 and 2001. The study demonstrated a 22% increase in the detection of prostate cancer at 7 years and a 17% increase at 10 years in the patient cohort undergoing annual digital rectal examination

(DRE) and PSA. Despite these findings, the number of deaths between the two study arms were not statistically significant suggesting that screening did not impart a survival benefit with short to intermediate follow-up. The European Randomized Study of Screening for Prostate Cancer (ERSPC) was a similarly designed prospective randomized trial that enrolled 162,387 men. The authors concluded that to prevent a single death from prostate cancer, 1410 men needed to be screened and 48 needed to be treated nevertheless this was a positive study in terms of demonstrating the survival imparted from prostate cancer screening.

Screening using PSA has evolved in recent years by looking at various PSA isoforms and exploring new serological and urinary biomarkers. The evaluation of unbound PSA or free PSA has been proposed in an attempt to improve cancer screening efforts while reducing the number of patients undergoing transrectal prostatic biopsies with its inherent risks, discomfort, and associated healthcare costs. Other novel markers have as well been considered including Prostate Cancer Antigen 3 (PCA3) which was first cited as a potential biomarker for prostate cancer in 1999. It differs from PSA in that it is acquired from the urine following a prostatic massage. Among prostate cancer patients, PCA3 has been found to be upregulated up to a 66-fold in 95% of patients. Although a large validation study has yet to be completed, PCA3 appears to show promise as an adjunctive screening tool to PSA. Additionally, there is an isoform of PSA called proPSA that is mostly found within the peripheral zone of the prostate and within the circulatory system. Multiple variants of this isoform exist with the [-2]proPSA showing the most compelling results pertaining to screening for prostate cancer. [-2]proPSA is the most prevalent form found within prostate cancer cells. Elevations of this variant have also been found to directly correlate with the underlying Gleason score of the tumor. Despite these promising data, the clinical use of these biomarkers remain to be defined until more robust clinical studies validate its superiority versus total serum PSA.

Evolving data pertaining to screening biomarkers and two recent large prospective clinical trials have fueled the controversy regarding screening guidelines and recommendations put forth by various medical governing bodies and organizations. According to the PLCO trial, harm associated directly with screening remains relatively low. DRE can lead to bleeding or significant discomfort/pain in 0.3 per 10,000 screened men. The blood procurement (i.e. phlebotomy) required in PSA screening imparts an associated risk of dizziness, bruising, or hematoma in 26.2 per 10,000 screened men along with 3 episodes of fainting per 10,000. Most importantly, complications from the resulting transrectal prostatic biopsy occurred in 68 per 10,000 cases which included infection, bleeding, and voiding difficulties. In addition, the overtreatment of clinically insignificant tumors which would likely never be biologically aggressive may for the most part only expose patients to the inherent risks and potential morbidities of localized prostate cancer treatments including incontinence and/or erectile dysfunction.

Four organizations currently provide some degree of guidance on the topic of screening. The American Urologic Association (AUA) and the American Cancer Society (ACS) both recommend giving men the option of screening starting at the age of 50 using the combination of PSA and DRE and starting earlier in higher risk men (e.g. patients with first and/or second degree relatives with prostate cancer, certain racial ethnicities such as African Americans). The National Comprehensive Cancer Network (NCCN) has some of the most definitive screening guidelines which include recommending a single total serum PSA test at the age of 40 followed by another PSA at the age of 45, with annual screening thereafter at the age of 50. Prostatic biopsies are recommended based on the NCCN guidelines when a total serum PSA is greater than 2.5 ng/mL. On the contrary, the United States Preventative Services Task Force (USPSTF) provide no guidelines stating that present research on the subject matter is inconclusive and in fact their position statement is against screening men over the age of 75.

3. Chemoprevention

Not surprisingly, along with the rise in the incidence of prostate cancer interest in prostate cancer prevention has come to the forefront. The Selenium and Vitamin E Cancer Prevention Trial (SELECT) is the largest chemoprevention trial in prostate cancer. They enrolled 35,534 participants that were randomized to three arms (one, both, or none of the supplements). Several smaller trials had previously shown a possible reduction in the incidence of prostate cancer among patients taking these proposed chemoprevention agents nevertheless it was felt a larger study was required to more definitely address this clinical question. Unfortunately, the final analysis of this study did not demonstrate a decrease in the risk of developing prostate cancer in either of the chemoprevention arms. In fact, a small increase in the diagnosis of prostate cancer was noted in the group taking vitamin E alone in addition to an increase in the incidence of diabetes among those taking selenium. At this time, the men in this trial have been instructed to discontinue taking these supplements and will be followed for the next three years to evaluate the long-term sequelae of this chemoprevention trial.

The concept of chemoprevention of prostate cancer has gained popularity in the last decade with the results of two large prospective studies (PCPT and REDUCE trials). Both of these trials assessed the impact of selective androgen blockade through 5-α reductase inhibition in an attempt to prevent prostate carcinogenesis. The two trials differed in their design, with the PCPT trial recruiting healthy men with no increased risk of developing prostate cancer whereas the REDUCE trial included men with a higher relative risk of developing prostate cancer. Both studies were positive in that they demonstrated a reduction in the overall incidence of prostate cancer among men receiving an oral 5-α reductase inhibitor.

The PCPT trial evaluated the specific effects of finasteride, with men receiving this agent being 24.8% less likely to develop prostate cancer. The trial however revealed the alarming concern of an increased incidence of higher grade tumors (Gleason 7-10 tumors) in the treatment arm. One proposed explanation for this was postulated to be the change in the appearance of the prostatic cytoarchitecture and cellular morphology as a result of the hormonal effects of finasteride. Another theory is that finasteride selectively inhibits lower grade tumors and shrinks the overall size of the prostatic gland resulting in an overall increase in the number of higher grade cancers detected within a now smaller gland.

The REDUCE trial differed from the PCPT trial in that the inclusion criteria were modified to target men with risk factors for developing prostate cancer as well as using a different 5-α reductase inhibitor (dutasteride) in the treatment arm. This trial included 8,200 men between the ages of 50 and 75 years of age. Men younger than 60 had a baseline total serum PSA between 2.5 and 10 ng/mL whereas older men had a total serum PSA value between 3.0 and 10 ng/mL. Additionally, the participants had a prostate biopsy within 6 months of enrollment demonstrating no evidence of cancer, atypical small acinar proliferation (ASAP), or high-grade prostatic intraepithelial neoplasia. Men were randomized to placebo or the dutasteride treatment arm. The study's primary treatment endpoint was the reduced risk of developing prostate cancer, with the dutasteride treatment arm having a 22.8% relative risk reduction and no increased incidence of higher Gleason grade tumors within the treatment arm.

4. Patient risk stratification

With the increased incidence of prostate cancer cases detected in recent years, a new therapeutic dilemma has arisen in that clinicians have contemplated whether a subset of tumors were clinically insignificant and could be surveilled rather than undergo definitive local therapy. In this regard, risk stratification models have been proposed as a means to tailor treatment recommendations based on the biological aggressivity and risk of progression of the tumor. The Partin tables were first proposed in 1993 in which they developed a cancer specific predictive model based on total serum PSA, biopsy Gleason score, and clinical stage. Patients and clinicians benefited from the use of the Partin tables to counsel and tailor patient treatment recommendations. The D'Amico risk stratification is a simplified version of the Partin tables dividing patients into one of three prognostic categories based on the same three pre-treatment diagnostic parameters (PSA, biopsy Gleason score, and clinical stage). Using the D'Amico risk groups, patients can be stratified into the low, intermediate, and high risk groups serving as an important clinical tool for guiding therapeutic options and suitability for clinical trials.

5. Treatment recommendations

The treatment modalities suitable for localized prostate cancer continue to evolve and expand, with novel technological advances. Dr. Walsh's pioneering work in the anatomical and surgical approach to the radical prostatectomy resulted in a dramatic decline in the reported morbidity of this procedure. Thereafter, Schuessler et al. published the first description of a laparoscopic radical prostatectomy in 1997 with the first case performed in 1991. This technique was however initially abandoned due to its steep learning curve and long operating times, without a clear benefit imparted to patients. With advances in laparoscopic skills and instrumentation, this minimally invasive approach was resurrected before being integrated with modern robotic assisted techniques. Today, nearly 85-90% of all radical prostatectomies are performed using a robotic assisted technique. The questions currently being raised with this technology relates to the expense of this procedure and whether it in fact imparts a clear benefit versus open surgery in terms of cancer control, continence, and potency preservation.

Radiotherapy for localized prostate cancer has evolved by leaps and bounds. External beam radiation therapy (XRT), brachytherapy, and high dose rate (HDR) implant therapy can all be utilized as first line treatment options for localized prostate cancer. Historically, XRT began as a four field box technique fractionating doses over several weeks. This was later replaced by three dimensional conformal radiation therapy and further refined using intensity modulated radiation therapy to limit the dose/toxicity delivered to surrounding tissues while maximizing the therapeutic effective dose delivered to the prostate.

Interstitial brachytherapy can be performed using three different radioisotopes (Iodine 125, Palladium 103, and Cesium 131). Each of these isotopes have different half-lives although all three have reported similar cancer specific outcomes. Interstitial brachytherapy as a monotherapy has become a viable treatment alternative to radical prostatectomy or XRT among patients in the low to intermediate D'Amico risk groups. Using this technique, radioactive seeds are implanted within the prostate under transrectal ultrasound guidance through the perineum and under general anesthesia. Contraindications to interstitial brachytherapy include patients with prostate sizes greater than 60 grams, a previous transurethral resection of the prostate, or significant baseline voiding complaints. The prostate size limitation imparted by brachytherapy result from the fact: (1) large prostates are unable to be completely treated due to the interference by the pubic bone during implantation and (2) patients with large prostates being at increased risk of post-implantation urinary retention. Despite these limitations, brachytherapy remains a popular treatment modality among low D'Amico risk patients, with comparable oncological outcomes to other treatment modalities.

In addition to surgery and radiotherapy, novel ablative therapies including cryotherapy and high-intensity focused ultrasound (HIFU) have emerged as primary local treatments to prostate cancer. Cryotherapy can be used as a primary treatment to localized disease but remains most frequently used as a salvage local therapy. HIFU has gained increasing popularity in recent years as a potential new local treatment for prostate cancer. HIFU was first proposed as a treatment option for prostate cancer in 1999 and entails the use of ultrasonic waves administered using a transrectal ultrasound probe technique. This approach provides an alternative to more traditional modalities such as surgery or radiotherapy. Although not FDA approved in the United States, this technology has been used in many European countries including France and Germany for several years. Long-term data evaluating the oncological outcome of HIFU and contrasting it to other currently available treatment modalities are lacking.

HIFU has also been evaluated as a form of focal therapy for prostate cancer. Unfortunately, data evaluating focal therapy in general have been disappointing. Up to 21% of patients treated by focal therapy may be undertreated according to a study by Katz el al. evaluating post-prostatectomy specimens. All patients in this study who met the original focal therapy criteria would have had a significant secondary tumor missed, with 58.3% of these patients having a final pathological Gleason score of ≥ 7 and 25% exhibiting a final pathological stage of pT3. Based on this and other compelling data, focal therapy appears to be an ineffective therapy in its current applications until we develop better imaging modalities for detecting clinically significant prostate cancer foci within an individual patient's prostate.

The use of neoadjuvant and adjuvant androgen deprivation therapy (ADT) has also been thoroughly investigated. The CaPSURE trial found a 2.6 fold increase in cardiovascular events in men treated with both ADT and RRP compared to RRP alone. Even though one could conceptually see how preoperative ADT would be beneficial, it has never been shown to improve the cancer specific outcomes of patients undergoing RRP (even amongst patients falling within the high risk D'Amico group).

Active surveillance has gained increasing popularity as a treatment alternative for a subset of patients with prostate cancer over the past decade. This has likely resulted from the previously mentioned stage migration of prostate cancer, with a significant proportion of patients presenting with clinically "insignificant" prostate cancer. Debate continues to ensue on the exact therapeutic role and which patients are ideally suited for active surveillance; nevertheless, its viability as a treatment alternative for a significant subset of prostate cancer patients is undeniable.

The management of locally advanced prostate cancer can constitute a therapeutic dilemma for clinicians. Treatment alternatives for these patients include: (1) XRT and adjuvant ADT for 2 to 3 years and (2) RRP +/-neoadjuvant/adjuvant chemohormonal therapy preferably as part of a clinical trial. Recent data from the Memorial Sloan Kettering Cancer Center on the surgical management of locally advanced and high-risk prostate cancer have been encouraging. In this study, 4,708 post-prostatectomy men were retrospectively evaluated and categorized as high-risk based on eight different definitions. Depending on the definition used, between 3 to 38% of these patients were considered high-risk. Interestingly, 22-63% of these men had pathologically organ confined cancer and a 5 year relapse-free probability of 49-80%. This suggests that men with traditionally high-risk disease may still be candidates for potentially curative surgical resection.

There have as well been major advances made in the management of hormone-refractory and metastatic prostate cancer. In this regard, taxotere remains the first line agent for the management of hormone refractory, metastatic prostate cancer. In addition, exciting new data pertaining to prostate cancer include vaccine therapy using Sipuleucel T, abiraterone, and cabazitaxel; all of which may potentially redefine our therapeutic approach to the management of advanced disease.

6. Conclusions

Significant advances have been made in the field of prostate cancer research and clinical/surgical care. Nevertheless, many unanswered questions remain. In addition, the true survival benefit imparted by prostate cancer screening remains a hotly debated issue within the scientific literature. Emerging prostate cancer tumor markers such as PCA3 and [-2]proPSA have not yet been shown to be superior to the current biomarker benchmark PSA. Advancements in laparoscopic technique and technology will hopefully continue to reduce the morbidity associated with radical prostatectomy. Lastly, new therapeutic agents have been discovered which have redefined the management of advanced prostate cancer. We hope the present chapter has highlighted some of the key clinical concepts and treatment principles pertaining to this highly prevalent malignancy.

The aim of the present textbook is to provide an in depth understanding of the intricacies encompassing the diagnosis and management of prostate cancer and encapsulate some of the current exciting areas of active clinical/translational research within our scientific community.

7. References

Andriole GL et al. (2009). Mortality Results from a Randomized Prostate-Cancer Screening Trial. *N Engl J Med*, Vol. 360, No .13, (Mar 2009), pp. 1310-1319

Andriole GL, Bostwick DG, Brawley OW, Gomella LG, Marberger M, Montorsi F, Pettaway CA, Tammela TL, Teloken C, Tindall DJ, Somerville MC, Wilson TH, Fowler IL, Rittmaster RS; REDUCE Study Group. (2010). The Effect of Dutasteride on the Risk of Prostate Cancer. *N Engl J Med*, Vol. 362, No. 13, (Apr 2010) pp. 1192-202

AUA Clincial Guidelines. (2009). Prostate-Specific Antigen Best Practices Statement

Chan TY, Mikolajczyk SD, Lecksell K et al. (2003). Immunohistochemical staining of prostate cancer with monoclonal antibodies to the precursor of prostate-specific antigen. *Urology*, Vol. 62, No. 1, (Jul 2003), pp. 177-81

Chapelon JY, Ribault M, Vernier F, Souchon R, Gelet A. (1999). Treatment of localised prostate cancer with transrectal high intensity focused ultrasound. *Eur J Ultrasound*, Vol. 9, No. 1, (Mar 1999), pp. 31-8

Civantos F, Soloway MS, Pinto JE. (1996). Histopathological effects of androgen deprivation in prostatic cancer. *Semin Urol Oncol*, Vol. 14, No. 2, (May 1996), pp. 22-31.

D'Amico AV, Whittington R, Malkowicz SB et al. (1998). Biochemical outcome after radical prostatectomy, external beam radiation therapy, or interstitial radiation therapy for clinically localized prostate cancer. *JAMA*, Vol. 280, No. 11, (Sept 1998), pp. 969-74

Hessels D, Klein Gunnewiek JM, van Oort I et al. (2003). DD3(PCA3)-based molecular urine analysis for the diagnosis of prostate cancer. *Eur Urol*, Vol. 44, No. 1, (July 2003), pp. 8-15

Jemal A, Tiwari RC, Murray T, et al. (2004). American Cancer Society: Cancer statistics 2004. *CA Cancer J Clin*, Vol. 54, No. 1, (Jan-Feb 2004), pp. 8-29

Katz B, Srougi M, Dall'oglio M, Nesrallah AJ, Sant'anna AC, Pontes J Jr, Reis ST, Sañudo A, Camara-Lopes LH, Leite KR. (2011). Are we able to correctly identify prostate cancer patients who could be adequately treated by focal therapy? *Urol Oncol*, (Mar 2011), Ahead of publication.

Klein EA, Thompson IM, Lippman SM, Goodman PJ, Albanes D, Taylor PR, Coltman C. (2001). SELECT: the next prostate cancer prevention trial. Selenum and Vitamin E Cancer Prevention Trial. *J Urol*, Vol. 166, No. 4, (Oct 2001), pp. 1311-5

Mikolajczyk SD, Millar LS, Wang TJ et al. (2000) A precursor form of prostate-specific antigen is more highly elevated in prostate cancer compared with benign transition zone prostate tissue. *Cancer Res*, Vol. 60, No. 3, (Feb 2000), pp. 756-9

Partin AW, Yoo J, Carter HB, Pearson JD, Chan DW, Epstein JI, Walsh PC. (1993). The use of prostate specific antigen, clinical stage and Gleason score to predict pathological stage in men with localized prostate cancer. *J Urol*, Vol. 150, No. 1, (Jul 1993), pp. 110-4

Schuessler WW, Schulam PG, Clayman RV, Kavoussi LR. (1997). Laparoscopic radical prostatectomy: initial short-term experience. *Urology*, Vol. 50, No. 6, (Dec 1997), pp. 854-7

Smith RA, Cokkinides V, Eyre HJ. (2006). American Cancer Society guidelines for the early detection of cancer, 2006. *CA Cancer J Clin*, Vol 56, No. 1, (Jan-Feb 2006), pp. 11-25

Sokoll LJ, Wang Y, Feng Z et al. (2008). [-2]proenzyme prostate specific antigen for prostate cancer detection: a national cancer institute early detection research network validation study. *J Urol*, Vol. 180, No. 2, (Aug 2008), pp. 539-43

Thompson IM, Goodman PJ, Tangen CM, et al. (2003). The influence of finasteride on the development of prostate cancer. *N Engl J Med*, Vol.349, No. 3, (July 2003), pp. 215-224

Tsai HK, D'Amico AV, Sadestsky N et al. (2007). Androgen deprivation therapy for localized prostate cancer and the risk of cardiovascular mortality. *J Natl Cancer Inst*, Vol. 99, No. 20, (Oct 2007), pp. 1516-24

U.S. Preventive Services Task Force Grade Definitions After May 2007. (May 2008). Available from: http://www.uspreventiveservicestaskforce.org/uspstf/gradespost.htm

Walsh PC, Donker PJ. (1982). Impotence following radical prostatectomy: insight into etiology and prevention. *J Urol*, Vol. 128, No. 3, (Sept 1982), pp. 492-7

Yossepowitch O, Eggener SE, Bianco FJ Jr, Carver BS, Serio A, Scardino PT, Eastham JA. (2007). Radical Prostatectomy for Clinically Localized, High Risk Prostate Cancer: Critical Analysis of Risk Assessment Methods. *J Urol*, Vol. 178, No 2, (Aug 2007), pp. 493-9

Part 2

Methods in Cancer Biology

Prostate Cancer, the Long Search for Etiologic and Therapeutic Factors: Dietary Supplementation Avoiding Invasive Treatment

Thomas Tallberg[1] and Faik Atroshi[2]

[1]*The Institute for Bio-Immunotherapy, Helsinki*
[2]*Pharmacology & Toxicology, ELTDK, University of Helsinki*
Finland

1. Introduction

The lack of a comprehensive aetiology for prostate cancer (CaP), and the need for an effective and inexpensive biological treatment modality, devoid of side-effects has resulted in a multitude of therapeutic trials. None of these has been very satisfying, and they have vaned from focal to invasive therapies for CaP. The progress has been delayed and hampered by the lack of any thorough effort to elucidate the cause of the disease. Such efforts would have speeded up the introduction of more rational therapy modalities. The different incidence of CaP in populations aroused our interest to proceed in a more physiologic way to empirically test different functional f factors, since they are non-toxic, although such an approach is consuming time. It was ethical to test the effect of these natural alimentary components, and follow the patients´ reaction and laboratory responses. Huggins and Hodges[1] had already, in 1941, decisively proven that CaP was a hormone dependent disease, although castration alone was not curative. In 1945 Huggins and Scott performed bilateral adrenalectomies[2] after the glands were found to produce DHEA, which could be transformed into testosterone, regarded to have caused recurrent disease. All patients died in a short time postoperatively. However, Huggins did not recognize that this showed the central position the adrenals had in regulating prostate cancer. In this paper we shall review some cases of prostate cancer treated patients. For these we especially follow the shift in FSH, LH, PRL, DHEA, DHEAS, SHBG, plus PSA. The involvement of adrenal glands became evident with an orchiectomized prostate cancer patient with excessively high FSH 120 IU/L and immeasurable PSA. In MRI (magnetic resolution imaging) there was no pituitary adenoma which could explain this high level, but both his adrenal glands were evenly hypertophic. Upon laparatomy the enlargement was due to bilateral zona reticularis (ZR) cell proliferation, while the adrenals other cell structures were normal. These bluish cells with strong green fluorescence had via the hypothalamus stimulated the pituitary to greatly increase FSH and LH, see Case A below with normal laboratory ranges displayed (the row at the top in all cases).

The Importance of adrenal ZR cells is unveiled by: A) their marked proliferation after orchiectomy; B) lack of ZR cells in castrated male pigs [eunuchs]; C) markedly decreased number of ZR cells in patients succumb-bing to CaP; D) the hormonal effect in extracts made from ZR cells of castrated boars; E) rapid lethal out-come if CaP patients after *orchiectomy* are also *adrenalectomized*. This operation was conclusively remo-ving the adrenal lifesaving functions of unknown fictive factors; Cycloprostatins No. I (increasing FSH-) & No. II (increasing PRL-levels).

FSH	LH	PRL	DHEA	DHEAS	Testost	Inhibin	Activin	S-Ferrit	SHBG	PSA
IU/L	IU/L	mU/L	nmol/L	μmol/L	nmol/L	pg/ml	pg/ml	μg/L	nmol/L	μg/L
1-9	2.5-12	50-300	3.0-17.0	0.5-8.0	9-38	~60	300-500	16-253	15-55	<4.0
120	53.8	228	3.2	1.9	0.8	<7.8	330	65	48	<1

Case A.

Cancer can be regarded as a complex metabolic deficiency disease. Nutritional therapy has few negative side effects, as it is a non-invasive treatment. In traditional Chinese medicine feeding patients with exotic herbs could help in curing them. At that time it was impossible to analyse the precise functional factors ingested, but we seem now to have reached an academic form of traditional Chinese medicine since we can include specific pure alimentary components to construct a supportive curative diet. Spontaneous regression of cancer is rare[3], and has been called "The metabolic triumph of the host"[4]. It implies that these patients by chance have ingested a complicated combination of bio-modulating natural components to regain the internal balance in their diseased body. The curative effect does not seem to involve apoptosis[5]. These observations signify that the complex metabolic deficiency triggering cancer, and also genetic weaknesses, can be compensated by feeding patients specific functional alimentary components. Strivings to delineate such metabolic factors has finally, after over 35 years, resulted in the present possibility to improve cancer therapies in a physiologic way - by dietary supplementation. This finding naturally also backs screening tests, since overtreatment can now be avoided. The aim of this long empiric study was actually to decrease the need for expensive invasive treatments, which are all marred by grave side-effects. We will in this article give a short resume´ of how these multiple biological factors were found, over the last decades.

Our cancer therapies usually only try to remove the symptoms by surgery or irradiation, but not to correct the actual aetiology, although the most important aim for cancer treatments should be to strive to avoid recurrent disease. Therefore there is a natural motivation to apply active bio-immunotherapy in many cancer forms. Present treatments are like treating a scurvy patient by extracting his loose teeth but not giving him vitamin-C!

Prostate cancer (CaP) is the most common form of malignancy in men. We find 5,000 cases per year in Finland, with 800 men succumbing to CaP in great pain due to multiple bone metastases. In China and India one million men are diagnosed with CaP every year about 15% dying of it. Last year approximately 300,000 cases were found in the European Union while 200,000 patients were diagnosed in the USA, and 27,000 died of CaP. The yearly casualty rate in Germany is 12,000 men, while in England 10,000, and they pass on in a very painful way from bone metastases. They should all have a chance to be clinically tested whether they have a satisfactory positive response from this physiologic treatment modality before they are remitted to different invasive therapies, which are all expensive, not physiologic, and cause grave side-effects.

Over the years, to facilitate the search, we developed working hypotheses to outline the meta-bolic regulating codes for our three main forms of cancer[5], schematically presented in Fig 1. The diseased body can take up these multiple components and restore the multi-

Prostate Cancer, the Long Search for Etiologic and Therapeutic Factors: Dietary Supplementation Avoiding Invasive Treatment

15

factorial balance securing normal health. Basically the elementary compounds are composed by natural organic and inorganic and neurogenic lipid molecules forming the correction of multifactorail deficiency disease/cancer. These components are; amino acids, essential trace-element ions, vitamins and lipids.

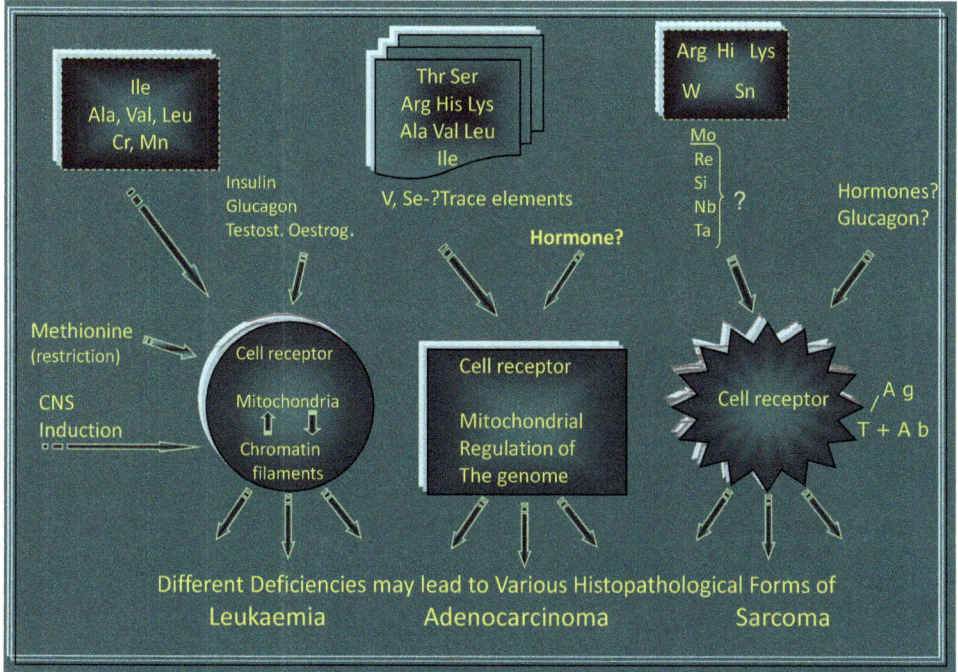

Fig. 1. The hypothetic cell regulatory code for our three main forms of cancer; leukaemia, adenocarcinoma, sarcoma. The combined effect of amino acids, trace element ions and lipids involved in the inductional control mitochondrial Regulation, epigenesist, immune reactions secure normal health.

The incidence of CaP has increased world-wide, and already 5000 new cases were diagnosed in Finland last year, and 800 died in intensive pain due to incurable bone metastases. In China and India 1 million cases are detected yearly, while 300,000 in the European Union, and 200,000 in USA, of which 40,000 and 27,000 respectively succumb to this painful disease. This high incidence has naturally led to a lot of therapeutic trials. None of these treatments for CaP has been completely satisfactory.

An economical, biological treatment modality which does not cause side-effects seems therefore to be urgently needed. This suggested physiologic dietary therapy is inexpensive devoid of side-effects and has the potential to contribute significantly to a comprehensive response to cancer. Curative clinical results obtained by feeding patients with exotic herbs in traditional Chinese medicine have given a positive clinical results, and must be regarded as a clear signal that mammals have a physiologic capacity to reverse malignant cells back into healthy transcription without apoptosis. In modern biotherapy this biological effect can be simulated by a balanced oral intake of the numerous missing alimentary components, in pure form. They act as a specific functional food. The regulating code is certainly more complex than the iodine deficiency causing endemic goitre. Our studies have indicated that co-operation by several organs is involved with the adrenal glands in a central position[6,7]. Figure 2. These unknown human adrenal biological factors are harboured in zona reticularis cells and they can be activated by feeding the alimentary components,[8] listed in Table 1.

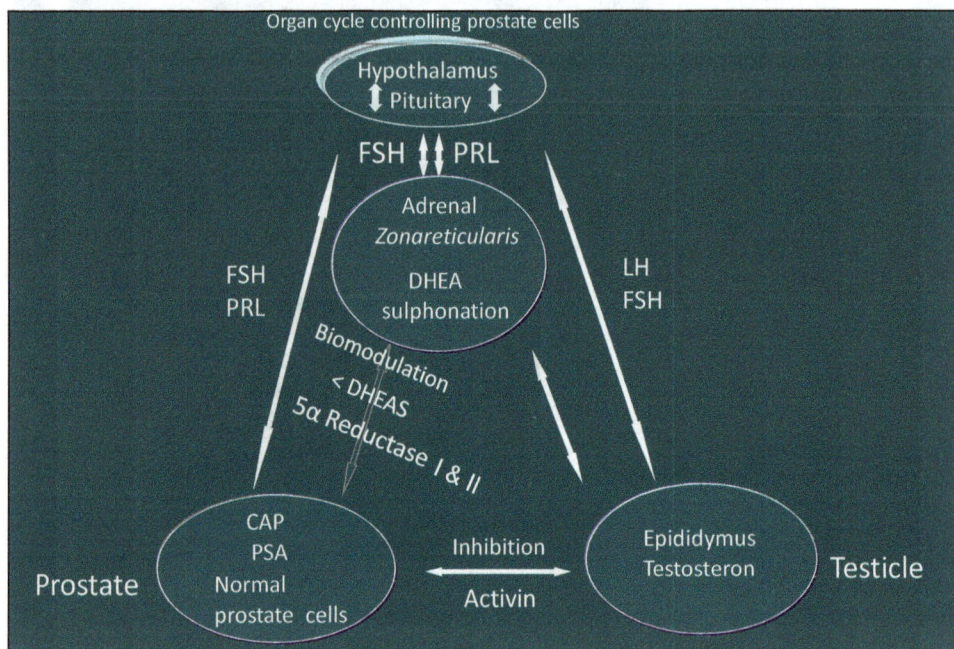

Organ cycle controlling prostate cells

Hypothalamus
Pituitary

FSH PRL

Adrenal
Zonareticularis

FSH
PRL

DHEA
sulphonation

LH
FSH

Biomodulation
< DHEAS
5α Reductase I & II

CAP
PSA
Normal
prostate cells

Prostate

Inhibition

Activin

Epididymus
Testosteron

Testicle

Fig. 2. A schematic "organ cycle" controlling cancer of prostate gland. Adrenal zonareticularis (ZR) cells are in a central position responsible for keeping prostate cells in normal function.

1.1 Present prostate cancer treatments

Prostatectomy, External Beam Radiation therapy (EBRT), Brachytherapy (intensity modulated), Three – Dimensional conformal, Low-Dose Brachytherpy, Cryotherapy, Local therapy, Lumpectomy, Systemic Therapy LHRH analogue implants, ADT androgen depletion therapy, Watchful Waiting,High-intensity focused ultrasound (HIFU) therapy, Vascular - Targeted (VTP), Photodynamic Therapy (PTD) using light-sensitive agents with local laser activation, leading to cell-destruction, Nonspecific dietary therapy (except a la, Tallberg), BMI risk, 5-alpha I & II reductase inhibition (Dutasterid, Proscar, Finasterid), Robotic-Assisted Radical Prostatectomy, Hyperthermia, Immune therapy, Life-style Trial, etc.

1.2 Adverse effects of treatments

Anaemia, Cognitive decline, Depression, Erectile dysfunction /libido loss, Fatigue / General weakness, Gastrointestinal symptoms, Gynecomastia, Bone fractures, hormonally related, Hot flashes, Lipid abnormalities, Osteoporosis, Weight gain/redistribution, Muscle wasting,

Increased fat deposition, General decrease in quality of life, and Marital Problems due to the hormone therapy, Stress, etc.

1.3 Clinical results

A regression of cancer reveal that cancer this complex chronic metabolic deficiency disease, may be cured by non-toxic dietary restoration of the healthy internal bodily milieu of the patient 5[4,5]. Specific mitochondria restore tumour cells to normal healthy transcription without apoptosis or cell destruction[6]. The incentive to try to delineate certain of the physiologic factors entailed in malignant transformation of patients suffering from CaP was bearing successful clinical results obtained with bio-immunotherapy for renal cancer[9], cutaneous and choroideal melanoma[8] in bio-immunotherapy. A positive clinical effect implicated a combined effect caused by specific metabolic dietary substitution, supported by specific active immunological stimulation of the patients' immune defense. The vaccine made from the patient´s own tumour tissue will be directed against autologous antigenic markers, representing the finger print of pertinent tumour markers[9]. For prostate cancer active immunotherapy *is not prescribed* since PSA is a serine protease metabolite, and not a true tumour marker. PSA could decline during immunization but the PSA antibody titer had not sufficient capacity and therefore PSA regained pathologic levels after 8 months[10].

2. Dietary amino acids in attempts to correct the metabolic deficiency causing cancer

The causes of CaP seem rather to be environmental than genetic, and dietary habits have a pronounced effect on prostate cancer incidence. The low incidence of CaP in Japan and Italy may be linked to the local ingestion of the amino acid serine (Ser) contained in soy and parmesan in Italy, further supported by the vitamin-like substance lycopene contained in tomatoes. The original idea that cancer represented a deficiency disease affecting amino acids was presented by Dr Howard Beard, already in 1941- 42[11,12]. He could cause impressive regression of established sarcoma in rats from daily injections of the three basic amino acids (Arg, His, Lys). Our efforts were, therefore, based on studies on the effect of natural non-toxic alimentary components. The effect, based on our rat leukaemia model, showed that the regulatory code was completely different from that of sarcoma. In both experimental models there was, however, a trend effect caused by feeding rats with Threonine (Thr) and Serine (Ser). Our efforts were therefore based on studies on the effect of natural non-toxic alimentary components.

The effect, based on our rat leukaemia model, showed that the regulatory code was completely different from that of sarcoma. If patients ingest the natural amino acid Ser, PSA which actually is a serine protease - the PSA activity declines. The Ser absorbed into the patients´ blood decreases PSA, through substrate inhibition. This is more physiologic and effective than the tyrosinase inhi-bition caused by Glivec. This stimulated our interest to advance in a more physiologic and rational way, selectively feeding patients natural alimentary factors and analysing the effect on CaP, although it would take a long time to delineate pertinent physiologic metabolic factors, linked to the hormonal balance. Huggins and Hodges had decisively proved that CaP was a hormone depen-dent disease, although castration as a single treatment was not curative[1].

Spontaneous cures of cancer are so rare because the etiological dietary deficiency leading to cancer is more complex than the simple lack of iodine causing endemic goitre. The statistical chance of getting multiple components in the right proportion, and long enough, to compensate a longstanding metabolic deficiency is extremely small without external active help. These positive findings based on dietary effects should lead us to a new paradigm for cancer therapies founded on restoring the physiological internal balance of the body. It has really improved our under-standing and biological means for treatment and prophylaxis of malignant cell proliferation. We are optimistically reforming prevailing toxic clinical treatment modalities, based on mistaken paradigm to kill all cancer cells with cytostatics instead of trying to regain the curative healthy internal balance.

The lack of an effective biological non-invasive treatment alternative, has led to the risk of over-treating patients. Our standard therapies are un-physiologic, and few methods are curative if app-lied in an advanced stage of CaP. The lack of aetiological understanding has led to a multitude of not well founded therapeutic trials. The progress has been hampered by the lack of thorough strivings to elucidate the cause of the disease. Such efforts would have made it possible more rapidly to find rational therapy modalities. The aim of our study, for over 35 years, has therefore been to clarify aetiology and prognostic traits in patients' suffering from different stages of pros-tate cancer. A better understanding of the causes for CaP could improve biological treatments and dietary schedules[13]. Presently, there is a new incentive for screening, since there is now an applicable biological treatment for CaP. In an early stage, while it still is possible to get a positive clinical response[14], patients should be tested for their response to this physiologic treatment modality.

2.1 The importance of administering trace-element ions

In Dr.H. Beards original studies[11,12] causing complete regression of experimental rat sarcoma from daily injections of 18 mg of all three basic amino acids (Arg, His, Lys). Regression of sarcoma stemmed from a complex formed between the basic amino acids and wolfram (W) ions. A related signal system was found with experimental leukaemia. In mammals the required trace-element ions were different, Cr and Mn formed the regulating signal with Ala, Ile, Leu, & Val preventing induction of leukaemia. In both these studies there was a positive trend effect with Serine and Threonine, hinting that the adeno-carcinoma regulatory code could comprise supplementation with Ser to male patients, while Threonine may be involved in female adeno-carcinoma. The PSA level decreased most likely due to substrate inhibition caused by the thus increased level of the natural amino acid Serine in the patients´ serum neutralizing his protease enzyme (PSA). We got very valuable support from Prof. Klaus Swartz the head of the only trace-element free laboratory in the world in Los Angeles. He kindly extrapolated from his rat experiments how much a minimal daily amount of essential trace-element ions a human 70 kg body would need. The mg amounts and ionic form listed in Table 1 are based on his suggestions.

An interesting observation was that Strontium may have been involved in regression of bone metastases. It was revealed when the ash a patient ingested, whose bone metastases had regressed, were analyzed for metals by proton-induced X-ray emission. It revealed that he had got 7mg of strontium (+ rubidium and 40 mg Zn daily), in addition to the trace-element ions we originally used (Table 1). Radioactive strontium was earlier used to scan bone-metastases. If repeatedly used it did not work because only ten percent of the i.v. bolus (of 85 mg) was actually radioactive. The non-active strontium molecules could block the tumour cell receptors and render the scanning unreliable. This is why we presently use technetium. It hinted that Sr played a role in the healing system of bone metastases in CaP

Prostate Cancer, the Long Search for Etiologic and Therapeutic Factors: Dietary Supplementation Avoiding
Invasive Treatment

19

patients[7,15]. Vanadine and Arginine (V & Arg) had previously been shown to arrest bone metastases in renal cancer cases[16].

Furthermore, Gly and Glu were fed to act as substrate inhibitors and prevent inflammatory reactions in the prostate gland (chronic Pin) caused by splitting the tri-peptide glutathione activating the inflammatory leukotriene cascade (Figure 3). Boron (B) is also an inhibitor of Gammaglutamyl transpeptidase which splits glutathione and may thus prevent sterile inflammatory reactions caused by the Leukotriene - B_4, C_4, D_4 & E_4 cascade - ending in the slow reacting substance of anaphylaxis (SRS-A)[17].

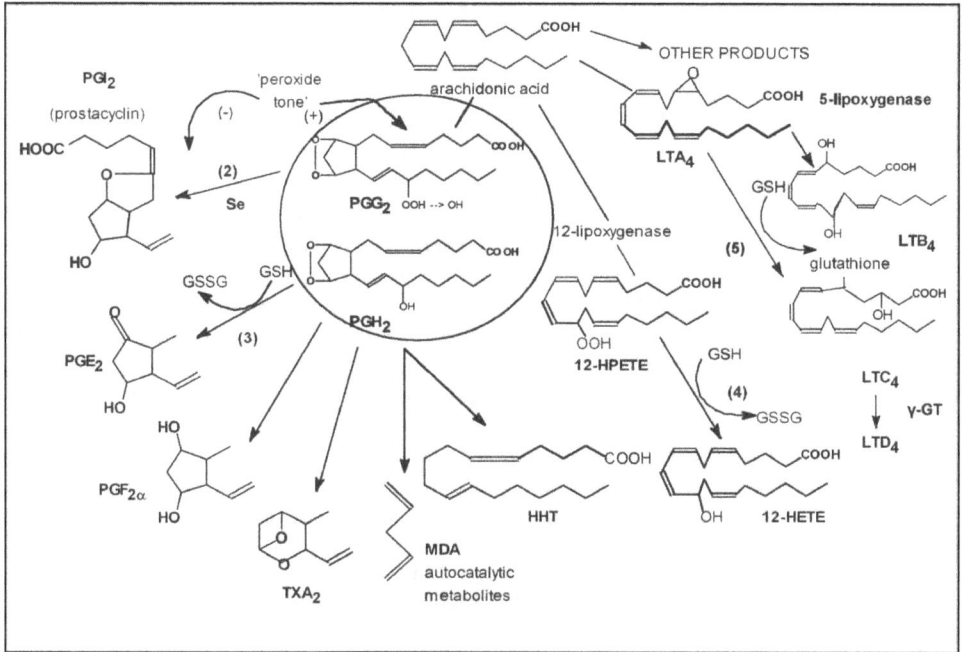

Fig. 3. Possible roles of the tri-peptide GSH in arachidonic acid metabolism (1 to 5). GSH reduces PGI_2 and increases PGE_2 formation. PGE_2-forming isomerases (3) require GSH as essential cofactor (cosubstrate). PGs are involved in the hyperalgesia of inflammation[31]

Molybdate (Mo) had an effect on the female menstrual cycle[13] to make it completely regular, and could perhaps activate a minute oestrogen production even in male patients. Due to side-effects oestrogen therapy for CaP has been stopped but a small physiologic stimulation may be beneficial? Vanadate together with Arg seemed to prevent and cure bone metastases in renal cancer patients and were therefore included as a possible natural co-factor complex related to the renal tissue.

2.2 The importance of administering lipids (CNS) to cancer patients

The enormous abundance of lipid molecules in the central nervous system (CNS) suggests that their role is not limited to be structural and energetic components of cells. Over the last decades, some lipids in the CNS have been identified as intracellular signalers, while others are known to act as neuromodulators of neurotransmission through binding to specific receptors. Neurotransmitters of lipidic nature, currently known as neurolipids, are synthesized during the metabolism of phospholipid precursors present in cell membranes. That central nervous lipid molecules were involved in keeping malignant cells in healthy transcription was observed already in the seventies[11]. CNS-lipid molecules were detected by thin layer chromatography to be present in the serum of cancer patients, following Herpes virus infections. The viral infection had caused lesions in the blood-brain barrier, and vital lipids had leaked out into the patients' blood. The minimal idea was to try to compensate this depletion by feeding patients with the lipids they had lost to corrected the depressed enzyme activity, on the patients' buffycoat cells in three days[17] and restored his natural immunity [lymphopoiesis] thanks to the activity of an un-identified titanium containing CNS-lipid molecule. The importance and vital function of millions of CNS-lipids the "lipidome" has constantly been overlooked. They have a variety of crucial functions, from embryogenesis to securing healthy mental and motor balance as presented earlier [13]. One of the most important factors is this Ti containing CNS-lipid, which stimulates the patients' immune reactions and alleviates neurologic pain. These CNS-lipids can be absorbed by nerves from the serum and normalize neuronal function. Millions of vital lipids present in the CNS can preserve the inductional control over all cells in a cancer patient. Pain is actually a warning signal that the nerve tissue cannot produce certain CNS-lipids, but when these become available through ingestion they circulate in the blood and are absorbed by the nerves, while decreasing the patients' distress. Following alimentary correction of the metabolic deficiency activated cell specific mitochondria can then be seen, by electron microscopy, to force cancer cells to regain a healthy form, without apoptosis[18, 19]. This Bio-Immunotherapy method has successfully been applied in randomized prospective studies in hundreds of patients suffering from melanoma (103 skin + 54 eye)[12], or metastasized renal cancer (127 cases)[15,16] a study was performed at Helsinki University[20].

3. Mitochondrial involvement linked to the healing reaction, without causing tumour cell lysis

The effect of specific dietary supplementation for prostate cancer is usually fairly rapid and seen in 6-8 weeks; the laboratory profile is shown here. These transformed mitochondria can be revealed since they become electron dense (black) because the enzymes in their crista gather significant amounts of metal ions [Cr, Fe, Zn, Ti, & Rb] when they become activated[6,18].

FSH	LH	PRL	DHEA	DHEAS	Testost	Inhibin	Activin	S-Ferrit	SHBG	PSA
IU/L	IU/L	mU/L	nmol/L	µmol/L	nmol/L	pg/ml	pg/ml	µg/L	nmol/L	µg/L
1-9	2.5-12	50-300	3.0-17.0	0.5-8.0	9-38	~60	300-500	16-253	15-55	<4.0
4.2	4.5	269	2.1	1.5	5.7			130	61	53.7
7.8	6.9	151	< 2.0	1.3	11.1			149	55	3.7

Case B. Typical laboratory profiles of a patient on specific functional dietary supplementation. FSH and Testosterone increase at the same time as PSA, DHEA, & DHEAS declines, indicating a good prognosis.

A biopsy taken from same lobe as previously showed a Gleason score of 7, revealed in EM that the tumour cell nucleus was surrounded by transformed mitochondria, Figure 4. Two

Prostate Cancer, the Long Search for Etiologic and Therapeutic Factors: Dietary Supplementation Avoiding Invasive Treatment

21

of them empty their electron dense activated enzymes into the nucleus when PSA had decreased to 3.7 µg/L, and he was clinically in good condition [Magnification x 10,000.]. They healed without apoptosis. If the initial PSA level is over 15 ng/mL the therapy has usually been started with combined hormone (e.g. LHRH Zoladex 3.6mg for months duration) supplemented by dietary measures. When PSA decreases rapidly as in Case B, following supplementation with both prostate powders (No1 & No2) in synergy with intermittent total anti-androgen blockade (Zoladex, 3.6mg + Androcur, 50mg x 2/day, for only 10 days) the PSA-level fell also rapidly from 34.3 ng/mL to 2.3 ng/mL in six weeks. In EM the tumour cell nucleus is often seen to be surrounded by transformed mitochondria which are electron dense, due to the increased content of Cr,Fe, Zn, Ti, & Rb [18] when the tumour progress is arrested Similar mitochondrial transformation with activation in the curing phase of mammalian malignant cells, triggered by this physiologic non-toxic biologic therapy has been seen in EM with experimental animal models (rat & horse[13]), in addition to episodes with human patients suffering from melanoma, and malignant histiocytoma[18,22]

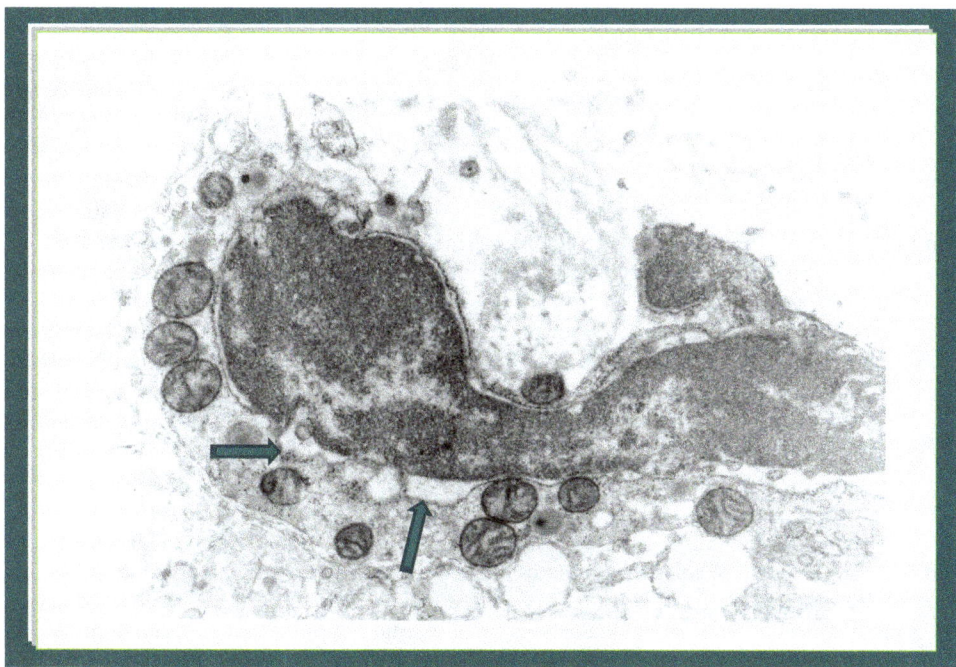

Fig. 4. Electron microscopy showing (magnification 10.000) with electron dense organ specific mitochondria Surrounding the tum cell nucleus when PSA normalized. Two mitochondria seem to empty their electron dense material into the nucleus when the patient was cured, without apoptosis.

4. Adverse effects caused by certain biological components

Alanine administration may increase the PSA-level and food items high in Ala should be avoided. Administration of DHEA 25mg per day is definitely contraindicated since it led to intensive pain and the patient died in three weeks from multiple bone metastases. Hormone refractory prostate cancer (HRPC) is not due to the emergence and selection of a hormone refractory cell clone. It seems to be the result of a too intensive LHRH treatment (continuous injections with 3 months duration) when the hormone therapy has been used to reach PSA nadir. Instead FSH and LH have decreased to <0.1 IU signaling adrenal feed-back exhaustion involving adrenal ZR cell function. The pituitary is not malfunctioning as PRL can increase to > 1000 mU/L. A brooding HRPC is seen when PSA, is forced to levels under 0.9 µg/L, due to excessive anti-androgen therapy, while PRL exceeds 600 mU/L indicating that the pituitary is not exhausted.

5. Attempts to actively increase FSH and PRL in patients, or the use of autologous vaccines failed

The positive prognostic effect of increased FSH- and prolactine (PRL) levels led to attempting active stimulation. Ingestion of extracts made from ZR cells of castrated male pigs can cause a marginal positive effect on FSH and PRL for a short time but no human forensic material was available for testing. Forensic human adrenal ZR-cell extracts should be tested as they probably contain these biologic stimulatory factors. If they could be characterized it could lead to a natural substitution therapy for CaP, like insulin is for diabetics.

Daily Injections with human FSH (75 -150 U/L) could increase the FSH-level for a short time, but would be impracticable in the long run, and too expensive. FSH-releasing factor was even less effective. Then again injection of human prolactin PRL or HCG had only a marginal effect on PSA. Attempts to externally increase FSH or PRL-levels did not seem to be functional. Physiologic stimulation directed at the adrenal glands appears to be the only practical therapeutic way.

Immunisation using autologous tumour polymer particles can decrease PSA-levels for some months but is not curative because PSA is only a metabolite, and not a regular tumour marker[10].

5.1 Description of some prognostic features in cases of specific dietary supplementation for CaP

The most important laboratory test to be taken immediately when CaP is suspected, or actually diagnosed, is to analyze the serum levels of FSH, LH, PRL, DHEA, DHEAS, SHBG, and f/t PSA. PSA as a single marker is not alone sufficient, since it can be held down by an increased FSH- or PRL-level. A high FSH-level and low DHEAS with decreasing PSA is a good prognostic sign, and this effect caused by alimentary supplementation is usually fairly rapid. In one patient of the earliest cases found by screening tests his PSA rose from 4.3 ng/mL to 6.4 in two months with a Gleason of 7. He was then routinely scheduled for prostatectomy. With informed consent he preferred to test this biological alternative, safeguarded by regular PSA controls, and immediate change back to the invasive treatment option if his PSA rose. On a double dietary daily dose and CNS-lipids, his PSA declined to 2.3 ng/mL in half a year, followed by diminished urinary distress, and without any side-effects. He opted then to take the prostate supplements only once a day. In half a year his PSA had once more started to rise and the double dose was reinitiated. The dose response was again positive, as his PSA-level declined to normal levels. His CaP became then stable for 6 years in continuous dietary therapy, but a slight increase in his PSA-level was seen (from 6 – 7 ng/mL over four months), when Arg substitution had been stopped for some time. This was to test if this component really was necessary to keep his PSA-level stable. The urologists persuaded him then immediately to accept prostatectomy, although we would have preferred to reinstate Arg to see if it would reduce PSA anew. His prostatectomy specimen showed that his Gleason score had declined to 4, and no growth of the prostate tumour tissue had occurred. This unnecessary operation stopped anyhow further biological treatment for CaP, as all tumour cells had been removed. We did not pay sufficient attention to the fact that this patient had, before his prostate cancer was diagnosed, also suffered from Crohn´s disease, however, most clinical symptoms had almost disappeared during his biological treatment for CaP[23]. Four years later his symptoms of Crohn´s disease of Crohn's had recurred, and he was consequently operated for colon cancer. This awoke our interest for sterile inflammatory diseases like, ulcerative colitis, rheuma, fibromyalgy, psoriasis polyarthritis[24] etc. The probable common denominator was the effect caused by supplementation with CNS-lipids which we had included to quell chronic prostatitis as a precancerous state for CaP. Administration of this lymphopoietic, Ti containing CNS-lipid molecule was aimed to normalize inflammatory reactions with the aid of this vitamin-like CNS factor, which now also seemed to affect other sterile inflammatory diatheses, as mentioned above.

In some patients the effect of a sole dietary supplementation is slow and protracted as shown in Case C. In this case ingestion of prostate powders (our cocktails) 1/day, alternatively 2/day, and CNS-lipids increased slowly the patients FSH- and LH-levels & constantly low DHEAS and rising testoteron while PSA is low, in the normal range. Dietary supplementation alone has kept him in stable disease, now for over five years. His starting Gleason score was 8.

	FSH	LH	PRL	DHEA	DHEAS	Testost	Inhibin	Activin	S-Ferrit	HBG	PSA
	IU/ L	IU/ L	mU/ L	nmol/ L	μmol/ L	nmol/ L	pg/ ml	pg/ ml	μg/ L	nmol/ L	μg/ L
	1-9	2.5-12	50-300	3.0-17.0	0.0-8.0	9-38	~60pg /ml	~500pg /ml	16-253	15-50	<4.0
2005	5.4	<0.01	48	5.5	1.5	4.9			455	77	<0.2
2006	8.4	2.5	83	3.2	1.2	5.6			376	82	<0.2
2007	13.8	6.2	114	3.5	1.0	10.2			313	61	0.22
2010	20.5	12.3	103	3.5	1.1				347	60	0.49

Case C.

A positive reparative reaction seems to be flagged by an increase in the FSH- LH- and prolactin (PRL) levels. Revelation of these unknown stimulatory factors could form a decisive prevention for the emergence of a "hormone refractory state", leading to improvement.

Case D. This patient was succumbing to CaP, 11.1996, [T4NxM1] with multiple bone met - 11/94] had orchiectomy -94, three years earlier. Initially PSA 92.6 decreased after orchiectomy 1994 to 5.7- 5.3 (-95) in combined bio-modulation but without Sr. He stopped the intake of all dietary components and became androgen independent (-96). PSA rose to

119 ng/mL, and he died showing extreme laboratory values, as measured from a blood sample taken the same day before his exitus.

FSH	LH	PRL	DHEA	DHEAS	Testost	Inhibin	Activin	S-Ferrit	SHBG	PSA
1-9	2.5-12	50-300	3.0-17.0	0.5-8.0	9-38	~60	300-500	16-253	15-55	<4
<0.1	<0.1	1060	7.2	6.8	0.6				2145	364

Case D.

The marked increase in PRL affirm that the pituitary function is not depressed and it is feverishly trying to save the patient, but without a concomitant FSH increase the case is lost.

His laboratory values have oscillated during all these years but conspicuously FSH has stayed high all the time indicating a continuous adrenal feed-back reaction which could involve in preventing recurrent disease.

FSH	LH	PRL	DHEA	DHEAS	Testost	Inhibin	Activin	S-Ferrit	SHBG	PSA
IU/L	IU/L	mU/L	nmol/L	μmol/L	nmol/L	pg/ml	pg/ml	μg/L	nmol/L	μg/L
1-9	2.5-12	50-300	3.0-17.0	0.5-8.0	9-38	~60	300-500	16-253	15-55	<4.0
67-30	37-16	159-95	< 2.0	< 0.8	1.0	< 7.8	330	109-99	58-61	< 0.1

Case E. CaP detected with PSA 30 μg/L with multiple bone metastases. Orchiectomy was performed 1992. Dietary bio-modulation + Strontium (7mg/day) started 1993. His periostal pain subsided in four months. All bone metastases disappeared 1996. He is now in excellent clinical condition 2011.

In patients with hurting bone metastases to get these to regress they may need to be orchiectomized if during the dietary substitution they have recurrent bone metastases. After castration the bone metastases could totally regress in half a year. This improved clinical result after recurrent CaP may signal that some factor in the testicular tissue is produced which during a prolonged biological therapy may arrest the positive effect of the full dietary substitution although it supplies many of the required factors; Sr, V, Ser, Arg etc. If this is required in selected cases for s cure it may be worth the castration, a fairly simple operation compared to prostatectomy, since the survival time of CaP with multiple hurting bone metastases is otherwise only 8 months ?.

Of the more than ten patients who were orchiectomized , all who not have got any adjuvant supportive dietary treatment have died. Some of them lived up to 8 years after castration, which is better than Huggins and Hodges got in the early forties. On the contrary, castrated patients who continuously have got our supportive metabolic functional alimentary factors are alive in good clinical condition, as well as those cases that have not been epidydectomized, but have been on dietary supplementation in synergy with short time intermittent hormone treatment. In certain cases the continuous hormone treatment with LHRH has been possible to stop completely, without leading to recurrent disease, with follow-up presently already over 5 years, as in Case B.

Prostate Cancer, the Long Search for Etiologic and Therapeutic Factors: Dietary Supplementation Avoiding Invasive Treatment

25

5.1.1 Short time intermittent hormone treatment blocks hormone refractory prostate cancer induction

Short time intermittent LHRH hormone treatment is definitely recommended as it has prevented the development of hormone refractory states.

FSH	LH	PRL	DHEA	DHEAS	Testost	Inhibin	Activin	S-Ferrit	SHBG	PSA
IU/L	IU/L	mU/L	nmol/L	µmol/L	nmol/L	pg/ml	pg/ml	µg/L	nmol/L	µg/L
1-9	2.5-12	50-300	3.0-17.0	0.0-8.0	9-38	~60pg/ml	~500pg/ml	16-253	15-50	<4.0
(Short time intermittent androgen ablation treatment with Zoladex 3.6mg + cyproteronacetate)										
15.2	16.1	993	3.8	2.4	6.4	75	410	1500	45	13.4
(Three months after Androcur 50mg x 2/day for 10 days to avoid flare-up after Zoladex 3.6mg injections.)										
4.2	7.3	1490	2.5	1.6	5.8	72	430	1100	2.5	
(Three months later when the activated adrenal feed-back has time to increase FSH and sometimes also PSA)										
15.2	17.7	1520	2.2		< 0.8	76	500	993	14.5	

Case F. Lab assay profiles during recommended short time intermittent LHRH treatment, Zoladex 3.6mg,+ Androcur 50mg X2/day with many months intervals, in synergy with specific dietary supplements.

Zoladex 3.6 mg inj can then be repeated, if also PSA has increased as in this case. If PSA stays low Zoladex would not need to be repeated as it stays low due to synergy with supplementation. One should not strive to reach a PSA nadir. Avoid injection of Zoladex 10.8mg every third month becau-se the adrenal feed-back will be exhausted, and FSH declines to < 1.0ng/mL. This is not due to pituitary dysfunction because PRL can start to increase when the body in vain is trying to defend itself (see Case C). This ominous turn is not due to selection of a hormone refractory cell clone, but to ZR exhaustion, as the adrenal glands have not been allowed to function during a necessary intermission in the hormone therapy. If the FSH-level is depressed to under 1 ng/mL it is a signal that the adrenal feed-back has been exhausted, but not the pituitary since PRL can be markedly increased (600 – 1060 mU/L), indicating a brooding HRPC.

Growth factors, activin & inhibin. Dramatic changes were seen after castration, during pregnancy and estrogen substitution therapy. CaP diagnosed by soft tissue biopsies had also specific profiles Inhibin and activin patterns changed dramatically in patients detected from soft tissue metastases, and not from biopsies of their prostate gland. A shift characterized by a very depressed inhibin level was seen in castrated patients, as well as during normal pregnancy, and in healthy females on estrogen substitution.

CaP patients diagnosed from the presence of *soft tissue metastases represent a special from* of prostate cancers (possibly neuroendocrine?). They may have markedly high serum activin-levels ((1890- 2180 pg/ml) paired with low inhibin-levels (25-34 pg/ml). Initially their serum ferritin levels are high (1164-2499 µg/ml), while DHEAS (< 0.8 – 1.8) and DHEA (2.2 - 2.4) are low. FSH-levels are normal or low (1.9 -5.1 IU/L) while LH-levels are undetectable (<0.1 IU/L). Case G. had a PSA-level of 10070 µg/L, while the other similar case showed a PSA of

246 µg/L. In both patients their PSA decreased to 5.3 µg/L, and 2.1 µg/L respectively in half a year, following intermittent short cycle LHRH therapy, in synergy with bio-modulating dietary measures. The high activin levels were not appreciably affected by the therapy, while PSA was decreased markedly, to normal levels.

FSH	LH	PRL	DHEA	DHEAS	Testost	Inhibin	Activin	S-Ferrit	SHBG	PSA
IU/L	IU/L	mU/L	nmol/L	µmol/L	nmol/L	pg/ml	pg/ml	µg/L	nmol/L	µg/L
1-9	2.5-12	50-300	3.0-17.0	0.0-8.0	9-38	~60pg/ml	~500pg/ml	16-253	15-50	<4.0
5.1	<0.1		2.4	1.8	<0.8	25	2900	1164		10070.0
combined hormone and dietary therapy led to CR of metastases (CR) and to normal PSA										
6.2	<0.1					22	2650	316		5.3

Case G. CaP was detected from neck metastases and he had also bone metastases. A special characteristic was extremely high activin- and PSA-levels 10,070 µg/L which decreased to 5.3 µg/L, in 6 months following combined intermittent short time LHRH plus dietary therapy. All soft tissue metastases regressed and he was in good health.

His extremely high activin 2900 and PSA-level of 10,070 µg/L, decreased in intermittent short time hormone therapy to 5.3 µg/L, in 6 months in combined LHRH + biological therapy. Patients don't die of high PSA, but of depressed FSH (< 0.1 ng/mL, due to adrenal feed-back exhaustion).

Orchiectomized CaP patients generate an increase in their FSH-levels to, 40 – 130 IU/L, in some months, but show also a characteristically manifestly *depressed serum inhibin level* *(<7.8 pg/ml)* while their activin level (~ 560 pg/ml) is normal. Surprisingly healthy *pregnant females revealed a similar change* in their inhibin / activin levels, with a correlation value of 1:70, until parturiency when the "growing cell-mass" – the healthy child is borne and the related value again becomes normal. Alarmingly also estrogen substitution (already 50 µg plasters) in postmenopausal women can show a similar dramatic change in their inhibin / activin correlation values. Such a provoked change in a females serum growth factor levels – usually actively made to *last more than nine months* by their gynaecologists – could easily fool the body that it should produce growing cells. This anomalous change may explain the observed increased breast-cancer and lymphoma incidence generated by estrogen substitution therapies in otherwise healthy females. The effect of *estrogen substitution therapy*, prescribed to any female patient, *should therefore obligatory be monitored by inhibin / activin assays*, to see *if it causes a reaction simulating pregnancy,* since it may physiologically be misinterpreted, and consequently generate proliferating (malignant?) cells.

The growth factor "activin" is appreciably increased (5-6x) in the serum of patients suffering from a rare special form of CaP, primarily diagnosed from soft tissue metastases, and not from the prostate gland. Strontium (Sr) is an essential component of the periost, and this trace-element is involved in curing bone metastases caused by ingestion of Sr 7mg/day. It has eradicated multiple metastases, now with a follow-up of over eighteen years - without recurrent disease. Ingestion of DHEA is contra-indicated since it can activate CaP. Autologous vaccines applied for CaP is not cura-tive and has only a short-time effect, since PSA is not a regular tumour marker but a metabolite.

5.2 Unfavorable clinical events

Excessive hormone treatment is unfavorable, e.g. LHRH analogue treatment using continuous injections with three months duration (> 10mg) in an effort to reach a PSA nadir exhausts the adrenal feed-back reaction and causes HRPC. FSH will then also decline to < 1.0 ng/mL. Excessive needle biopsies (12 -24 cores) may spread malignant CaP cells and could be the reason for the high recurrency rate of 35 -40 % following prostatectomies [25] . The use of specific serum markers [26] , MIR, PSA velocity etc. should decrease the need for un-necessary cores, and the few biopsies actually needed should be directed more precisely. The side effects with pain, and caused inflammations would diminish. This biological treatment schedule would anyway be the same disregarding the numbers of cancer focuses in the different lobes of the prostate gland.

The dietary effect which increases FSH is sometimes protracted. In Case E. it took 9 months of continuous prostate powder ingestion to cause an increase from 5.4 to 8.4, and after 5 years it had risen to 20.5 IU/L. The response to dietary therapy is **fairly progressive** so that one can judge, in months, if the patient will respond to this specific dietary supportive therapy based only on standard laboratory tests, FSH increases and DHEAS decreases etc. Initially increased FSH or PRL-levels are good prognostic signs and should always be analyzed when CaP is found by screening tests, since invasive treatments can be avoided. The human adrenal biological factors harbored in the zona reticularis (ZR), fictively called cycloprostatin I & II, should be purified from forensic healthy human adrenal material aided by assays for their stimulatory effect on the pituitary. The clinical use of such purified factors could form a biological compensatory medical treatment for CaP.

1.	Oral administration of each (2-5g/day) of respective L-amino acids; Arg, Asp, Glu, Gly, Lys, & Ser, all in connection with meals.
2.	Essential trace-element salts prescribed orally as biologically active ions, at dose levels of some milligrams (1-3mg/day); Chromium ($CrCl_2.6H_2O$) 6mg (=1.17 mg Cr), Molybdenum ($Na_2 MoO_4 .2 H_2 O$) 4mg ($\approx$ 2mg Mo), Rubidium ($RbCl_2 . 2 H_2O$) 1-10mg ($\approx$ 7mg Rb), Tinn ($SnCl_4.5H_2O$) 4mg (=1.35mg Sn), Strontium ($SrCl_2$) 1-7mg ($\approx$ 4mg Sr), Vanadine ($Na_2VO_4.4 H_2O$), 6mg (= 2.5 mg V), Wolfram ($Na_2WO_4. 2 H_2O$), 4mg (=2.3mg W), Zink (= Zn 30mg).
3.	Physiologic dosages of vitamins; A,B,C,D,E,K , folic acid and lycopene.
4.	To improve lymphopoiesis and the immune-defence of patients a diet containing prion-free neurologic lipids (micro-capsulated CNS-lipids).
5.	Dose-levels are adjusted based on the clinical response as measured during the therapy, and correlated to the patients´ body weight.
6.	Transformed organ specific mitochondria participate in the curing phase of CaP.

Table 1. As Cancer is a complex metabolic deficiency disease it is curable by dietary supportive measures.

5.2.1 Un-interrupted hormone therapy may cause HRPC, avoided by short time intermittent treatment

The effect of hormone therapy for CaP, in recommended intermittent short time pulses combined with metabolic bio-modulation activates a feed-back reaction recorded as characteristic changes in the laboratory response profile, with FSH, LH and/or PRL increase trailed by DHEAS and PSA decreases, a reaction in which adrenal ZR cells seem to have a central regulatory function. Orchiectomy will cause FSH to increase, further accentuated by prostatectomy. Prostate cancer patients die in a short time if orchiectomy is followed by adrenalectomy which attests the importance of functional adrenal glands. A dramatic rise in activin levels is recorded in a special form of CaP, diagnosed in biopsies from soft tissue metastases. Inhibin is again remarkably decreased following orchiectomy. A similar depressed inhibin level was surprisingly also seen in normal pregnancy, and during the popular estrogen substitution therapy. If estrogen substitution in postmenopausal females cause a growth factor shift mimicking pregnancy her body may not understand that cells, especially malignant cells, should not be allowed to multiply. The increased breast cancer incidence may possibly be connected with this unnatural shift in the levels of these, inhibin/activin, growth factors [13,15]. Patients on estrogen substitution should be tested for these growth factor levels to see if they inadvertently have been rendered to belong to a risk zone for malignant cell proliferation?

Complete regression of CaP shows that this complex posses chronic metabolic deficiency disease can be treated by non-toxic dietary restoration of the healthy internal milieu in the patient activating organ (cell) specific mitochondria to restore normal healthy transcription of malignant cells without apoptosis or cell destruction as seen in Figure 4. The improvement could be due to activation of cell/organ specific mitochondria which regulate the genome, and can force oncogen transcription back to a normal healthy form[21, 22]. This was first seen in rats in which induction of leukaemia was prevented by activated, electron dense cell-specific mitochondria functioning at body temperature [18]. They were found to lose their inductive regulatory potency if stored at +4 ^{0}C (because we are warm-bloodied?). The enzymes in mitochondrial crista were activated by metal ions; Cr. Fe, Zn, Ti, Rb, and this metal increase made them electron dense, and possible to observe by EM[22].

5.2.2 Mitochondria inducing healing, correcting mutations, activation of stem- cells & transplantation

Most of our standard treatments represent a poor practice alternative often in the form of a toxic therapy for a complex metabolic deficiency disease, and by only removing the symptoms, which make patients prone to suffer recurrent disease in 35 -40% even after prostatectomy. Patients who after the operation later on start to show a biochemical increase in PSA, supposedly due to a non-radical operation, or to the active spread of malignant cells by excessive biopsy cores (12-24). A chronic inflammatory (Pin) reaction may be induced by these bloody interventions, and any inflammatory reaction is potentially carcinogenic [23,24] , like we see e.g. as a sequel of the lack of a lymphopoietic central nervous lipid molecule - linked to titan - resulting in an aberrant immune-response as in; Crohn´s disease, ulcerative colitis, rheuma, psoriasis, & fibromyalgy [24,30] etc. This physiologic deficit can be compensated by the intake of CNS-lipids (and/or butter) [23,24,30]. If these lipid precursors are present in the patients´ blood the depletion caused by daily stress can be compensated during our sleep.

Prostate Cancer, the Long Search for Etiologic and Therapeutic Factors: Dietary Supplementation Avoiding
Invasive Treatment

29

A well directed biopsy core may suffice to evaluate the Gleason score. This functional dietary treatment will principally be the same disregarding the number of actual CaP focuses.

6. Conclusion

The primary effort of this long study was to characterize etiological factors for CaP before starting any big randomized series. Instructive features compiled from approximately 70 patients suffering from different forms and stages of CaP were followed-up for decades. This has resulted in a recommendation to apply these findings in a biological treatment modality. Understanding of the nature of that particular tumour it can help us to optimize therapy or to design therapeutic approaches. Patients after prostatectomy may not respond as well to dietary supplementation with activation of the adrenal ZR feed-back cycle, since this organ cycle may require or involve also normal pros-tate cells to be fully effective. Probably prostatectomy should not be performed before one has had time to evaluate the patients´ responses to this physiologic bio-modulating treatment. The positive clinical effect of continuous dietary treatment is prolonged, and is today already extending over 19 years in a case who initially suffered from multiple hurting bone metastases[13] . This beneficial adrenal fed-back activation has continuously been stimulated by ingestion of the biological factors listed in Table1.

An efficient biological treatment modality devoid of side effects and economical, will give scree-ning for CaP a new rational, since the progress of the disease can now be arrested and even bone metastases be cured in a physiologic way. The dispute over the marginal improvement in survival rates between patients on Watchful Waiting over cases that are prostatectomized could be missed by the fact that neither group has received any biological supportive treatment to compensate the actual aetiological metabolic deficiency. And thus the surgical removal of symptoms of CaP (i.e. prostatectomy) does not censure the aetiological deficiency[7, 15].

The importance of mitochondrial function, linked to the memory of the nucleotide sequence in the chromosomes they have created [21] can explain how identical mutations in both chromosomes can lead to that 10% of the off-springs have lost the mutation, and are healthy. This does not require a change of Mendel´s law since mitochondrial memory could explain this surprising result as they correct the mutation during replication [28] ! Correction of the fault can occur when mitochondria have a memory of what they have created [21,27]. The interesting study by Hohlfelds group on paediatric skin burns may be explained by the possibility that cell specific mitochondria transgressed from the male skin transplant they used into the female receptor-cells, whereby the full genome present in any of her cells could transform into her own skin – a "transplant" which cannot be rejected. This represents a further step of refined "stem-cell" activation, which is not hemmed by restrictions presently affecting stem cell studies [28] . To efficiently learn to use *cell-specific mitocho-ndria and epigenesis* in biology and medicine will be the scientific challenge of this century!

7. Aknowledgements

We thank all co-workers, mentioned in the references, for their continuous efforts to shape this vital biologic treatment modality. These studies have for decades been supported by grants from the Albert Lindsay von Julin Foundation.

8. References

[1] Huggins, C.; Hodges, C.V.: Studies on prostate cancer: I. Effect of castration, estrogen, and androgen injection on serum phosphatases in metastatic carcinoma of the prostate. Cancer Research 1 (1941) 293-97.

[2] Huggins, C.; Scott, W.W. Bilateral adrenalectomy in prostate cancer. Ann Surg. 1945: 22, 1031-41.

[3] Everson T.C. Spontaneous regression of cancer. Ann NY Acad Sci. 1964:114; 721-35.

[4] Cole W.M. Spontaneous regression of cancer. The metabolic triumph of the host. Ann NY Acad Sci 1974:239; 111-15.

[5] Tallberg T. Cancer treatment, based on active nutritional bio-modulation, hormonal therapy and specific autologous immunotherapy. J Aust Coll Nutr & Env Med. 1996: 15 No.1, 5-23.

[6] Tallberg T. Biological cancer therapy, its effect on inductional control, triggered by hormones and mediated by transformed mitochondria. J Austr Coll Nutr & Env Med. 1998: 17; 17-24.

[7] Tallberg Th. Studies on cancer of the Prostate Gland, a search for Aetiological and Prognostic Factors. J Aust Coll Nutr & Env Med. 2003:22 No.2; 11-16

[8] Tallberg T. A Possibility to Prevent Recurrent Melanoma, Renal, Breast and Prostate Cancer Utilizing Inexpensive Powders Containing Specific Dietary Supplementary Factors. J Aust Coll Nutr & Env Med. 2005:24 No.3; 3-9.

[9] Tallberg T. Development of a combined biological and immunological cancer therapy modality. J Aust Coll Nutr & Env Med. 2003: 22 No.1, 1-20.

[10] Tallberg Th., Klippel K.F. Effect on PSA from combined therapy with LHRH-analogue, specific immune- therapy, and active biomodulation. Fourth Eur Urol Winter forum. Abstr. Davos Feb.19-25th 1995.

[11] Beard H.H. The effect of parental injection of synthetic amino-acids upon appearance, growth and dissapperance of emge sarcoma in rats. Arch Biochem. 1942:1; 177-85.

[12] Beard H.H. Effect of subcutaneous injection of individual amino-acids upon the appearance, growth and disappearance of Emge sarcoma in rats. Exp Med Surg. 1943:1; 123-35.

[13] Tallberg Th. Regulation of cancer by therapeutic vaccination and dietary bio-modulation involving organ specific mitochondria. Int J Biotechnology. 2007: 9, ¾; 391-410.

[14] Thomas Tallberg and Mervi Dabek. Prostate Cancer, Aetiological, Therapeutic, Prognostic and Prophylactic Factors. Anticancer Research. 2008 :28 No.5C; Abstr.658, 3507-3508.

[15] Tallberg Th., M. H. Dabek. Dietary substitution therapy of prostate cancer patients: A possible nonivasive treatment. Int J Trends in Med. 2011: 1; 21-27.

[16] Tallberg Th., Tykkä H., Mahlberg K. et al. Active specific immunotherapy with supportive measures in the treatment of palliatively nephrectomised, renal adenocarcinoma. 1985: 11; 233-43.

[17] Tallberg Th., Tykkä H., Halttunen P. et al. Cancer immunity. The effect in cancer immunotherapy of polymerized autologous tumour tissue and supportive measures. 1979: 39; Suppl. 151. 1-35.

[18] Tallberg, T., Stenbäck, H., Hallamaa, R., Dabek, J., Johansson, E., Kallio, E. Studies on mitochondrial regulation of the genome. Deutsche Zschr Onkol. (German J Oncol) 2002: 34; 128 -39.

[19] Tallberg Th., Hallamaa R. Cancer Regulated by Organ-Specific Mitochondria Via Lipidomics, Genomics and Proteomics. Anticancer Res. 2008: 72 No.5C; Abstr.659

[20] Tykkä H. Active specific immunotherapy with supportive measures in the treatment of advanced palliatively nephrectomised renal adenocarcinoma. A controlled clinical study. Scand J Urol Nephrol 1981, pp. 1- 107.

[21] Tallberg Th. Mitochondria seem to regulate the genome in the chromosomes they have phylogenetically created. Trends in Biomedicine in Finland 2000: ISBN 951-98382-1-X, pp. 36-38.

[22] Tallberg Th., Stenbäck H., Dabek J., Palkama A. Complete disappearance of human malignant histioc- cytoma cells following dietary biotherapy, leading to activation of inductional control mediated by mitochomdria. J Austr Coll Nutr & Env Med. 1996: 15 No 2 ; 5-10.

[23] Tallberg Th. Lipidomics, the function of vital lipid molecules forming our brain and spinal cord. J Trends in Biomed. 2008: 3 No1; 6-19.

[24] Tallberg Th. Biological dietary treatment of inflammatory bowel disease. The XL Nordic Meeting of Gastroenterolgy 8-11 June 2009, Stavanger, Norway Abstr P12.

[25] Capitanio U., Ahyal S., Graefen M. et al. Assessment of Biological Recurrence Rate in Patients With Pathological Confined Prostate Cancer. Urology 2008:72 (6); 1208-1213.

[26] Leman L.S., Cannon G.W., Trock B.J. et al. EPCA-2: A Highly Specific Serum Marker for Prostate Cancer. Urology 2007:69 (4), 714-720.

[27] Hohlfeld, J., de Buys Rossingh, A., Hirt-Burry, N., Chaubert, P., Gerber, S., Scaletta, C., and Hohlfeld, P. Tissue engineered fetal skin constructs for paediatric burns´. Lancet 2005 (Research Letters), August 18, DOI: 10.1016/50140-6736(05)67107-3, pp.1-3.

[28] Lolle, S.L., Young, J.M., and Pruit, R.E. Genom-wide non-mendellan inheritance of extra-genomic information in Arabidopsis´, Nature 2005:434;505-509.

[29] Tallberg Th. Constrains linked to stem cell research, as compared with the refined medical regulation of cell-induction caused by organ/cell specific mitochondria. BIT´s 3rd Annual Protein and Peptide Conference (PepCon-2010), Cancer Research, March21-23, 2010.

[30] Tallberg Th., Dabek J., Hallamaa R., and Atroshi F. Lipidomics: The function of Vital Lipids in Embryogenesis Preventing Autism Spectrum Disorders, Treating Sterile Inflammatory Diatheses with a lymphopoietic Central Nervous System Component. J Lipids: Volume 2011, Article ID 137175, 6 pages. doi:10.1155/2011/137175.

[31] Atroshi F., Sankari S., Työppönen J. and Parantainen J. Inflammation related changes in trace elements, GSH-metabolism, prostaglandins and sialic acid. In: Trace Elements in Man and Animals 6 (Hurly LS ; Keen CL; Lonnerdal Bo, & Rucker RB, Editors), Plenum Press, New York & London, 1988, pp.97-99.

3

Effective Methodologies for Statistical Inference on Microarray Studies

Makoto Aoshima and Kazuyoshi Yata
Institute of Mathematics, University of Tsukuba, Ibaraki
Japan

1. Introduction

A common feature of high-dimensional data such as genetic microarrays is that the data dimension is extremely high, however the sample size is relatively small. This type of data is called the high-dimension, low-sample-size (HDLSS) data. Such HDLSS data present with substantial challenges to reconsider existing methods in the multivariate statistical analysis. Unfortunately, it has been known that most conventional methods break down in HDLSS situations and alternative methods are often highly sensitive to the curse of dimensionality.

In this chapter, we present modern statistical methodologies that are very effective to draw statistical inference from HDLSS data. We focus on a series of effective HDLSS methodologies developed by Aoshima and Yata (2011) and Yata and Aoshima (2009, 2010a,b, 2011a,b). We demonstrate how those methodologies perform well and bring a new insight into researches on prostate cancer.

In Section 2, we first consider Principal Component Analysis (PCA) for microarray data to visualize a data structure having tens of thousands of dimension by projecting on a few dimensional PC space. We note that classical PCA cannot sufficiently visualize a latent structure of microarray data because of the curse of dimensionality. We overcome the difficulty with the help of the *cross-data-matrix (CDM) methodology* that was developed by Yata and Aoshima (2010a,b).

Next, in Section 3, we consider an effective clustering for microarray data. We apply the CDM methodology to estimating the principal component (PC) scores. We show that a clustering method given by using a CDM-based first PC score effectively classifies individuals into two groups. We demonstrate accurate clustering by using prostate cancer data given by Singh et al. (2002).

Further, in Section 4, we consider an effective classification for microarray data. We pay special attention to the quadratic-type classification methodology developed by Aoshima and Yata (2011). We give a sample size determination for the classification so that the misclassification rates are controlled by a prespecified upper bound. We examine how the classification methodology performs well by using some microarray data sets.

Finally, in Section 5, we consider a variable selection procedure to select a set of significant variables from microarray data. In most gene expression studies, it is important to select relevant genes for classification so that researchers can identify the smallest possible set of genes that can still achieve good predictive performance. We implement the two-stage variable selection procedure, developed by Aoshima and Yata (2011), that provides screening of variables in the first stage. We select a significant set of associated variables from among a set of candidate variables in the second stage. We show that the selection procedure assures a high accuracy by eliminating redundant variables. We identify predictive genes to classify patients according to disease outcomes on prostate cancer.

2. PCA for high-dimension, low-sample-size data

Suppose we have a $p \times n$ data matrix $X = [x_1, ..., x_n]$ with $p > n$, where $x_k = (x_{1k}, ..., x_{pk})^T$, $k = 1, ..., n$, are independent and identically distributed as a p-dimensional distribution having mean μ and positive-definite covariance matrix Σ. The eigen-decomposition of Σ is given by $\Sigma = H \Lambda H^T$, where Λ is a diagonal matrix of eigenvalues $\lambda_1 \geq \cdots \geq \lambda_p (> 0)$ and $H = [h_1, ..., h_p]$ is a matrix of corresponding eigenvectors. Then, $Z = \Lambda^{-1/2} H^T (X - [\mu, ..., \mu])$ is considered as a $p \times n$ sphered data matrix from a distribution with zero mean and the identity covariance matrix. Here, we write $Z = [z_1, ..., z_p]^T$ and $z_j = (z_{j1}, ..., z_{jn})^T$, $j = 1, ..., p$. We assume that the fourth moments of each variable in Z are uniformly bounded and $||z_j|| \neq 0$ for $j = 1, ..., p$, where $|| \cdot ||$ denotes the Euclidean norm. We note that the multivariate distribution assumed here does not have to be a normal distribution, $N_p(\mu, \Sigma)$, and the random variables in Z do not have to be regulated by a ρ-mixing condition. We consider a general setting as follows:

$$\lambda_j = a_j p^{\alpha_j} \ (j = 1, ..., m) \quad \text{and} \quad \lambda_j = c_j \ (j = m+1, ..., p). \tag{1}$$

Here, $a_j (> 0)$, $c_j (> 0)$ and $\alpha_j (\alpha_1 \geq \cdots \geq \alpha_m > 0)$ are unknown constants preserving the ordering that $\lambda_1 \geq \cdots \geq \lambda_p$, and m is an unknown positive integer. The model (1) is an extension of a multi-component model or spiked covariance model given by Johnstone and Lu (2009). This is a quite general model for high-dimensional data. For example, a mixture model given by (6) in Section 3 is one of the examples that have the model (1) as in (7). One would also find the model (1) in a highly-correlated, high-dimensional data analysis such as graphical models, high dimensional regression models, and so on.

Let $X_o = X - [\bar{x}, ..., \bar{x}]$, where $\bar{x} = \sum_{i=1}^{n} x_i / n$. The sample covariance matrix is given by $S = (n - 1)^{-1} X_o X_o^T$ and its dual matrix is defined by $S_D = (n - 1)^{-1} X_o^T X_o$. Note that S_D and S share non-zero eigenvalues. Let $\hat{\lambda}_1 \geq \cdots \geq \hat{\lambda}_{n-1} (\geq 0)$ be the eigenvalues of S_D. Let us write the eigen-decomposition of S_D by $S_D = \sum_{j=1}^{n-1} \hat{\lambda}_j \hat{u}_j \hat{u}_j^T$, where $\hat{u}_j$'s are the corresponding eigenvectors of $\hat{\lambda}_j$ such that $||\hat{u}_j|| = 1$ and $\hat{u}_i^T \hat{u}_j = 0 \ (i \neq j)$.

2.1 Naive PCA in HDLSS situations
Yata and Aoshima (2009) gave sufficient conditions to claim the consistency property for the sample eigenvalues: For $j = 1, ..., m$, it holds that

$$\frac{\hat{\lambda}_j}{\lambda_j} \xrightarrow{p} 1 \tag{2}$$

under the conditions:

   (YA-i) $p \to \infty$ and $n \to \infty$ for j such that $\alpha_j > 1$;

   (YA-ii) $p \to \infty$ and $p^{2-2\alpha_j}/n \to 0$ for j such that $\alpha_j \in (0, 1]$.

Here, $\xrightarrow{p}$ denotes the convergence in probability. If z_{jk}, $j = 1, ..., p$ ($k = 1, ..., n$) are independent, the above conditions are improved by the necessary and sufficient conditions as follows:

(YA-i') $p \to \infty$ and $n \to \infty$ for j such that $\alpha_j > 1$;

(YA-ii') $p \to \infty$ and $p^{1-\alpha_j}/n \to 0$ for j such that $\alpha_j \in (0, 1]$.

For the details including the limiting distribution of $\hat{\lambda}_j$, see Yata and Aoshima (2009). If the population distribution is $N_p(\mu, \Sigma)$, one may consider that z_{jk}, $j = 1, ..., p$ ($k = 1, ..., n$) are independent. When $\alpha_j > 1$, the sample size n is free from p in (YA-i) or (YA-i'). However, when $\alpha_j \in (0, 1]$, one would find difficulty in naive PCA in view of (YA-ii) or (YA-ii') in HDLSS data situations. Let us see a simple case that $p = 10000$, $\lambda_1 = p^{1/2}$ and $\lambda_2 = \cdots = \lambda_p = 1$. Then, we observe from (YA-ii) that it should be $n >> p^{2-2\alpha_1} = p = 10000$. It is somewhat inconvenient for the experimenter to handle PCA in HDLSS data situations.

2.2 Beyond naive PCA

Yata and Aoshima (2010a,b) created an effective methodology called the *cross-data-matrix (CDM) methodology* to handle HDLSS data situations: Let $n_{(1)} = [n/2] + 1$ and $n_{(2)} = n - n_{(1)}$, where $[x]$ denotes the largest integer less than x. Suppose that we have a $p \times n$ data matrix,

$$X = [x_1, ..., x_n] = [x_{11}, ..., x_{1n_{(1)}}, x_{21}, ..., x_{2n_{(2)}}]. \tag{3}$$

We define $p \times n_{(i)}$ data matrices, X_1 and X_2, by $X_i = [x_{i1}, ..., x_{in_{(i)}}]$, $i = 1, 2$. Note that X_1 and X_2 are independent. Let $X_{oi} = X_i - [\bar{x}_i, ..., \bar{x}_i]$, $i = 1, 2$, where $\bar{x}_i = \sum_{j=1}^{n_{(i)}} x_{ij}/n_{(i)}$. We define a cross data matrix by $S_{D(1)} = ((n_{(1)} - 1)(n_{(2)} - 1))^{-1/2} X_{o1}^T X_{o2}$ or $S_{D(2)} = ((n_{(1)} - 1)(n_{(2)} - 1))^{-1/2} X_{o2}^T X_{o1}$ ($= S_{D(1)}^T$). Note that rank$(S_{D(1)}) \le n_{(2)} - 1$. When we consider the singular value decomposition of $S_{D(1)}$, it follows that $S_{D(1)} = \sum_{j=1}^{n_{(2)}-1} \tilde{\lambda}_j \tilde{u}_{j(1)} \tilde{u}_{j(2)}^T$, where $\tilde{\lambda}_1 \ge \cdots \ge \tilde{\lambda}_{n_{(2)}-1} (\ge 0)$ denote singular values of $S_{D(1)}$, and $\tilde{u}_{j(1)}$ (or $\tilde{u}_{j(2)}$) denotes a unit left- (or right-) singular vector corresponding to $\tilde{\lambda}_j$ ($j = 1, ..., n_{(2)} - 1$).

[Cross-data-matrix (CDM) methodology]

(Step 1) Define a cross data matrix by $S_{D(1)} = ((n_{(1)} - 1)(n_{(2)} - 1))^{-1/2} X_{o1}^T X_{o2}$.

(Step 2) Calculate the singular values, $\tilde{\lambda}_j$'s, of $S_{D(1)}$ for the estimation of λ_j's.

Note that $S_{D(1)} S_{D(1)}^T = \sum_{j=1}^{n_{(2)}-1} \tilde{\lambda}_j^2 \tilde{u}_{j(1)} \tilde{u}_{j(1)}^T$. Thus one can calculate the singular values, $\tilde{\lambda}_j$'s, by the positive square-root of the eigenvalues of $S_{D(1)} S_{D(1)}^T$. The CDM methodology assures the following properties. For the details, see Yata and Aoshima (2010a,b).

Theorem 2.1. *For $j = 1, ..., m$, it holds that*

$$\frac{\tilde{\lambda}_j}{\lambda_j} \xrightarrow{p} 1 \tag{4}$$

under the conditions:

(i) $p \to \infty$ and $n \to \infty$ for j such that $\alpha_j > 1/2$;

(ii) $p \to \infty$ and $p^{2-2\alpha_j}/n \to 0$ for j such that $\alpha_j \in (0, 1/2]$.

Corollary 2.1. *Assume further in Theorem 2.1 that* z_{jk}, $j = 1, ..., p$ ($k = 1, ..., n$) *are independent. Then, for* $j = 1, ..., m$, *we have (4) under the conditions:*

(i) $p \to \infty$ *and* $n \to \infty$ *for j such that* $\alpha_j > 1/2$;

(ii) $p \to \infty$ *and there exists a positive constant* ε_j *satisfying* $p^{1-2\alpha_j}/n < p^{-\varepsilon_j}$ *for j such that* $\alpha_j \in (0, 1/2]$.

Theorem 2.2. *Let* $Var(z_{jk}^2) = M_j$ $(< \infty)$ *for* $j = 1, ..., m$ ($k = 1, ..., n$). *Assume that* λ_j ($j \leq m$) *has multiplicity one. Then, under the conditions (i)-(ii) in Theorem 2.1, it holds for* $j = 1, ..., m$, *that*

$$\sqrt{\frac{n}{M_j}} \left(\frac{\tilde{\lambda}_j}{\lambda_j} - 1 \right) \Rightarrow N(0, 1), \tag{5}$$

where "$\Rightarrow$" denotes the convergence in distribution and $N(0, 1)$ denotes a random variable distributed as the standard normal distribution.

Corollary 2.2. *Assume further in Theorem 2.2 that* z_{jk}, $j = 1, ..., p$ ($k = 1, ..., n$) *are independent. Then, for* $j = 1, ..., m$, *we have (5) under the conditions:*

(i) $p \to \infty$ *and* $n \to \infty$ *for j such that* $\alpha_j > 1/2$;

(ii) $p \to \infty$ *and* $p^{2-4\alpha_j}/n \to 0$ *for j such that* $\alpha_j \in (0, 1/2]$.

Remark 2.1. When the population distribution is $N_p(\mu, \Sigma)$, one has that $M_j = 2$ for $j = 1, ..., p$.

Remark 2.2. The condition (ii) given by Theorem 2.1 (or Theorem 2.2) is a sufficient condition for the case of $\alpha_j \in (0, 1/2]$. If more information is available about the population distribution, the condition (ii) can be relaxed to give consistency under a broader set of (p, n). For example, when the population distribution is $N_p(\mu, \Sigma)$, the asymptotic properties are claimed under a broader set of (p, n) given by (ii) of Corollary 2.1 (or Corollary 2.2).

Remark 2.3. In view of Theorem 2.1 compared to (2), the CDM methodology successfully relaxes the condition for the case that $\alpha_j > 1/2$. The conditions given by Theorem 2.1 are not continuous in α_j at $\alpha_j = 1/2$. On the other hand, the conditions given by Corollaries 2.1 and 2.2 are continuous in α_j.

When we apply the CDM methodology, we simply divided X into $x_1, ..., x_{n_{(1)}}$ and $x_{n_{(1)}+1}, ..., x_n$ in (3). In general, there exist ${}_nC_{n_{(1)}}$ ways to divide X into X_1 and X_2. The CDM methodology can be generalized as follows:

[Generalized cross-data-matrix (GCDM) methodology]

(Step 1) Set iteration number T. Set $t = 1$.

(Step 2) Randomly split $x_1, ..., x_n$ into $X_1 = [x_{1(1)}, ..., x_{1(n_{(1)})}]$ and $X_2 = [x_{2(1)}, ..., x_{2(n_{(2)})}]$.

(Step 3) Define a cross data matrix by $S_{D(1)t} = ((n_{(1)} - 1)(n_{(2)} - 1))^{-1/2} X_{o1}^T X_{o2}$, where $X_{oi} = X_i - [\bar{x}_i, ..., \bar{x}_i]$, $i = 1, 2$, and $\bar{x}_i = \sum_{j=1}^{n_{(i)}} x_{i(j)}/n_{(i)}$.

(Step 4) Calculate the singular values, $\tilde{\lambda}_{1t} \geq \cdots \geq \tilde{\lambda}_{n_{(2)}-1t}(\geq 0)$, of $S_{D(1)t}$.

(Step 5) If $t < T$, put $t = t + 1$ and go to Step 2; otherwise go to Step 6.

(Step 6) Estimate λ_j by $\tilde{\lambda}_{j(T)} = \sum_{t=1}^{T} \tilde{\lambda}_{jt}/T$ for each j.

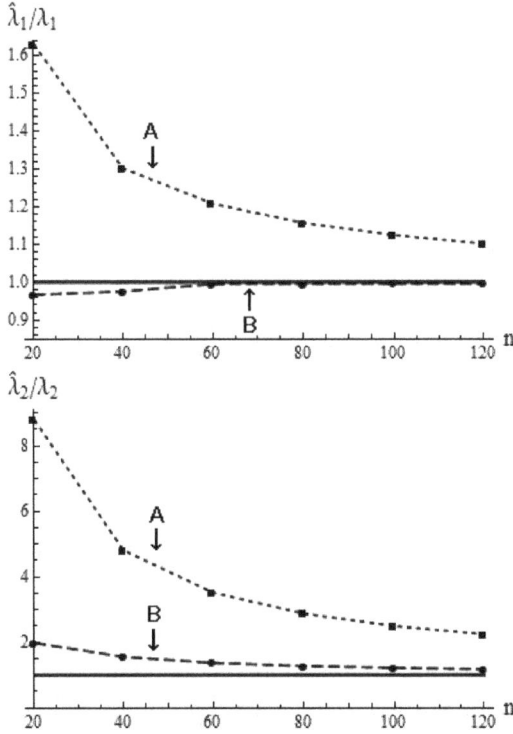

Fig. 1. The behaviors of A: $\hat{\lambda}_j / \lambda_j$ and B: $\tilde{\lambda}_j / \lambda_j$ for the first eigenvalue (upper panel) and second eigenvalue (lower panel) when the samples, of size $n = 20(20)120$, were taken from $N_p(\mathbf{0}, \boldsymbol{\Sigma})$ with $p = 1600$.

2.3 Performances

We observed that naive PCA requires the sample size n depending on p for $\alpha_i \in (1/2, 1]$ in (2). On the other hand, the CDM methodology allows the experimenter to choose n free from p for the case that $\alpha_i > 1/2$ as in Theorem 2.1 or Corollary 2.1. The CDM methodology might make it possible to give feasible estimation of eigenvalues for HDLSS data with extremely small n compared to p.

We first considered a normal distribution case. Independent pseudorandom normal observations were generated from $N_p(\mathbf{0}, \boldsymbol{\Sigma})$ with $p = 1600$. We considered $\lambda_1 = p^{2/3}$, $\lambda_2 = p^{1/3}$ and $\lambda_3 = \cdots = \lambda_p = 1$ in (1). We used the sample of size $n = 20(20)120$ to define the data matrix $X : p \times n$ for the calculation of S_D in naive PCA, whereas we divided the sample into $X_1 : p \times n_{(1)}$ and $X_2 : p \times n_{(2)}$ for the calculation of $S_{D(1)}$ in the CDM methodology. The findings were obtained by averaging the outcomes from 1000 ($= R$, say) replications. Under a fixed scenario, suppose that the r-th replication ends with estimates of λ_j, $\hat{\lambda}_{jr}$ and $\tilde{\lambda}_{jr}$ ($r = 1, ..., R$), given by naive PCA and the CDM methodology. Let us simply write $\hat{\lambda}_j = R^{-1} \sum_{r=1}^{R} \hat{\lambda}_{jr}$ and $\tilde{\lambda}_j = R^{-1} \sum_{r=1}^{R} \tilde{\lambda}_{jr}$. We considered two quantities, A: $\hat{\lambda}_j / \lambda_j$ and B: $\tilde{\lambda}_j / \lambda_j$. Figure 1 shows the behaviors of both A and B for the first two eigenvalues. By observing the behavior of A, naive PCA seems not to give a feasible estimation within

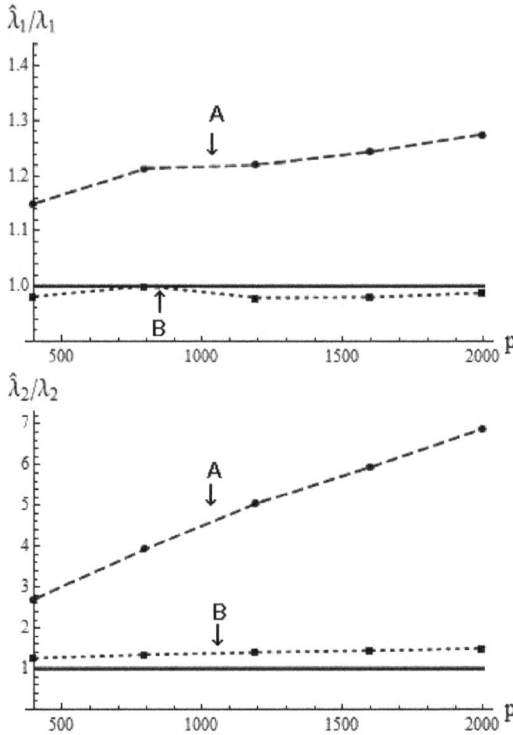

Fig. 2. The behaviors of A: $\hat{\lambda}_j / \lambda_j$ and B: $\tilde{\lambda}_j / \lambda_j$ for the first eigenvalue (upper panel) and second eigenvalue (lower panel) when the samples, of size $n = 60$, were taken from $t_p(\mathbf{0}, \mathbf{\Sigma}, \nu)$ with $\nu = 15$ and $p = 400(400)2000$.

the range of n. The sample size n was not large enough to use the eigenvalues of S_D for such a high-dimensional space. On the other hand, in view of the behavior of B, the CDM methodology gave a reasonable estimation surprisingly well for such HDLSS data sets. The CDM methodology seems to perform excellently as expected theoretically.

Next, we considered a non-normal distribution case. Independent pseudorandom observations were generated from a p-variate t-distribution, $t_p(\mathbf{0}, \mathbf{\Sigma}, \nu)$, with mean zero, covariance matrix $\mathbf{\Sigma}$ and degree of freedom $\nu = 15$. We considered the case that $\lambda_1 = p^{2/3}$, $\lambda_2 = p^{1/3}$ and $\lambda_3 = \cdots = \lambda_p = 1$ in (1) as before. We fixed the sample size as $n = 60$. We set the dimension as $p = 400(400)2000$. Similarly to Figure 1, the findings were obtained by averaging the outcomes from 1000 replications. Figure 2 shows the behaviors of two quantities, A: $\hat{\lambda}_j / \lambda_j$ and B: $\tilde{\lambda}_j / \lambda_j$, for the first two eigenvalues. Again, the CDM methodology seems to perform excellently as expected theoretically. One can observe the consistency of $\tilde{\lambda}_j$ for all $p = 400(400)2000$. We conducted simulation studies for other settings as well and verified the superiority of the CDM methodology to naive PCA in various HDLSS data situations.

3. Clustering for high-dimension, low-sample-size data

Suppose we have a mixture model to classify a data set into two groups. We assume that the observation is sampled with mixing proportions w_j's from two populations, Π_1 and Π_2, and the label of the population is missing. We consider a mixture model whose p.d.f. (or p.f.) is given by

$$f(x) = w_1\pi_1(x; \mu_1, \Sigma_1) + w_2\pi_2(x; \mu_2, \Sigma_2), \tag{6}$$

where w_j's are positive constants such that $w_1 + w_2 = 1$ and $\pi_i(x; \mu_i, \Sigma_i)$'s are p-dimensional p.d.f. (or p.f.) of Π_i having mean vector μ_i and covariance matrix Σ_i. Let μ and Σ be the mean vector and the covariance matrix of the mixture model. Then, we have that $\mu = w_1\mu_1 + w_2\mu_2$ and $\Sigma = w_1w_2(\mu_1 - \mu_2)(\mu_1 - \mu_2)^T + w_1\Sigma_1 + w_2\Sigma_2$. We suppose that x_k, $k = 1, ..., n$, are independently taken from (6) and define a $p \times n$ data matrix $X = [x_1, ..., x_n]$. Let $\Delta = ||\mu_1 - \mu_2||^2$. Let λ_{11} and λ_{21} be the largest eigenvalues of Σ_1 and Σ_2. We assume that $\Delta = cp^\beta$, where c and β are positive constants. We assume that $\lambda_{11}/\Delta \to 0$ and $\lambda_{21}/\Delta \to 0$ as $p \to \infty$. Then, as for the largest eigenvalue, λ_1, of Σ and the corresponding eigenvector, h_1, we have that

$$\frac{\lambda_1}{w_1w_2\Delta} \to 1 \quad \text{and} \quad \text{Angle}(h_1, (\mu_1 - \mu_2)/\Delta^{1/2}) \to 0. \tag{7}$$

We note from (7) that the mixture model given by (6) holds the model (1) about Σ. Let s_{1k} denote the first principal component (PC) score of x_k ($k = 1, ..., n$). Then, from Yata and Aoshima (2010b), it holds as $p \to \infty$ that

$$\frac{s_{1k}}{\sqrt{\lambda_1}} \xrightarrow{p} \begin{cases} \sqrt{w_2/w_1} & \text{when } x_k \in \Pi_1, \\ -\sqrt{w_1/w_2} & \text{when } x_k \in \Pi_2. \end{cases}$$

Thus one would be able to classify the data set $\{x_1, ..., x_n\}$ into two groups if s_{1k} is effectively estimated in HDLSS data situations. In this section hereafter, we borrow symbols from Section 2.

3.1 Effective estimation for PC scores

In general, the j-th PC score of x_k is given by $h_j^T(x_k - \mu) = z_{jk}\sqrt{\lambda_j} (= s_{jk}$, say). Yata and Aoshima (2009) considered a sample eigenvector by $\hat{h}_j = ((n-1)\hat{\lambda}_j)^{-1/2}X_o\hat{u}_j$ and an naive estimator of the j-th PC score of x_k by $\hat{h}_j^T(x_k - \bar{x}) = \hat{u}_{jk}\sqrt{(n-1)\hat{\lambda}_j} (= \hat{s}_{jk}$, say), where $\hat{u}_j^T = (\hat{u}_{j1}, ..., \hat{u}_{jn})$. Note that $\hat{h}_j$ can be calculated by using a unit-norm eigenvector, $\hat{u}_j$, of S_D whose size is much smaller than S especially for a HDLSS data matrix. Now, we apply the CDM methodology to the PC score in order to improve the naive estimator. Recall that $\tilde{u}_{j(1)}$ (or $\tilde{u}_{j(2)}$) is a unit left- (or right-) singular vector corresponding to the singular value $\tilde{\lambda}_j$ ($j = 1, ..., n_{(2)} - 1$) of $S_{D(1)} = ((n_{(1)} - 1)(n_{(2)} - 1))^{-1/2}X_{o1}^T X_{o2}$.

[CDM methodology for PC scores]

(Step 1) Calculate the singular vectors $\tilde{u}_{j(i)}$'s, $i = 1, 2$, of $S_{D(1)}$.

(Step 2) Adjust the sign of $\tilde{u}_{j(2)}$ by $\tilde{u}_{j(2)} = \text{Sign}(\tilde{u}_{j(1)}^T X_{o1}^T X_{o2} \tilde{u}_{j(2)}) \tilde{u}_{j(2)}$. After the modification, let $\tilde{u}_{j(i)}^T = (\tilde{u}_{j1(i)}, ..., \tilde{u}_{jn_{(i)}(i)})$, $i = 1, 2$.

(Step 3) Calculate $\tilde{s}_{jk(i)} = \tilde{u}_{jk(i)} \sqrt{(n_{(i)} - 1)\tilde{\lambda}_j}$, $k = 1, ..., n_{(i)}$; $i = 1, 2$. Estimate the j-th PC score of x_k by $\tilde{s}_{jk} = \tilde{s}_{jk(1)}$, $k = 1, ..., n_{(1)}$ and $\tilde{s}_{jk+n_{(1)}} = \tilde{s}_{jk(2)}$, $k = 1, ..., n_{(2)}$.

One can calculate the singular vector $\tilde{u}_{j(i)}$'s by the eigenvectors of $S_{D(i)} S_{D(i)}^T$. Let $\text{MSE}(\tilde{s}_j) = n^{-1} \sum_{k=1}^n (\tilde{s}_{jk} - s_{jk})^2$ denote the sample mean-square error of the j-th PC score. Note that $\text{Var}(s_{jk}) = \lambda_j$. Then, Yata and Aoshima (2010b) gave the following properties on the CDM-based PC scores.

Theorem 3.1. *Assume that λ_j ($j \leq m$) has multiplicity one. Then, it holds that*

$$\frac{\text{MSE}(\tilde{s}_j)}{\lambda_j} \xrightarrow{p} 0 \qquad (8)$$

under the conditions (i)-(ii) in Theorem 2.1. If z_{jk}, $j = 1, ..., p$ ($k = 1, ..., n$) are independent, we have (8) under the conditions (i)-(ii) in Corollary 2.1.

Theorem 3.2. *Assume that λ_j ($j \leq m$) has multiplicity one. Then, for any k ($= 1, ..., n$), it holds that*

$$\lambda_j^{-1/2} \tilde{s}_{jk} \xrightarrow{p} z_{jk} \qquad (9)$$

under the conditions (i)-(ii) of Theorem 2.1. If z_{jk}, $j = 1, ..., p$ ($k = 1, ..., n$) are independent, we have (9) under the conditions (i)-(ii) of Corollary 2.2.

The CDM-based PC score can be generalized as follows:

[GCDM methodology for PC scores]

(Step 1) Set iteration number T. Set $t = 1$.

(Step 2) Randomly split $x_1, ..., x_n$ into $X_1 = [x_{1(1)}, ..., x_{1(n_{(1)})}]$ and $X_2 = [x_{2(1)}, ..., x_{2(n_{(2)})}]$.

(Step 3) Define a cross data matrix by $S_{D(1)t} = ((n_{(1)} - 1)(n_{(2)} - 1))^{-1/2} X_{o1}^T X_{o2}$, where $X_{oi} = X_i - [\bar{x}_i, ..., \bar{x}_i]$, $i = 1, 2$, and $\bar{x}_i = \sum_{j=1}^{n_{(i)}} x_{i(j)}/n_{(i)}$. Calculate the singular values, $\tilde{\lambda}_{1t} \geq \cdots \geq \tilde{\lambda}_{n_{(2)}-1t} (\geq 0)$, and the corresponding singular vectors, $\tilde{u}_{j(i)t}$'s, $i = 1, 2$, of $S_{D(1)t}$. If $t = 1$, go to Step 5; otherwise go to Step 4.

(Step 4) Adjust the sign of $\tilde{u}_{j(1)t}$ by $\tilde{u}_{j(1)t} = \text{Sign}(\tilde{u}_{j(1)t}^T \tilde{u}_{j(1)1}) \tilde{u}_{j(1)t}$.

(Step 5) Adjust the sign of $\tilde{u}_{j(2)t}$ by $\tilde{u}_{j(2)t} = \text{Sign}(\tilde{u}_{j(1)t}^T X_{o1}^T X_{o2} \tilde{u}_{j(2)t}) \tilde{u}_{j(2)t}$. After the modification, let $\tilde{u}_{j(i)t}^T = (\tilde{u}_{j(1i)t}, ..., \tilde{u}_{j(n_{(i)}i)t})$, $i = 1, 2$.

(Step 6) Calculate $\tilde{s}_{j(ki)t} = \tilde{u}_{j(ki)t} \sqrt{(n_{(i)} - 1)\tilde{\lambda}_{jt}}$, $k = 1, ..., n_{(i)}$; $i = 1, 2$, and adjust the subscript k of $\tilde{s}_{j(ki)t}$ as $\tilde{s}_{jkt}$ corresponding to x_k.

(Step 7) If $t < T$, put $t = t + 1$ and go to Step 2; otherwise go to Step 8.

(Step 8) Estimate the j-th PC score of x_k by $\tilde{s}_{jk(T)} = \sum_{t=1}^T \tilde{s}_{jkt}/T$ for each j and k.

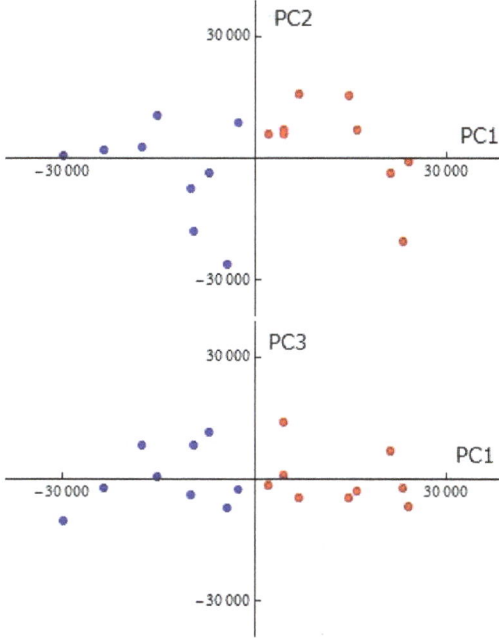

Fig. 3. Scatterplots of PC scores by PC1 and PC2 (upper panel) or PC1 and PC3 (lower panel) by using the GCDM methodology. There are 9 samples from Normal Prostate (blue point) and 9 samples from Prostate Tumors (red point).

3.2 Demonstration

We analyzed gene expression data about prostate cancer given by Singh et al. (2002). Refer to Pochet et al. (2004) for details of the data set. The data set consisted of 12600 ($= p$) genes and 34 microarrays in which there were 9 samples from Normal Prostate and 25 samples from Prostate Tumors. As for Prostate Tumors, we chose the first 9 samples and set 18 ($= n$) microarrays in which there were 9 samples from Normal Prostate and 9 samples from Prostate Tumors. We assumed the mixture model given by (6) for the data set. We defined the data matrix by X : 12600×18. We set $(n_{(1)}, n_{(2)}) = (9, 9)$ and $T = 1000$. We focused on the first three PC scores. We randomly divided X into X_1 : 12600×9 and X_2 : 12600×9, and calculated $\tilde{s}_{jkt}$, $k = 1, ..., 18$, for $j = 1, 2, 3$. According to the GCDM methodology, we repeated this operation $T = 1000$ times and obtained $\tilde{s}_{jk(T)}$, $k = 1, ..., 18$; $j = 1, 2, 3$, as an estimate of the j-th PC score of x_k. We also obtained $(\tilde{\lambda}_{1(T)}, \tilde{\lambda}_{2(T)}, \tilde{\lambda}_{3(T)}) = (2.77 \times 10^8, 1.62 \times 10^8, 6.34 \times 10^7)$. Figure 3 gives the scatterplots of the first three PC scores on the (PC1, PC2) plane or the (PC1, PC3) plane. As observed in Figure 3, Normal Prostate (blue point) and Prostate Tumors (red point) seem to be separated clearly. It is obvious especially for the first PC score (PC1) line. All the first PC scores of the samples from Normal Prostate are negative, whereas those from Prostate Tumors are positive. This observation is theoretically supported by the arguments in Section 3.1.

4. Classification for high-dimension, low-sample-size data

Suppose we have independent and p-dimensional populations, Π_i, $i = 1, 2$, having *unknown* mean vector $\mu_i = (\mu_{i1}, ..., \mu_{ip})^T$ and *unknown* positive-definite covariance matrix Σ_i for each i. *We do not assume that* $\Sigma_1 = \Sigma_2$. The eigen-decomposition of Σ_i $(i = 1, 2)$ is given by $\Sigma_i = H_i \Lambda_i H_i^T$, where Λ_i is a diagonal matrix of eigenvalues $\lambda_{i1} \geq \cdots \geq \lambda_{ip} > 0$ and $H_i = [h_{i1}, ..., h_{ip}]$ is an orthogonal matrix of corresponding eigenvectors. Having recorded i.i.d. samples, $x_{i1}, ..., x_{in_i}$, from each Π_i, we have a $p \times n_i$ $(p > n_i)$ data matrix $X_i = [x_{i1}, ..., x_{in_i}]$, where $x_{ij} = (x_{i1j}, ..., x_{ipj})^T$, $j = 1, ..., n_i$. We assume $n_i \geq 4$, $i = 1, 2$. Then, $Z_i = \Lambda_i^{-1/2} H_i^T (X_i - [\mu_i, ..., \mu_i])$ is considered as a $p \times n_i$ sphered data matrix from a distribution with zero mean and the identity covariance matrix. Here, we write $Z_i = [z_{i1}, ..., z_{in_i}]$ and $z_{ij} = (z_{i1j}, ..., z_{ipj})^T$, $j = 1, ..., n_i$. Note that $E(z_{ijl}^2) = 1$ and $E(z_{ijl}z_{ij'l}) = 0$ for $i = 1, 2$; $j (\neq j') = 1, ..., p$; $l = 1, ..., n_i$. We assume that $\lambda_{ip} > 0$ $(i = 1, 2)$ as $p \to \infty$ and the fourth moments of each variable in Z_i are uniformly bounded. In this section, we assume the following assumption for Π_i's:

(A-i) $z_{ijl}, j = 1, ..., p$, are independent for $i = 1, 2$.

One of the population distributions satisfying (A-i) is $N_p(\mu_i, \Sigma_i)$. We also assume the following condition for Σ_i's as necessary:

(A-ii) $\dfrac{\text{tr}(\Sigma_i^t)}{p} < \infty$ $(t = 1, 2)$ and $\dfrac{\text{tr}(\Sigma_i^4)}{p^2} \to 0$ as $p \to \infty$ for $i = 1, 2$.

Remark 4.1. If all λ_{ij}'s are bounded, (A-ii) trivially holds. For a spiked model such as $\lambda_{ij} = a_{ij}p^{\alpha_{ij}}$ $(j = 1, ..., m_i)$ and $\lambda_{ij} = c_{ij}$ $(j = m_i + 1, ..., p)$ with positive constants a_{ij}'s, c_{ij}'s and α_{ij}'s, (A-ii) holds under the condition that $\alpha_{ij} < 1/2$, $j = 1, ..., m_i (< \infty)$; $i = 1, 2$. As an interesting example, (A-ii) holds for $\Sigma_{i'} = c_{i'}(\rho_{i'}^{|i-j|^{q_{i'}}})$, $i' = 1, 2$, where $c_{i'}$'s, $q_{i'}$'s and $\rho_{i'}$'s(< 1) are positive constants.

4.1 Discriminant rule for HDLSS data

Let x_0 be an observation vector on an individual belonging to Π_1 or to Π_2. Having recorded $x_{i1}, ..., x_{in_i}$ from each Π_i, we estimate μ_i and Σ_i by $\bar{x}_{in_i} = \sum_{j=1}^{n_i} x_{ij}/n_i$ and $S_{in_i} = \sum_{j=1}^{n_i} (x_{ij} - \bar{x}_{in_i})(x_{ij} - \bar{x}_{in_i})^T/(n_i - 1)$. Aoshima and Yata (2011) considered a discriminant rule that classifies x_0 into Π_1 if

$$\frac{p||x_0 - \bar{x}_{1n_1}||^2}{\text{tr}(S_{1n_1})} - \frac{p||x_0 - \bar{x}_{2n_2}||^2}{\text{tr}(S_{2n_2})} - p \log \left\{ \frac{\text{tr}(S_{2n_2})}{\text{tr}(S_{1n_1})} \right\} - \frac{p}{n_1} + \frac{p}{n_2} + \gamma < 0 \qquad (10)$$

and into Π_2 otherwise. Here, $-p/n_1 + p/n_2$ is a bias-correction and γ is a tuning parameter. We denote the error rate of misclassifying an individual from Π_1 (into Π_2) or from Π_2 (into Π_1) by $e(2|1)$ or $e(1|2)$. Let $\Delta = ||\mu_1 - \mu_2||^2$ and $\Delta_{\Sigma_i} = (\text{tr}(\Sigma_1) - \text{tr}(\Sigma_2))^2/\text{tr}(\Sigma_i)$, $i = 1, 2$. Let us write that $\Delta_i = \Delta + \Delta_{\Sigma_i}/2$, $i = 1, 2$, and $\Delta_\star = \min_{i=1,2} \Delta_i$. Aoshima and Yata (2011) gave the following property.

Theorem 4.1. *Assume (A-i)-(A-ii). Under the condition that* $\max_{i=1,2}\{\text{tr}(\Sigma_i^2)\}/(\Delta_\star^2 \min_{i=1,2}\{n_i\}) \to 0$ *as* $p \to \infty$, *for the discriminant rule given by (10) with* $\gamma = 0$, *it holds as* $p \to \infty$ *that*

$$e(2|1) \to 0 \quad and \quad e(1|2) \to 0. \qquad (11)$$

Remark 4.2. Assume (A-i)-(A-ii). Let us consider a case that $\text{tr}(\Sigma_1)/\text{tr}(\Sigma_2) \neq 1$ as $p \to \infty$. Then, it follows that $\min_{i=1,2} \Delta_{\Sigma_i}/p > 0$ as $p \to \infty$. Since it holds $\max_{i=1,2}\{\text{tr}(\Sigma_i^2)\}$ $/(\Delta_\star^2 \min_{i=1,2}\{n_i\}) \to 0$ as $p \to \infty$, we can claim (11) in the case.

Remark 4.3. Let $n_{i(1)} = [n_i/2] + 1$ and $n_{i(2)} = n_i - n_{i(1)}$ for each Π_i $(i = 1,2)$. We omit the subscript i for a while. For each Π, split $x_1, ..., x_n$ into $X_1 = [x_{11}, ..., x_{1n_{(1)}}]$ and $X_2 = [x_{21}, ..., x_{2n_{(2)}}]$. Let $X_{o1} = X_1 - [\bar{x}_1, ..., \bar{x}_1]$ and $X_{o2} = X_2 - [\bar{x}_2, ..., \bar{x}_2]$, where $\bar{x}_1 = \sum_{j=1}^{n_{(1)}} x_{1j}/n_{(1)}$ and $\bar{x}_2 = \sum_{j=1}^{n_{(2)}} x_{2j}/n_{(2)}$. Define $S_{n(1)} = (n_{(1)} - 1)^{-1}X_{o1}X_{o1}^T$ and $S_{n(2)} = (n_{(2)} - 1)^{-1}X_{o2}X_{o2}^T$. Note that $\text{tr}(S_{n(1)}S_{n(2)}) = \text{tr}(S_{D(1)}S_{D(1)}^T) = \sum_{j=1}^{n_{(2)}-1} \tilde{\lambda}_j^2$. Then, we have that $E(\text{tr}(S_{n(1)}S_{n(2)})) = \text{tr}(\Sigma^2)$. As for $\text{tr}(\Sigma_i^2)$, Yata (2010) considered an unbiased estimator, $\text{tr}(S_{in_i(1)}S_{in_i(2)})$, as an application of the CDM methodology given by Yata and Aoshima (2010a,b).

Remark 4.4. We note that $\Delta_\star$ is estimated by

$$||\bar{x}_{1n_1} - \bar{x}_{2n_2}||^2 - \sum_{i=1}^{2} \text{tr}(S_{in_i})/n_i + \frac{|\text{tr}(S_{1n_1}) - \text{tr}(S_{2n_2})|^2}{2\max_{i=1,2} \text{tr}(S_{in_i})} \ (= \hat{\Delta}_\star, \text{ say}).$$

We analyzed gene expression data given by Armstrong et al. (2001) in which data set consisted of 12582 ($= p$) genes. We had two populations about leukemia subtypes, i.e., Π_1: acute lymphoblastic leukemia (ALL, 24 samples) and Π_2: acute myeloid leukemia (AML, 28 samples). We set $n_1 = n_2 = 10$. Then, we constructed the discriminant rule given by (10) with $\gamma = 0$. From Remarks 4.3 and 4.4, we calculated $\max_{i=1,2}\{\text{tr}(S_{in_i(1)}S_{in_i(2)})\} = 3.16 \times 10^{19}$ and $\hat{\Delta}_\star = 2.67 \times 10^{10}$, so that $\max_{i=1,2}\{\text{tr}(S_{in_i(1)}S_{in_i(2)})\}/(\hat{\Delta}_\star^2 \min_{i=1,2}\{n_i\}) = 0.0044$. Thus, one may conclude that $\max_{i=1,2}\{\text{tr}(\Sigma_i^2)\}/(\Delta_\star^2 \min_{i=1,2}\{n_i\})$ must be sufficiently small. Hence, from Theorem 4.1, the discriminant rule given by (10) with $\gamma = 0$ was expected to hold (11). In Table 1, we investigated the performance of the discriminant rule by using test data sets consisting of $24 - n_1 = 14$ remaining samples from Π_1 and $28 - n_2 = 18$ remaining samples from Π_2. We observed that the discriminant rule showed $e(1|2) = 0$ and $e(2|1) = 0$ successfully as expected by theory.

	(10) with $\gamma = 0$
$1-\bar{e}(2|1)$	14/14 (=1.0)
$1-\bar{e}(1|2)$	18/18 (=1.0)

Table 1. The correct discrimination rates for test data sets consisting of 14 samples from Π_1 and 18 samples from Π_2.

4.2 Sample size determination for classification

One would be interested in designing the discriminant rule given by (10) so as to hold both $e(2|1) \leq \alpha$ and $e(1|2) \leq \beta$ when $\Delta_\star \geq \Delta_L$, where α, $\beta \in (0, 1/2)$ and Δ_L (> 0) are prespecified constants. We assume $\Delta_L = o(p^{1/2})$. Aoshima and Yata (2011) showed the following property.

Theorem 4.2. *Assume that* $\text{tr}(\Sigma_1)/\text{tr}(\Sigma_2) \to 1$ *as* $p \to \infty$. *Let*

$$\omega(x_0) = \frac{p||x_0 - \bar{x}_{1n_1}||^2}{\text{tr}(S_{1n_1})} - \frac{p||x_0 - \bar{x}_{2n_2}||^2}{\text{tr}(S_{2n_2})} - p\log\left\{\frac{\text{tr}(S_{2n_2})}{\text{tr}(S_{1n_1})}\right\} - \frac{p}{n_1} + \frac{p}{n_2}.$$

Then, under the regularity conditions, it holds as $p \to \infty$ *and* $n_1, n_2 \to \infty$ *that*

$$\frac{w(x_0) + \Delta_2(\mathrm{tr}(\Sigma_2)/p)^{-1}}{2\sqrt{(\mathrm{tr}(\Sigma_1)/p)^{-2}\mathrm{tr}(\Sigma_1^2)/n_1 + (\mathrm{tr}(\Sigma_2)/p)^{-2}\mathrm{tr}(\Sigma_1\Sigma_2)/n_2}} \Rightarrow N(0,1) \quad \text{when } x_0 \in \Pi_1;$$

$$\frac{w(x_0) - \Delta_1(\mathrm{tr}(\Sigma_1)/p)^{-1}}{2\sqrt{(\mathrm{tr}(\Sigma_2)/p)^{-2}\mathrm{tr}(\Sigma_2^2)/n_2 + (\mathrm{tr}(\Sigma_1)/p)^{-2}\mathrm{tr}(\Sigma_1\Sigma_2)/n_1}} \Rightarrow N(0,1) \quad \text{when } x_0 \in \Pi_2.$$

Let $\sigma = \max\{\mathrm{tr}(\Sigma_1^2)^{1/2}, \mathrm{tr}(\Sigma_2^2)^{1/2}\}$. We find the sample size for each Π_i $(i = 1, 2)$ as

$$n_i \geq \frac{(z_\alpha + z_\beta)^2 \sigma}{\Delta_L^2} \mathrm{tr}(\Sigma_i^2)^{1/4} \sum_{j=1}^{2} \mathrm{tr}(\Sigma_j^2)^{1/4} \quad (= C_i, \text{ say}), \tag{12}$$

where z_α is the upper α point of $N(0,1)$. Note that $C_i = O(p/\Delta_L^2)$ for $i = 1, 2$, under (A-ii). Thus under $\Delta_L \to \infty$ as $p \to \infty$, it holds that $C_i/p \to 0$ as $p \to \infty$. Then, Aoshima and Yata (2011) gave the following theorem.

Theorem 4.3. *Assume (A-i)-(A-ii). Let* $\gamma = (\mathrm{tr}(S_{1n_1} + S_{2n_2})/(2p))^{-1}\Delta_L(z_\beta - z_\alpha)/(z_\alpha + z_\beta)$ *in (10). Then, under the regularity conditions, for the discriminant rule given by (10) with (12), it holds as* $p \to \infty$ *that*

$$\limsup e(2|1) \leq \alpha \quad \text{and} \quad \limsup e(1|2) \leq \beta$$

when $\Delta_\star \geq \Delta_L$.

Remark 4.5. One can design Δ_L by using the two sample test given by Aoshima and Yata (2011). Under the regularity conditions, it holds that

$$\frac{||\bar{x}_{1n_1} - \bar{x}_{2n_2}||^2 - \sum_{i=1}^{2} \mathrm{tr}(S_{in_i})/n_i - \Delta}{\sqrt{\widehat{Var}(||\bar{x}_{1n_1} - \bar{x}_{2n_2}||^2)}} \Rightarrow N(0,1)$$

as $p \to \infty$ and $n_i \to \infty$, $i = 1, 2$, where

$$\widehat{Var}(||\bar{x}_{1n_1} - \bar{x}_{2n_2}||^2) = 2\frac{\mathrm{tr}(S_{1n_1(1)}S_{1n_1(2)})}{n_1(n_1 - 1)} + 2\frac{\mathrm{tr}(S_{2n_2(1)}S_{2n_2(2)})}{n_2(n_2 - 1)} + 4\frac{\mathrm{tr}(S_{1n_1}S_{2n_2})}{n_1 n_2}.$$

Note that $E(||\bar{x}_{1n_1} - \bar{x}_{2n_2}||^2 - \sum_{i=1}^{2} \mathrm{tr}(S_{in_i})/n_i) = \Delta$. Thus it follows that

$$P\left(\frac{||\bar{x}_{1n_1} - \bar{x}_{2n_2}||^2 - \sum_{i=1}^{2} \mathrm{tr}(S_{in_i})/n_i}{\sqrt{\widehat{Var}(||\bar{x}_{1n_1} - \bar{x}_{2n_2}||^2)}} - z_{\alpha'} \leq \frac{\Delta}{\sqrt{\widehat{Var}(||\bar{x}_{1n_1} - \bar{x}_{2n_2}||^2)}}\right) \to 1 - \alpha'$$

with $\alpha' \in (0, 1/2)$. From the fact that $\Delta_\star \geq \Delta$, we design a lower bound of $\Delta_\star$ by

$$\Delta_L = ||\bar{x}_{1n_1} - \bar{x}_{2n_2}||^2 - \sum_{i=1}^{2} \mathrm{tr}(S_{in_i})/n_i - z_{\alpha'}\sqrt{\widehat{Var}(||\bar{x}_{1n_1} - \bar{x}_{2n_2}||^2)}$$

for sufficiently small α'.

Since Σ_i's are unknown, it is necessary to estimate C_i's in (12) with some pilot samples. We proceed the following two steps:

[Two-stage procedure for classification]

(Step 1) Choose a pilot sample size, $m (\geq 4)$, such as $m/C_i \in (0,1)$, $i = 1, 2$, as $p \to \infty$. Take pilot samples of size m from each Π_i and define $X_i = [x_{i1}, ..., x_{im}]$, $i = 1, 2$. Let $m_{(1)} = [m/2] + 1$ and $m_{(2)} = m - m_{(1)}$. For each Π_i, divide X_i into $X_i = [X_{i1}, X_{i2}]$ with $X_{i1} : p \times m_{(1)}$ and $X_{i2} : p \times m_{(2)}$, and calculate

$$S_{im(1)} = \frac{(X_{i1} - [\bar{x}_{im_{(1)}}, ..., \bar{x}_{im_{(1)}}])(X_{i1} - [\bar{x}_{im_{(1)}}, ..., \bar{x}_{im_{(1)}}])^T}{m_{(1)} - 1}$$

and (13)

$$S_{im(2)} = \frac{(X_{i2} - [\bar{x}_{im_{(2)}}, ..., \bar{x}_{im_{(2)}}])(X_{i2} - [\bar{x}_{im_{(2)}}, ..., \bar{x}_{im_{(2)}}])^T}{m_{(2)} - 1},$$

where $\bar{x}_{im_{(1)}} = \sum_{j=1}^{m_{(1)}} x_{ij}/m_{(1)}$ and $\bar{x}_{im_{(2)}} = \sum_{j=m_{(1)}+1}^{m} x_{ij}/m_{(2)}$. Define the total sample size for each Π_i by

$$N_i = \max \left\{ m, \left[\frac{(z_\alpha + z_\beta)^2 \hat{\sigma}}{\Delta_L^2} \operatorname{tr}(S_{im(1)} S_{im(2)})^{1/4} \sum_{j=1}^{2} \operatorname{tr}(S_{jm(1)} S_{jm(2)})^{1/4} \right] + 1 \right\}, \quad (14)$$

where $\hat{\sigma} = \max\{ \operatorname{tr}(S_{1m(1)} S_{1m(2)})^{1/2}, \operatorname{tr}(S_{2m(1)} S_{2m(2)})^{1/2} \}$.

(Step 2) Take additional samples x_{ij}, $j = m+1, ..., N_i$, of size $N_i - m$ from each Π_i. By combining the initial samples and the additional samples, calculate $\bar{x}_{iN_i} = \sum_{j=1}^{N_i} x_{ij}/N_i$ and $S_{iN_i} = \sum_{j=1}^{N_i} (x_{ij} - \bar{x}_{iN_i})(x_{ij} - \bar{x}_{iN_i})^T/(N_i - 1)$, $i = 1, 2$. Then, we classify x_0 into Π_1 if

$$\frac{p\|x_0 - \bar{x}_{1N_1}\|^2}{\operatorname{tr}(S_{1N_1})} - \frac{p\|x_0 - \bar{x}_{2N_2}\|^2}{\operatorname{tr}(S_{2N_2})} - p\log\left\{ \frac{\operatorname{tr}(S_{2N_2})}{\operatorname{tr}(S_{1N_1})} \right\} - \frac{p}{N_1} + \frac{p}{N_2} + \hat{\gamma} < 0 \quad (15)$$

and into Π_2 otherwise, where $\hat{\gamma} = (\operatorname{tr}(S_{1N_1} + S_{2N_2})/(2p))^{-1} \Delta_L (z_\beta - z_\alpha)/(z_\alpha + z_\beta)$.

Aoshima and Yata (2011) gave the following theorem.

Theorem 4.4. *Assume (A-i)-(A-ii). Then, under the regularity conditions, for the discriminant rule given by (15) with (14), it holds as $p \to \infty$ that*

$$\limsup e(2|1) \leq \alpha \quad \text{and} \quad \limsup e(1|2) \leq \beta$$

when $\Delta_\star \geq \Delta_L$.

Remark 4.6. One may take different pilot-sample-sizes, $m_i (\geq 4)$, such as $m_i/C_i \in (0,1)$ as $p \to \infty$ for $i = 1, 2$. Then, the assertion in Theorem 4.4 is still claimed.

Remark 4.7. Assume (A-i)-(A-ii). Then, it holds as $p \to \infty$ that $N_i/C_i \xrightarrow{p} 1$ for $i = 1, 2$, which are in the HDLSS situation in the sense that $N_i/p \xrightarrow{p} 0$, $i = 1, 2$, under $\Delta_L \to \infty$ as $p \to \infty$.

4.3 Demonstration

We analyzed gene expression data given by Chiaretti et al. (2004) in which data set consisted of 12625 ($= p$) genes and 128 samples. Note that the expression measures were obtained by using the three-step robust multichip average (RMA) preprocessing method. Refer to Pollard et al. (2005) as well for the details. The data set had two tumor cellular subtypes, Π_1: B-cell (95 samples) and Π_2: T-cell (33 samples). We set $\alpha = 0.1$, $\beta = 0.02$ and $m = 6$. Our goal was to construct a discriminant rule ensuring that both $1 - e(2|1) \geq 0.9$ and $1 - e(1|2) \geq 0.98$ when $\Delta_\star \geq \Delta_L$, where Δ_L is designed later.

First, we took the first 6 samples from each Π_i as a pilot sample. According to Remark 4.5, we calculated $||\bar{x}_{1m} - \bar{x}_{2m}||^2 - \sum_{i=1}^{2} \text{tr}(S_{im})/m = 1890$ and $\widehat{Var}(||\bar{x}_{1m} - \bar{x}_{2m}||^2) = 87860$. By setting $\alpha' = 0.01$ so that $z_{\alpha'} = 2.33$, we designed a lower bound of $\Delta_\star$ by

$$\Delta_L = ||\bar{x}_{1m} - \bar{x}_{2m}||^2 - \sum_{i=1}^{2} \text{tr}(S_{im})/m - z_{\alpha'}\sqrt{\widehat{Var}(||\bar{x}_{1m} - \bar{x}_{2m}||^2)} = 1200.$$

According to (14), the total sample size for each Π_i was given by

$$N_1 = \max\left\{6, \left[\frac{(z_\alpha + z_\beta)^2 \hat{\sigma}}{\Delta_L^2}\text{tr}(S_{1m(1)}S_{1m(2)})^{1/4}\sum_{j=1}^{2}\text{tr}(S_{jm(1)}S_{jm(2)})^{1/4}\right] + 1\right\} = 10,$$

$$N_2 = \max\left\{6, \left[\frac{(z_\alpha + z_\beta)^2 \hat{\sigma}}{\Delta_L^2}\text{tr}(S_{2m(1)}S_{2m(2)})^{1/4}\sum_{j=1}^{2}\text{tr}(S_{jm(1)}S_{jm(2)})^{1/4}\right] + 1\right\} = 6.$$

So, we took the next 4 ($= N_1 - m$) samples from Π_1. On the other hand, since $N_2 = m$, we did not take additional samples from Π_2. We had $\hat{\gamma} = (\text{tr}(S_{1N_1} + S_{2N_2})/(2p))^{-1}\Delta_L(z_\beta - z_\alpha)/(z_\alpha + z_\beta) = 58.1$. Then, we constructed the discriminant rule given by (15) ensuring that both $1 - e(2|1) \geq 0.9$ and $1 - e(1|2) \geq 0.98$ when $\Delta_\star \geq 1200$.

We compared the constructed discriminant rule with two other discriminant rules, DLDR and DQDR, that were given by Dudoit et al. (2002) as follows: Diagonal linear discriminant rule (DLDR) classifies x_0 into Π_1 if

$$(x_0 - (\bar{x}_{1N_1} + \bar{x}_{2N_2})/2)^T S_{diag}^{-1}(\bar{x}_{2N_2} - \bar{x}_{1N_1}) < 0$$

and into Π_2 otherwise, where $S_{diag} = \text{diag}(s_{1N}, ..., s_{pN})$ having $s_{jN} = \sum_{i=1}^{2}\sum_{l=1}^{N_i}(x_{ijl} - \bar{x}_{ijN_i})^2$ $/(N_1 + N_2 - 2)$ and $\bar{x}_{ijN_i} = \sum_{l=1}^{N_i} x_{ijl}/N_i$. On the other hand, diagonal quadratic discriminant rule (DQDR) classifies x_0 into Π_1 if

$$(x_0 - \bar{x}_{1N_1})^T S_{diag(1)}^{-1}(x_0 - \bar{x}_{1N_1}) - (x_0 - \bar{x}_{2N_2})^T S_{diag(2)}^{-1}(x_0 - \bar{x}_{2N_2}) - \log\left\{\frac{\det(S_{diag(2)})}{\det(S_{diag(1)})}\right\} < 0$$

and into Π_2 otherwise, where $S_{diag(i)} = \text{diag}(s_{(i)1N_i}, ..., s_{(i)pN_i})$ having $s_{(i)jN_i} = \sum_{l=1}^{N_i}(x_{ijl} - \bar{x}_{ijN_i})^2 /(N_i - 1)$. We constructed the three discriminant rules by using the common data sets of sizes $(N_1, N_2) = (10, 6)$. In Table 2, we investigated those performances by using the remaining samples of sizes $(95 - N_1, 33 - N_2) = (85, 27)$ as test data sets. We observed that the discriminant rule given by (15) showed an adequate performance.

	(15)	DLDR	DQDR
$1-\overline{e}(2|1)$	75/85 (=0.882)	63/85 (=0.741)	76/85 (=0.894)
$1-\overline{e}(1|2)$	27/27 (=1.0)	24/27 (=0.889)	24/27 (=0.889)

Table 2. The correct discrimination rates, by (15), DLDR and DQDR, for test data sets consisting of 85 samples from Π_1 and 27 samples from Π_2.

5. Variable selection for high-dimension, low-sample-size data

Suppose we have two independent and p-dimensional populations, Π_i, $i = 1, 2$, having *unknown* mean vector $\boldsymbol{\mu}_i = (\mu_{i1}, ..., \mu_{ip})^T$ and *unknown* positive-definite covariance matrix $\boldsymbol{\Sigma}_i$ for each i. *We do not assume* $\boldsymbol{\Sigma}_1 = \boldsymbol{\Sigma}_2$. We consider an effective methodology to select a significant set of associated variables from among high-dimensional data sets. That is, we consider testing the following hypotheses simultaneously:

$$H_{0j} : \mu_{1j} = \mu_{2j} \quad \text{vs.} \quad H_{1j} : \mu_{1j} \neq \mu_{2j} \quad \text{for } j = 1, ..., p. \tag{16}$$

Our interest is to select a set of significant variables such that $\boldsymbol{D} = \{j : \mu_{1j} \neq \mu_{2j}\}$. Assume that $|\boldsymbol{D}| = S$ for some $S \geq 1$, where $|\boldsymbol{D}|$ denotes the number of elements in set $\boldsymbol{D}$. A variable selection procedure $\hat{\boldsymbol{D}}$ maps the data into subsets of $\{1, ..., p\}$. We are interested in designing $\hat{\boldsymbol{D}}$ ensuring that both the asymptotic *family-wise error rate* (FWER) is 0, i.e.,

$$P(|\boldsymbol{D}^c \cap \hat{\boldsymbol{D}}| \neq 0) \to 0, \tag{17}$$

and the asymptotic *average power* (AP) is 1, i.e.,

$$\frac{|\boldsymbol{D} \cap \hat{\boldsymbol{D}}|}{S} \xrightarrow{p} 1 \quad \text{when } \min_{j \in \boldsymbol{D}} |\mu_{1j} - \mu_{2j}|^2 > \delta, \tag{18}$$

where $\delta \ (> 0)$ is a prespecified constant. When S is bounded $(< \infty)$, one can modify (18) by

$$P(\boldsymbol{D} \subseteq \hat{\boldsymbol{D}}) \to 1 \quad \text{when } \min_{j \in \boldsymbol{D}} |\mu_{1j} - \mu_{2j}|^2 > \delta.$$

We note that the assertion (18) does not consider the case when $\min_{j \in \boldsymbol{D}} |\mu_{1j} - \mu_{2j}|^2 = \delta$.

5.1 Variable selection procedure for HDLSS data

Let $\sigma_i = \max_{1 \leq j \leq p} \sigma_{(i)j}$ $(i = 1, 2)$, where $\sigma_{(i)j}$, $j = 1, ..., p$, are diagonal elements of $\boldsymbol{\Sigma}_i$. We assume that $\sigma_{(i)j} < \infty$ for $i = 1, 2$; $j = 1, ..., p$, and $E_\theta\{\exp(t|x_{ijl} - \mu_{ij}|/\sigma_{(i)j}^{1/2})\} < \infty$, $i = 1, 2$; $j = 1, ..., p$, for some $t > 0$. Then, for testing the hypotheses (16), we take samples,

$x_{i1}, ..., x_{in_i}$, of size

$$n_i \geq \frac{(\log p)^{1+\zeta}}{\delta} \tag{19}$$

from each Π_i $(i = 1, 2)$, where $\zeta \in (0, 1]$ is a chosen constant. Let $x_{il} = (x_{i1l}, ..., x_{ipl})^T$, $l = 1, ..., n_i$. Calculate $T_{j(\mathbf{n})} = \bar{x}_{1jn_1} - \bar{x}_{2jn_2}$ for $j = 1, ..., p$, where $\bar{x}_{ijn_i} = \sum_{l=1}^{n_i} x_{ijl}/n_i$ for each Π_i. Then, test the hypothesis for $j = 1, ..., p$, by

$$\text{rejecting } H_{0j} \iff |T_{j(\mathbf{n})}| > \sqrt{\delta}. \tag{20}$$

Let $\hat{D} = \{j \mid \text{rejecting } H_{0j}\}$. Then, from Theorem 5.1 given in Aoshima and Yata (2011), we can claim the following theorem.

Theorem 5.1. *The test given by (20) with (19) has as $p \to \infty$ that*

$$P(|D^c \cap \hat{D}| \neq 0) \to 1;$$

$$\frac{|D \cap \hat{D}|}{S} \xrightarrow{p} 1 \quad \text{when} \quad \min_{j \in D} |\mu_{1j} - \mu_{2j}|^2 > \delta. \tag{21}$$

One would be interested in a two-stage variable selection procedure so as to provide screening of variables in the first stage. We consider selecting a significant set of associated variables from among a set of candidate variables in the second stage. Aoshima and Yata (2011) proposed the following effective methodology:

[Two-stage variable selection procedure]

(Step 1) Choose a pilot sample size m such as $m = O(\log p)$ and $m \to \infty$ as $p \to \infty$. Take pilot samples x_{il}, $l = 1, ..., m$, of size m from each Π_i $(i = 1, 2)$. Calculate $T_{j(m)} = \bar{x}_{1jm} - \bar{x}_{2jm}$ for $j = 1, ..., p$, where $\bar{x}_{ijm} = \sum_{l=1}^{m} x_{ijl}/m$ for each Π_i. Then, provide screening of variables by

$$\tilde{D} = \{j \mid |T_{j(m)}| > \sqrt{\delta}\} \tag{22}$$

for a set of candidate variables. Let $\tilde{S} = |\tilde{D}|$. Define the additional sample size for each Π_i by

$$N = \left[\frac{\max\{(\log \tilde{S})^{1+\xi}, (\log p)^\varepsilon\}}{\delta} \right] + 1, \tag{23}$$

where $\xi \in (0, 1]$ and $\varepsilon \in (0, 1]$ are chosen constants.

(Step 2) Regarding $j \in \tilde{D}$, take new samples x_{ijl}, $l = m + 1, ..., m + N$, of size N from each Π_i. Calculate $T_{j(N)} = \bar{x}_{1j(N)} - \bar{x}_{2j(N)}$, where $\bar{x}_{ij(N)} = \sum_{l=m+1}^{m+N} x_{ijl}/N$, $j \in \tilde{D}$ for each Π_i. Then, test the hypothesis by

$$\text{rejecting } H_{0j} \iff |T_{j(N)}| > \sqrt{\delta} \tag{24}$$

for $j \in \tilde{D}$, and define

$$\hat{D} = \{j \in \tilde{D} \mid \text{rejecting } H_{0j}\}. \tag{25}$$

Select the variables regarding $\hat{D}$.

From Theorem 5.2 in Aoshima and Yata (2011), we can claim the following theorem.

Theorem 5.2. *The two-stage variable selection procedure, (22) and (25), given by (24) with (23) has (21) as $p \to \infty$.*

5.2 Demonstration

We analyzed the gene expression data of Prostate Cancer that were given by Singh et al. (2002). The data took a pre-processing given by Jeffery et al. (2006). The data set consisted of 12600 ($= p$) genes and two groups, Π_1: Normal Prostate (50 samples) and Π_2: Prostate Tumors (52 samples).

5.2.1 Variable selection procedure

We set $\delta = 1.5$. Our goal was to find variables j's such that $|\mu_{1j} - \mu_{2j}|^2 > 1.5$. We chose the pilot sample size for each Π_i as $m = 18 (= O(\log p))$. Then, we took the first 18 samples from each Π_i as pilot samples, which are given in Table 3.

$j \backslash l$	Π_1: Normal Prostate		Π_2: Prostate Tumors	
	1 $\cdots$	18	1 $\cdots$	18
1	6.776 $\cdots$	7.017	6.888 $\cdots$	6.905
$\vdots$	$\vdots$	$\vdots$	$\vdots$	$\vdots$
12600	3.050 $\cdots$	3.612	3.097 $\cdots$	3.549

Table 3. Pilot samples, x_{ijl} ($p = 12600$, $m = 18$)

We considered screening variables by $\tilde{D} = \{j| |\bar{x}_{1jm} - \bar{x}_{2jm}|^2 > 1.5\}$. Then, we obtained a set of candidate variables as $\tilde{D} = \{192, 198, 200, ..., 12153, 12156, 12432\}$ with $\tilde{S} = |\tilde{D}| = 160$. We set $(\xi, \varepsilon) = (1.0, 1.0)$. According to (23), the additional sample size for each Π_i was given by

$$N = \left[\frac{\max\{(\log \tilde{S})^{1+\xi}, (\log p)^{\varepsilon}\}}{\delta} \right] + 1 = 18.$$

Regarding $j \in \tilde{D}$, we took additional samples x_{ijl}, $l = m+1, ..., m+N$, of size $N = 18$ from each Π_i, which are given in Table 4.

$j \backslash l$	Π_1: Normal Prostate		Π_2: Prostate Tumors	
	19 $\cdots$	36	19 $\cdots$	36
192	9.859 $\cdots$	8.973	9.338 $\cdots$	10.212
198	8.622 $\cdots$	7.077	6.120 $\cdots$	7.724
$\vdots$	$\vdots$	$\vdots$	$\vdots$	$\vdots$
12432	9.884 $\cdots$	9.091	8.00 $\cdots$	9.388

Table 4. Additional samples, $x_{ijl}, j \in \tilde{D}$ ($\tilde{S} = 160$, $N = 18$)

We selected significant variables by $\hat{D} = \{j \in \tilde{D}| \text{ rejecting } H_{0j}\} = \{j \in \tilde{D}| |\bar{x}_{1j(N)} - \bar{x}_{2j(N)}|^2 > 1.5\}$ and finally obtained

$$\hat{D} = \{556, 7412, 8662, 11552\} \tag{26}$$

with $\widehat{S} = |\widehat{D}| = 4$. For $j \in \widehat{D}$, we calculated $\bar{x}_{ijm+N} = \sum_{l=1}^{m+N} x_{ijl}/(m+N)$ for each Π_i and obtained estimates of $\mu_{1j} - \mu_{2j}$ for $j \in \widehat{D}$ as

$$\{\bar{x}_{1jm+N} - \bar{x}_{2jm+N}|\ j \in \widehat{D}\} = \{-1.511, -1.472, -1.79, -2.148\}.$$

The required sample-size in the two-stage variable selection procedure was $m + N = 36$ for each Π_i. On the other hand, the required sample-size in the single variable selection procedure given by (20) with (19) was $n_i \geq (\log p)^{1+\zeta}/\delta = 59.43$ with $\zeta = 1.0$. The two-stage variable selection procedure allows the experimenter to reduce the cost of sampling in the second stage.

5.2.2 Classification after variable selection

In Section 4, we considered a two-stage discriminant procedure in HDLSS data situations. In some cases the experimenter would encounter the situation that the required sample size, N_i, is much larger than the available sample size if $\Delta_\star = ||\mu_1 - \mu_2||^2 + (\mathrm{tr}(\Sigma_1) - \mathrm{tr}(\Sigma_2))^2/\max_{i=1,2}\{2\mathrm{tr}(\Sigma_i)\}$ is much smaller than $\mathrm{tr}(\Sigma_i^2)$'s. In that case, we recommend that the experimenter should consider the classification based only on the selected variables. We selected a set of significant variables by $\widehat{D} = \{556, 7412, 8662, 11552\}$ that was given in (26). We set $n_1 = n_2 = m + N = 36$, where m and N were given in Section 5.2.1. Let us write the selected 4-variable data as $x_{il} = (x_{i556l}, x_{i7412l}, x_{i8662l}, x_{i11552l})^T$, $i = 1, 2$, for the l-th sample. Then, we considered a typical quadratic discriminant rule that classifies x_0 into Π_1 if

$$(x_0 - \bar{x}_{1n_1})^T S_{1n_1}^{-1}(x_0 - \bar{x}_{1n_1}) - \log\left\{\frac{\det(S_{2n_2})}{\det(S_{1n_1})}\right\} < (x_0 - \bar{x}_{2n_2})^T S_{2n_2}^{-1}(x_0 - \bar{x}_{2n_2}), \quad (27)$$

and into Π_2 otherwise, where x_0 is an observation vector with respect to the 4 variables on an individual belonging to Π_1 or to Π_2, $\bar{x}_{in_i} = \sum_{l=1}^{n_i} x_{il}/n_i$ and $S_{in_i} = \sum_{l=1}^{n_i}(x_{il} - \bar{x}_{in_i})(x_{il} - \bar{x}_{in_i})^T/(n_i - 1)$, $i = 1, 2$.

We compared the discriminant rule given by (27) after variable selection with those given by (10) with $\gamma = 0$, DLDR and DQDR. Note that the three competitors were constructed by using the original (12600-variable) data without variable selection. In Table 5, we investigated those performances by using test data sets consisting of $50 - n_1 = 14$ remaining samples from Π_1 and $52 - n_2 = 16$ remaining samples from Π_2. We observed that the discriminant rule given by (10) with $\gamma = 0$ showed a bad performance for x_0 classified into Π_1: Normal Prostate. We inspected the condition of Theorem 4.1 for the data sets and found that $\max_{i=1,2}\{\mathrm{tr}(S_{in_i(1)}S_{in_i(2)})\}/(\widehat{\Delta}_\star^2 \min_{i=1,2}\{n_i\}) = 0.15$ according to Remark 4.4 so that $\max_{i=1,2}\{\mathrm{tr}(\Sigma_i^2)\}/(\Delta_\star^2 \min_{i=1,2}\{n_i\})$ seems not to be sufficiently small. This may be a reason why Theorem 4.1 is not applicable to the present data sets. On the other hand, we observed that the discriminant rule given by (27) after variable selection showed a good performance when compared to the competitors. We recommend that the experimenter should consider

	(27) after variable selection	(10) with $\gamma = 0$	DLDR	DQDR
$1-\overline{e(2|1)}$	10/14 (=0.714)	4/14 (=0.286)	4/14 (=0.286)	4/14 (=0.286)
$1-\overline{e(1|2)}$	15/16 (=0.938)	15/16 (=0.938)	15/16 (=0.938)	15/16 (=0.938)

Table 5. The correct discrimination rates by (27) after variable selection, (10) with $\gamma = 0$, DLDR and DQDR for test data sets consisting of 14 samples from Π_1 and 16 samples from Π_2.

the classification after variable selection if $\widehat{\Delta}_\star$ is not large enough to claim the condition of Theorem 4.1 or to claim the assertion in Theorem 4.4 within the available sample size.

6. Acknowledgments

Research of the first author was partially supported by Grant-in-Aid for Scientific Research (B) and Challenging Exploratory Research, Japan Society for the Promotion of Science (JSPS), under Contract Numbers 22300094 and 23650142. Research of the second author was partially supported by Grant-in-Aid for Young Scientists (B), JSPS, under Contract Number 23740066.

7. References

[1] Aoshima, M. & Yata, K. (2011). Two-stage procedures for high-dimensional data, *Sequential Analysis* (Editor's Special Invited Paper), to appear.

[2] Armstrong, S.A., Staunton, J.E., Silverman, L.B., Pieters, R. den Boer, M.L., Minden, M.D., Sallan, S.E., Lander, E.S., Golub, T.R. & Korsmeyer, S.J. (2001). MLL translocations specify a distinct gene expression profile that distinguishes a unique leukemia, *Nature Genetics*, Vol. 30, 41-47.

[3] Chiaretti, S., Li, X., Gentleman, R., Vitale, A., Vignetti, M., Mandelli, F., Ritz, J. & Foa, R. (2004). Gene expression profile of adult T-cell acute lymphocytic leukemia identifies distinct subsets of patients with different response to therapy and survival, *Blood*, Vol. 103, 2771-2778.

[4] Dudoit, S., Fridlyand, J. & Speed, T. P. (2002). Comparison of discrimination methods for the classification of tumors using gene expression data, *Journal of American Statistical Association*, Vol. 97, 77-87.

[5] Jeffery, I.B., Higgins, D.G. & Culhane, A.C. (2006). Comparison and evaluation of methods for generating differentially expressed gene lists from microarray data, *Bioinformatics*, Vol. 7, 359.

[6] Johnstone, I.M. & Lu, A.Y. (2009). On consistency and sparsity for principal components analysis in high dimensions, *Journal of American Statistical Association*, Vol. 104, 682-693.

[7] Pochet, N., De Smet, F., Suykens, J.A. & De Moor, B.L. (2004). Systematic benchmarking of microarray data classification: assessing the role of non-linearity and dimensionality reduction, *Bioinformatics*, Vol. 20, 3185-3195.

[8] Pollard, K.S., Dudoit, S. & van der Laan, M.J. (2005). Multiple testing procedures: R multtest package and applications to genomics, In: Gentleman, R., Carey, V., Huber, W., Irizarry, R. & Dudoit, S. (ed.) Bioinformatics and Computational Biology Solutions Using R and Bioconductor. Springer, New York, pp 249-271.

[9] Singh, D., Febbo, P.G., Ross, K., Jackson, D.G., Manola, J., Ladd, C., Tamayo, P., Renshaw, A.A., D'Amico, A.V., Richie, J.P., Lander, E.S., Loda, M., Kantoff, P.W., Golub, T.R. & Sellers, W.R. (2002). Gene expression correlates of clinical prostate cancer behavior, *Cancer Cell*, Vol.1(2), 203-209.

[10] Yata, K. (2010). Effective two-stage estimation for a linear function of high-dimensional Gaussian means, *Sequential Analysis*, Vol. 29, 463-482.

[11] Yata, K. & Aoshima, M. (2009). PCA consistency for non-Gaussian data in high dimension, low sample size context, *Communications in Statistics -Theory & Methods*, Special Issue Honoring Zacks, S. (ed. Mukhopadhyay, N.), Vol. 38, 2634-2652.

[12] Yata, K. & Aoshima, M. (2010a). Intrinsic dimensionality estimation of high-dimension, low sample size data with d-asymptotics, *Communications in Statistics -Theory & Methods*, Special Issue Honoring Akahira, M. (ed. Aoshima, M.), Vol. 39, 1511-1521.

[13] Yata, K. & Aoshima, M. (2010b). Effective PCA for high-dimension, low-sample-size data with singular value decomposition of cross data matrix, *Journal of Multivariate Analysis*, Vol. 101, 2060-2077.

[14] Yata, K. & Aoshima, M. (2011a). Inference on high-dimensional mean vectors with fewer observations than the dimension, *Methodology and Computing in Applied Probability*, in press.

[15] Yata, K. & Aoshima, M. (2011b). Effective PCA for high-dimension, low-sample-size data with noise reduction via geometric representations, *Journal of Multivariate Analysis*, revised.

4

Advanced Models for Target Validation & Drug Discovery in Prostate Cancer

Malin Åkerfelt, Ville Härmä and Matthias Nees
Medical Biotechnology Knowledge Centre
VTT technical Research Centre of Finland Turku
Finland

1. Introduction

Prostate cancer (PrCa) is one of the most prevalent malignant diseases among men in Western countries. Despite good initial treatment response is observed in the vast majority of PrCa patients, tumor relapse is observed in about 7-10% of patients undergoing standard anti-hormonal therapies with anti-androgens and/or GnRH antagonists. There is currently no cure for **castration-resistant prostate cancer** (**CRPC**), and median survival for these patients is only about 18 months. The high mortality rate of advanced cases is closely associated with invasive carcinomas and systemic metastasis, most frequently to the bone; and CRPC is almost always coincident with overexpression/amplification of the **androgen receptor (AR)** gene. CRPCs fail to respond to all currently prescribed first line anti-hormones such as flutamide, nilutamide or casodex (bicalutamide). The second line anti-tumor treatment against CRPC, frequently taxanes like docetaxel, is administered to patients after the first or second relapse. Taxanes are often supported by zoledronic acid targeting bone metastases. These drugs and drug combinations are in most cases initially effective, but rarely curative. Although taxanes do show potent anti-tumor effects, advanced PrCa patients develop resistance and only gain several months of survival time. For decades, no major improvements have been made in the therapy of advanced PrCa. However, this situation has dramatically changed over the last few years with a number of novel, promising drug concepts in the pipeline, some of which have already entered the market. It is not expected that these drugs will be curative, and relapses and therapy failures are expected to develop in these cases which may remain fatal. Therefore, the demands will remain high to develop yet better drugs, and more faithful models that reliably mimic at least some of the key aspects of advanced prostate cancers. These models are required to recapitulate the mechanisms leading to therapeutic resistance & failure also for new compounds and drug combinations entering the clinics now. There will remain a need to mimic which mechanisms either in the tumor cells or in the tumor-associated microenvironment may have contributed to the resistance. This consistent high demand in improved models will go hand in hand with a better understanding of the pros and cons of the various models available. Continued development of improved model systems for PrCa and in particular CRPC could lead to an informed ranking according to the maximal throughput in drug screens that can be achieved, balanced against their true informative value and relevance for recapitulating clinical PrCa. A systematic side-by-side comparison of available models, e.g. cell lines, organotypic three-dimensional cultures and co-cultures, xenografts, tissue recombination techniques and **genetically engineered mouse models** (**GEMMs**) is still missing. Furthermore, model development in PrCa is significantly lagging behind the advances in other fields, primarily breast cancer. Here, a considerably larger body of literature, methods, and better understanding of the pre-clinical models has been achieved, owing in part to innovative technologies such as 3D organotypic cultures and 3D tumor growth assays. Although prostate and breast cancer share many biological and histological properties and features, they remain fundamentally different diseases with different molecular pathways leading to transformation and progression. Modeling PrCa and in particular CRPC requires dedicated and specialized model development, coupled with a thorough characterization thereof.

In line with the relative lack of reliable PrCa models, and in contrast to other epithelial cancers, only a relative small number of molecular targets other than androgen receptor (AR) and AR-associated genes have been identified and validated in CRPCs (Feldman & Feldman, 2001). Even gene expression profiles of clinical prostate cancer samples were lagging behind studies related to e.g. breast cancers or gliomas, in particular characterization of advanced and metastatic lesions has been missing. Only recently, comprehensive large-scale transcriptome studies (> 250 clinical samples), combined with other levels of genetic analyses such as miRNA expression, next-generation sequencing, and analysis of mutations & copy number changes, have become available (Taylor et al., 2010). These studies will be invaluable for target identification and bioinformatic network analyses of PrCa's. Similarly, the identification of potent drugs that could block AR functions in CRPCs, such as novel synthetic anti-androgens, was mainly based on a relative small panel of largely reductionist models and cell lines (van Bokhoven et al., 2003a; 2003b). This situation has only slightly improved after the generation of a panel of new, more informative cell lines in the 1990's, and remains a key problem in PrCa research.

Additionally, many of the routine models for the pre-clinical phase of drug development are greatly insufficient, and fail to recapitulate key aspects of the molecular and biologic diversity of PrCa. For example, many PrCa cell lines actually lack expression of key molecular components such as AR or the critical ETS fusion factors. Furthermore, in particular in the early stages of pre-clinical research and cell-based screens, cell lines are routinely cultivated in monolayer on plastic. This does not support formation of **extracellular matrix (ECM)** nor relevant **cell-cell interactions** and epithelial **differentiation processes** to occur. Cell-cell-contacts formed by cells on plastic are of temporary nature, and fail to properly recapitulate differentiation and maturation programs intrinsic to epithelial cells. A key feature of both breast and PrCa is the capacity to undergo "acinar morphogenesis", i.e. the formation of functional glandular spheroids and tubular structures that connect such organoids. These are a key element of epithelial plasticity and contribute to cell motility and invasiveness (branching, spreading). No such features can be observed in monolayer cultures, depriving otherwise even potentially informative model systems of biological relevance. To overcome these shortcomings, organotypic cultures of breast and prostate cancer cell lines have been investigated since the early 1970's.

Cells can also be embedded in artificial or natural matrices or scaffolds. This provides an altogether different biology that has very little resemblance to the "floating" spheroids formed in non-adherent cultures, apart from the often equally rounded overall shape. Spheroid cultures or PrCa cells embedded in extracellular matrices have been systematically explored since 2001 (Bello-DeOcampo et al., 2001; Lang et al., 2001). This was again lagging behind the breast cancer field, in which such efforts were initiated in the 1990's (Streuli et al.,

1991; Weaver et al., 1995; Weaver et al., 1996). Later studies introduced a focus on tissue differentiation, morphogenesis and imaging (Debnath et al., 2003; Debnath & Brugge, 2005; Mailleux et al., 2008). The development of defined scaffolds/matrices is ongoing, although the most widely used material remains Matrigel. This is derived from a mouse sarcoma cell line that produces large amounts of laminin-rich ECM.

However, the most important shortcoming of currently available models for PrCa and CRPC is the lack of complexity that is recapitulated by mono-culture of a single cell type, usually the tumor cells. These do not act as singular entities and a carcinoma in fact represents a disturbed, but nevertheless complex tissue with its own regulation of tissue homeostasis. Tumor and stromal cells (in combination with ECM components such as laminins and collagens) are the main actors in tissue formation, followed by smooth muscle or myoepithelial cells and invading components of the immune system (Fig. 1). The development of co-culture systems of tumor cells with relevant tumor-associated or normal fibroblasts has not yet left the developmental phase. Despite a large number of different approaches, there is no consensus which of these models would be particularly informative and relevant. Most of the co-culture models may not be highly reproducible and remain only poorly standardized. Thus, more reliable models to study tumor-host interactions and the role of the stromal compartment in development and progression of PrCa are still much in demand. Also the role of tumor stroma in mouse xenografts is debated.

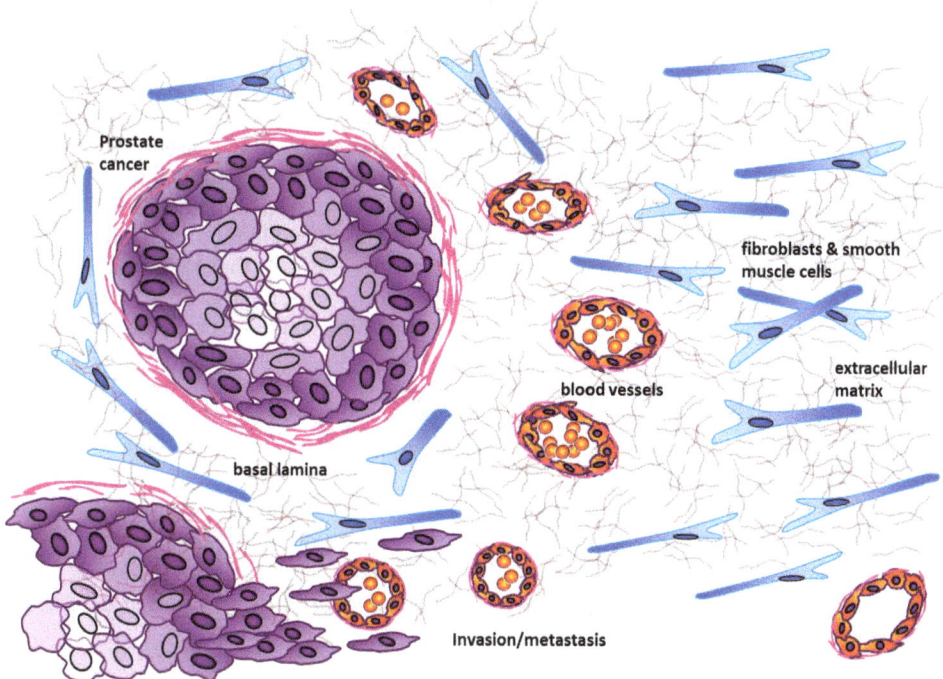

Fig. 1. Anatomy of prostate cancer. In low-grade tumors, cancer cells are still enclosed by intact basement membrane. The interstitial ECM is composed of fibrous proteins such as collagens, glycosaminoglycans and fibronectin. The cellular part is formed by fibroblasts, smooth muscle cells, myoepithelial cells, endothelial cells and invading actors of the immune system.

As a result, a lack of understanding of key molecular events in tumor progression to metastatic, invasive prostate cancers (CRPC) remains. Most models lack the required complexity, but also relevant high throughput capacities required for early stage pre-clinical research. Furthermore, most complex experimental systems are not cost effective. Many of the basic tools required for high content or **high-throughput cell-based screening (HTS)**, such as miniaturization, automation, and reliable readout systems are in a rudimentary state. Furthermore, those few model systems that allow higher throughput, may not be very representative for prostate cancer biology and differentiation. Such experimental systems are typically based on floating "prostaspheres" or organoids/microtissues; these, however, do not undergo significant differentiation processes. Only very few, matrix-embedded organotypic models are available for HTS. Apart from the lack of biological relevance of many experimental systems, it also remains generally difficult to transfer informative model systems across different laboratories. Together, these eminent insufficiencies may explain why preclinical studies are too often poorly predictive for the outcome of clinical trials, and why many of these trials eventually fail – typically in stage II or III. Generally, for a new compound to be synthesized and approved on the market it takes about 10 years or more, costing billions of dollars, and the number of FDA approved drug has steadily decreased during the last few years. At this point of the clinical drug discovery pipeline, a large sum of money has already been invested. Parts of it could have been saved, provided the target validation strategy had been more informative and pre-clinical models utilized had been more predictive. **Therefore, it is critical for future drug development to integrate multiple efforts, models and target validation strategies into a more comprehensive approach.** Only a broader spectrum of biologically relevant models allows thorough exploration of key mechanisms involved in therapy failure, and to focus on the major pathways involved in progression to CRPC. Furthermore, it will be mandatory to include the essential aspects of tumor-host cell interactions and tumor cell heterogeneity. This chapter will give an overview of the most relevant cell-based model systems currently available. We will mainly focus on in vitro cell culture models with an excursion into the wide field of orthotopic and subcutaneous xenografts. Only some selected examples for GEMMs that have been recently developed will be addressed here, in close connection to the cancer mechanisms and pathway they are modeling. Excellent reviews on mouse models of PrCa in general (Hensley & Kyprianou, 2011; Park et al., 2010) and GEMMS in particular (Jeet et al., 2010; Wang, 2011) have been published recently. According to this, we felt an overview of the status of ex vivo models may be timely, as this field is rapidly evolving and has not been widely reviewed. The most urgent unmet needs apply for the research related to fatal, under-treated CRPC. Our focus will therefore be mainly on the molecular pathways involved in progression to CRPC. Our aim is to discuss how advanced models may help to address improve target validation and drug discovery particularly in CRPC.

2. Target Validation: Modelling pathways and mechanisms in castration-resistant prostate cancer (CRPC)

2.1 Modeling AR modifications in CRPC

AR functions remain critical in essentially all CRPCs. AR is the target of genetic DNA amplifications leading to its overexpression (Koivisto et al., 1997; Visakorpi et al., 1995), as well as function-modifying point mutations. DNA amplifications targeting the AR locus result in overexpression of AR in up to 30% of the patients. Gain-of-function mutations of

AR (20-30% of patients) enable AR to bind a broad spectrum of steroidal and non-steroidal molecules as agonists (Koivisto et al., 1999; van de Wijngaart et al., 2010). Functionally relevant AR modifications include also changes in co-regulatory molecules such as nuclear co-activators and repressors. Additionally, alterations of signaling cascades that lead to activation of AR independent of ligand(s) have been described (reviewed in (Scher & Sawyers, 2005). In combination, these modifications are the most critical molecular mechanism that renders CRPCs independent of physiological levels of androgens. CRPCs thrive on significantly reduced levels of androgens or utilize alternative ligands that are more readily available. In some cases, AR mutations may render PrCa cells completely independent of external ligand supplies and the tumors develop an entirely independent, self-sufficient AR signaling axis – although AR still remains the main target. Ligand-independent and ligand-mediated functional activation of AR is reflected by phoshorylation, subsequent nuclear import (Jenster et al., 1993), and transcriptional activation of AR target genes such as **PSA (prostate-specific antigen)**. While PSA and other classic AR-controlled genes remain mostly driven by AR, the overall spectrum of AR-responsive genes is often greatly altered and expanded in advanced cancers (Wang et al., 2009a). This observation has only recently changed the basic understanding of CRPC biology.

Upon failure of primary therapy, anti-androgens such as casodex, flutamide or nilutamide fail to block AR and/or start promoting cell proliferation instead. These antagonists often convert to agonists (activators) of AR signaling, a poorly understood mechanistic complication (Dahut & Madan, 2010) - for which few experimental model systems exist. Many AR mutations described in patients confer gain-of-function properties. In the clinics, the conversion of anti-androgens and tumor relapse is reflected in a sudden steep increase of PSA levels. Nevertheless, PSA rise as such is only poorly indicative of patient survival and fails to predict response or failure of therapy. Instead of PSA, scintigraphy and PET imaging have turned out to be more reliable. However, the most promising method may be the detection of **circulating tumor cells (CTCs)** (Attard et al., 2009; Danila et al., 2010; Danila et al., 2011). CTCs typically contain the same cancer-relevant mutations as the primary tumor, e.g. amplified/mutated AR. These features can be utilized for further characterization and fine tuning of diagnostic tools (Attard et al., 2010; Zhang et al., 2010). However - the role of CTCs in forming distant metastases and relapse is only poorly understood. No good models are available that would dynamically mimic the systemic spread of PrCa cells. For example, xenografts rarely produce metastatic lesions to the bone, which represents the most frequent metastatic site in humans. Additionally, detection of small metastatic lesions by in vivo imaging is technically difficult (van Weerden et al., 2009), and may require removal of the primary tumor to allow monitoring the metastases. In vivo imaging may also suffer from extremely dynamic cell behavior in vivo: small lesions spontaneously disappear and reoccur at other locations, with few lesions able to successfully maintain themselves. It remains unclear how well these animal models represent the acute human problem of developing metastatic CRPC (Eaton et al., 2010). Major improvements in the use of light-emitting cell lines and more sensitive detection methods may help to overcome these difficulties in the future. Even more important would be the generation of reliable cell line models that effectively form metastatic lesions in mouse models – ideally utilizing mechanisms similar to human systemic spread.

Until very recently, little progress was made in the development of novel anti-androgens. The most exciting new entities, MDV3100, its derivative RD162 and TAK-700, were recently demonstrated as superior to casodex in castration-resistant LNCaP-AR xenograft models. Both MDV3100 and TAK-700 were also successful in clinical studies (Attard et al., 2011;

Chen et al., 2009; Massard & Fizazi, 2011; Tran et al., 2009). A phase I/II multi-center first-in-man trial of MDV3100 was recently completed (Scher et al., 2010), and a regulatory phase III trial with advanced PrCa patients previously failing taxane therapy has started in 2010. According to preliminary clinical data, MDV3100 does not quickly develop agonism to AR in CRPCs, and shows a more consistently and robust antagonist activity clearly superior to casodex. The still limited potential of these drugs is reflected in the possibility to generate MDV3100 resistant cell clones, e.g. *in vivo* by continued daily treatment of mice followed by serial passage of LNCaP/AR xenografts, or *in vitro* by using VCaP cells and long term drug exposure. In the majority of these resistant clones, AR expression is maintained. This is likely to happen in relapsed tumors from future clinical use. As expected, MDV3100-resistant CRPC cells remain dependent on continued AR signaling as demonstrated by siRNA knockdown: Not even the most advanced novel drugs are capable of breaking this addiction. In conclusion, novel drugs like Orteronel (TAK-700) and MDV3100 are unlikely to be curative, and will result in relapse and further progression with yet unknown frequency and time course. To explore the putative molecular mechanisms of MDV3100 or TAK-700 resistance in the future will require a very systematic approach and the use of a comprehensive panel of complementary models. There will also be a need to systematically address the impact of the tumor microenvironment and the stromal counterpart, using organotypic and co-culture models. These interactions are expected to considerable contribute to the development of late stage drug resistance, compared to treatment of primary tumors.

CRPC tumors may gain the capability to metabolically synthesize sufficient levels of androgens, which renders the tumors completely independent of endocrine hormone supplies (testis, adrenal gland). The drug **abiraterone acetate**, recently approved by the FDA for treatment of advanced CRPC, (Agarwal et al., 2010; de Bono et al., 2011; Molina & Belldegrun, 2011), blocks the formation of androgens by inhibiting CYP17A1 (17α-hydroxylase/17, 20 lyase). This metabolic enzyme is involved in the formation of DHEA and androstenedione. These intermediates are then further metabolized to testosterone (Attard et al., 2009a; Attard et al., 2009b). Like MVD3100 and TAK-700, abiraterone showed promising results in phase I-III clinical trials (Ryan et al., 2010; Shah & Ryan, 2010; Sharifi, 2010), but the response rate is equally incomplete and was approved by the FDA in April 2011. Abiraterone is also expected to result in resistances, with mechanisms that are very likely to involve the tumor microenvironment (stromal cells, endocrine factors and myoepithelial/smooth muscle cells). For example, the stromal cells may actually be responsible for developing resistance, subsequently providing significant levels of androgens to nearby tumor cells.

Nevertheless, recent success stories only illustrate that AR remains the fundamental target in PrCa, essentially throughout all stages of progression. Nevertheless, the novel drugs also demonstrate that it is possible to temporarily block AR or androgen functions even in CRPC. How well these new drugs will improve the efficacy of CRPC treatment, will be shown in the future. Understanding both the mechanisms of action & pathways leading to the expected resistance in tumor cells will require more than ever the use of a panel of advanced prostate cancer models. More detailed understanding of AR-related signaling pathways and an improved, contextual target validation will have the potential to significantly improve therapy and patient outcome. Ideally, this will include exploring the potency of combination therapies with older concepts, such as ketoconazole (Figg et al., 2010; Peehl et al., 2002; Ryan et al., 2010) or prednisone (Danila et al., 2010).

The insight that PrCa progression to CRPC is intricately associated with hyperactive androgen signaling was recently demonstrated by the generation of a mouse model based on an activating AR mutation (T877A), which was overexpressed in prostatic epithelial cells by targeted somatic mutagenesis. ARpe-T877A mice formed hypertrophies and eventually carcinomas (Takahashi et al., 2011). Tumor progression was greatly enhanced by overexpression of Wnt-5a that served as an activator. These findings suggest that mutant AR alone may already provide tumor-promoting properties which are further potentiated by additional genetic alterations. Such novel and exciting transgenic mouse models for PrCa may become very powerful tools in future pre-clinical trials (Jeet et al., 2010; Wang, 2011).

2.2 Modeling ETS fusion transcripts in PrCa & CRPC

AR may be the key player in PrCa progression but is certainly not acting in isolation. This was recently demonstrated by the discovery of TMPRSS2-ETS factor fusion genes that can be attributed to 40-60% of all PrCa (Tomlins et al., 2005; Tomlins et al., 2006; Tomlins et al., 2007; Tomlins et al., 2008). Other ETS fusion factors such as ETV1 and ETV4 (Hermans et al., 2008a; Hermans et al., 2008b) were soon following. The panel of ETS fusion rearrangements and driver genes/promoters is still growing, although the most frequent and relevant translocation is the TMPRSS2-ERG event. The occurrence of TMPRSS2-ETS factor fusion events is considered an important initiating event in PrCa tumor progression (Mosquera et al., 2008; Perner et al., 2007; Saramaki et al., 2008), but is not sufficient to fully transform benign prostate cells. This has been demonstrated by the fact that ETS fusion genes also act as tumor-initiating factors in transgenic mouse models (Brenner et al., 2011; Carver et al., 2009a; Carver et al., 2009b), but generally require cooperative oncogenic events such as haplo-insufficiency or complete loss of PTEN and activation of c-Myc (Sun et al., 2008) for progression to invasive carcinomas. Apart from the tumors, ETS fusion gene transcripts have also been detected in clinical pre-malignant lesions such as **HGPIN (high grade prostatic intraepithelial neoplasias)**. Surprisingly, TMPRSS2-ERG expression is frequently associated with a favorable prognosis (Hermans et al., 2009; Saramaki et al., 2008). Thus, ETS factor fusion genes events may represent cancer-initiating events, but might not critically contribute to tumor progression and CRPC. Also in clinical PrCa, ETS factors may need to cooperate with additional oncogenic events such as PI3Kinase pathway activation, loss of one allele of PTEN and AR amplification (King et al., 2009; Squire, 2009; Yu et al., 2010), which are considered key factors for tumor progression. However, this topic remains controversial: Duplication of the TMPRSS2-ERG fusion gene locus was associated with worsened prognosis and progression towards advanced CRPC (Attard et al., 2008; Attard et al., 2010). This also makes sense, as ETS fusion events are strictly androgen-responsive and require functional AR, which links ETS factors intimately to AR biology. Accordingly, TMPRSS2-ERG fusion gene expression is massively re-activated in CRPC tumors (Cai et al., 2009), concomitant with the over-expression of androgen-dependent genes like PSA. Thus, appropriate models for CRPC and the role of AR should not underestimate the contribution of ETS fusion genes, and their function cannot be clearly functionally separated from AR signaling. Only a small fraction of PrCa cell lines that contain actively transcribed ETS fusion transcripts have been described, such as the VCaP and DuCaP lines (Korenchuk et al., 2001). These cell lines harbor the characteristic AR amplification. Both VCaP and DuCaP, established from different metastatic lesions of the same patient, represent excellent models for both CRPC and ETS-factor positive PrCa. Nevertheless, these cell lines do not readily form metastatic lesions in xenograft mouse models (Havens et al., 2008; Loberg et al., 2007;

van Golen et al., 2008) nor do they belong to the most straightforward cell lines to grow in the laboratory – which somewhat limits their value. More advanced, aggressive models for CRPC based on VCaP cells have been generated using mouse xenografts (Loberg et al., 2006a; Loberg et al., 2006b). Apart from VCaP, only the NCI-H660 cell line contains another TMPRSS2-ERG fusion event (Mertz et al., 2007). But NCI-H660 is not a typical "luminal" PrCa cell line and lacks expression of AR, which renders this model rather irrelevant for many aspects of CRPC. This line was initially described as a small-cell lung carcinoma before it was reclassified as the metastasis of a prostate small-cell carcinoma. NCI-H660 may represent a model for the neuroendocrine differentiation phenotype, which is sometimes observed in PrCa. Furthermore, the classic castration-resistant, androgen-responsive LNCaP cell line contains a rearranged ETV1 fusion gene. However, ETV1 is not functionally expressed and LNCaP therefore not a very relevant model for ETS factor biology. Loss of ETV1 expression may indicate that this gene is not required for progression to CRPC. In summary, it is surprising that ETS fusion events appear to be under-represented in established PrCa cell lines. This observation may be related to particular difficulties to establish ETS-factor positive PrCa lines from clinical tumor material. The diagnosis of ETS factor fusion genes in PrCa have only now begun to affect clinical practice and diagnostics (Laxman et al., 2008; Tomlins et al., 2009), although detection of fusion events may soon become a routine technique (Hu et al., 2008; Jhavar et al., 2008; Mao et al., 2008). As of yet, the discovery of ETS fusion genes has also not resulted in many novel and useful therapeutic concepts (Björkman et al., 2008), although the first functional insights may yet have to be followed up and clinically translated (Gupta et al., 2010; Mohamed et al., 2011; Yu et al., 2010). A lack of appropriate models that faithfully mimic the biology of ETS fusions in the context of PrCa and CRPC may have contributed to the relative slow progress in this field.

2.3 Modeling molecular pathways beyond AR: PTEN, PI3 kinase and AKT

Alternative pathways for ligand-independent activation of AR are discussed as key mechanisms in at least a subset of CRPC. However, the kinases suggested to be involved, their clinical relevance, and the number of cases affected are still highly debated. Insights from large-scale tumor sequencing efforts such as the Sanger Institute (COSMIC database of somatic mutations in cancer; http://www.sanger.ac.uk/perl/genetics/CGP/cosmic) have identified candidate genes that are most frequently mutated in PrCa. According to this database (Status July 2011), p53 mutations are the most frequently found somatic alterations (19%), followed by PTEN (14%), and KRAS mutations (7%). Mutations in all three ras genes (HRAS, KRAS, NRAS) together account for about 13% of PrCa cases. Other frequent mutations, pointing essentially to the same key molecular pathways involved in prostate cancer progression, are EGFR (7%), beta-catenin (CTNNB1; 6%), Retinoblastoma (RB, 6%) and B-raf (4%). The frequencies for PTEN are significantly higher if genetic deletions (LOH) and rearrangements are also taken into account. Loss of one allele of PTEN is the most frequent genetic alteration in primary PrCa, while loss of both PTEN alleles is frequently observed in advanced CRPC. This genetic background information is critical to evaluate the biological relevance of models for PrCa and CRPC.

PTEN (phosphatase and tensin homolog deleted on chromosome 10) and the downstream PI3 Kinase (PI3K) and AKT pathways are closely linked to CRPC. PTEN loss and perturbation of these pathways have been implicated in early stage prostate carcinogenesis (Zong et al., 2009) as well as late stage CRPC (Verhagen et al., 2006; Vlietstra et al., 1998).

PTEN negatively regulates the activity of AKT and PI3K pathways. Loss of one or both alleles of PTEN increases the intracellular levels of the second messenger PIP3 and results in constitutive activation of AKT. PI3K promotes the activation of AKT at Thr^{308} via the kinase PDK1, followed by a second phosphorylation step by PDK2 at Ser^{473}. AKT then translocates into the nucleus and triggers many cell survival mechanisms, promotes cell cycle progression, and possibly invasion (reviewed in (Sarker et al., 2009)). Oncogenic, activating AKT mutations and gene amplifications have been described (Boormans et al., 2010). AKT's role as a primary survival factor may significantly contribute to the development of CRPC and therapy failure. Furthermore, PI3K and AKT are important pathways for the maintenance of PrCa stem cell populations (Dubrovska et al., 2009; Korkaya et al., 2009; Sarker et al., 2009) and stem cell survival. The PI3K pathway cooperates with other important proto-oncogene such as c-Myc (Clegg et al., 2011) in PrCa and model systems, and promotes cancer progression in both. Receptor tyrosine kinases (RTKs) like EGF Receptor, Her2/ERBB2, c-MET or IGF1R, as well as non-RTK's, also result in the activation of PI3K and AKT. Therefore, frequent observation of EGFR mutations in PrCa's functionally contributes to the same clinically relevant pathways, as do s Ras and B-raf mutations, which are downstream signaling cascades. PTEN loss, AKT and PI3K pathways have been functionally associated with ligand-independent AR activation mechanisms, but conclusive validation and precise functional details e.g. in clinical tumors are clearly missing. AKT may interact with and contribute to the ligand-independent phosphorylation of AR in CRPCs (Shen & Abate-Shen, 2007). Gain of function mutations in the PI3K pathway, primarily mutations of PIK3CA, are also the most frequent genetic mutation in breast cancers (Samuels et al., 2004), and occur sporadically in PrCa (< 1%).

Tissue-specific knock-out of a single allele of PTEN in mice promotes the formation of hyperplastic lesions but not carcinogenesis, (Korsten et al., 2009; Liao et al., 2010c). Haplo-insufficiency of PTEN strongly requires cooperation with additional tumorigenic events such as TMPRSS2-ERG fusion genes (Carver et al., 2009b; King et al., 2009; Squire, 2009), loss of NKX3.1 (Song et al., 2009), p53 mutations (Abou-Kheir et al., 2010; Couto et al., 2009), STAT3 (Blando et al., 2011), and AR overexpression. Loss of PTEN in the mouse prostate epithelium is generally insufficient to generate malignant lesions in transgenic mouse models (Couto et al., 2009), and typically results only in the formation of pre-malignant hyperplastic lesions. Interestingly, PTEN inactivation in mouse models without supporting additional events may primarily result in a specific form of senescence, which can be readily overcome by p53 knock-down (Alimonti et al., 2010). The resulting tumor cells show a dramatically increased stem- or progenitor cell and self-renewing potential (Dubrovska et al., 2009; Korkaya et al., 2009; Mulholland et al., 2009). It is also possible to isolate PTEN (-/+) mouse PrCa cell lines from primary tumors for molecular follow-up studies (Jiao et al., 2007; Liao et al., 2010c), and to further genetically modify these cells for generating androgen-independent CRPC lines. This includes the stromal compartment, which can also be extracted from transgenic mice and used for sophisticated tissue recombination and grafting experiments (Liao et al., 2010a; Liao et al., 2010b). Tissue recombination, e.g. combining mouse urogenital mesenchyme cells, or tumor-associated fibroblasts are a powerful model to explore tumor-host interactions and tumor microenvironment (Liao et al., 2010a). Cells from genetically engineered mouse models (GEMMs) can be further propagated in spheroid or 3D cultures, which may enhance the stem cell character of the resulting clones (Liao et al., 2010b).

The requirement for additional oncogenic events is also exemplified in mice in which loss of PTEN is combined with over-expression of the TMPRSS2-ERG fusion oncogene (Carver et al., 2009b) or loss of NKX3.1 (Song et al., 2009). NKX3.1 (-/-) PTEN (+/-) mice spontaneously develop androgen-independent lesions following castration (Abate-Shen et al., 2003; Gao et al., 2006; Kim et al., 2002; Ouyang et al., 2005), which renders this model particularly interesting for CRPC. Despite the availability of several mouse models generated by targeted knock-down of PTEN, only a few of these have resulted in castration-resistant tumors that represent human CRPC. In some instances, the physical or chemical castration of mice has been used to generate CRPCs (Banach-Petrosky et al., 2007; Shen & Abate-Shen, 2007). However, it is unclear how relevant this approach is as the endocrine production of androgens is different in mice and men. Furthermore, carcinomas will ideally form only after a very long time period, related to the natural aging process of the mouse (> 12 months). This represents a logistic restriction for the availability of such tumors/cell lines for larger scale experimentation.

Simultaneously, addressing the most AR-associated pathways (PI3K, AKT, mTOR) is incomplete without simultaneously incorporating upstream aspects of RTK signaling on these pathways and AR. The most relevant RTKs are most likely EGFR, ERBB2/Her2, IGF1R and the c-MET/HGF Receptors. In connection with AKT and PI3K activation, these RTK's and signaling modifiers like IGFBP2 (Mehrian-Shai et al., 2007) are important for the development and progression of PrCa; however their mutation spectrum and relevance in PrCa and CRPC is not very well established. Most critically, there are no PrCa animal models available yet that would systematically address these signaling mechanisms for generation of GEMMs. Oncogenic signaling and crosstalk through different RTK's, the variable functions and shifting roles of RTK's during therapy, tumor cell selection and the development of resistance, are likely to represent key mechanisms for target validation in anti-cancer therapy. Among the kinase receptors, the c-MET/HGF receptor pathway represents a particularly interesting target for CRPC and there is a need to recapitulate its molecular role by advanced model systems. Like EGFR, c-MET signaling appears to play a key role in many aspects of PrCa pathology (Szabo et al., 2011; Tu et al., 2010), particularly in regulating tumor cell motility, invasion and metastases (Pisters et al., 1995) as well as **epithelial-to-mesenchymal transition (EMT)**. Furthermore, c-Met/HGF signaling is possibly involved in the maintenance of cancer-initiating (stem-) cells and stem cell proliferation (Eaton et al., 2010; Pfeiffer et al., 2011).

2.4 Modeling tumor cell heterogeneity and mechanisms involved in cancer initiating or stem cells

An increasing amount of evidence implies a role for many additional mechanisms in progression to therapy-resistant cancers. This includes the overexpression of anti-apoptotic genes (Bcl-2 or Mcl-1, BIRC5/survivin), induction of the MDR (multi drug resistance) transmembrane pumps, activation of NF-κB, STAT2/3, and integrin-linked survival pathways (Weaver et al., 2002). These pathways may be critical for at least subsets of CRPCs. Cells that utilize additional survival mechanisms successfully may be strongly selected for under the conditions of anti-cancer treatment, and are likely to contribute to resistant cell clones. They are also likely to contribute to the generation of tumor cell heterogeneity before, during and after anti-cancer therapy. A spectrum of cellular factors like aneuploidy, differentiation and epigenetics are apparent in tumor tissues. Both genetic and non-genetic heterogeneities are likely to contribute to the clonal selection of resistant tumor cells and/or tumor stem cell populations (Brock et al., 2009; Shackleton et al., 2009). Additional levels of heterogeneity are added by the cell populations from the tumor microenvironment (fibroblasts, myoepithelial cells), the immune system (monocytes, macrophages), and endothelial cells. During anti-cancer treatment, the hierarchical organization of tumors and their homeostatic regulation changes significantly. Together with the generation of genetically different clones, both aspects give rise to increasingly tumorigenic tumor cells & therapy resistance. The tumor context, tumor-host interactions and co-evolution with stromal components (Karnoub et al., 2007; Weinberg, 2008) are therefore critical aspects to understand clonal evolution and the nature of the resistant cells (Sawyers, 2007). However, there is a fundamental lack of reliable model systems to monitor dynamic changes in tumor & stromal heterogeneity (Marusyk & Polyak, 2010). The need for better systems to monitor epithelial plasticity is evident (van der Pluijm, 2011; Wang & Shen, 2011).

Alternatively, it has been suggested that residual disease and tumor relapse may be largely based on the long-term survival of **cancer-initiating cells (CICs)** or **cancer stem cells (CSCs)**. These rare and mitotically rather inactive cell populations have been suggested to persist during therapy, while the bulk tumor mass may yet be largely diminished. Stem cell populations may be intrinsically more resistant to chemotherapy (Diehn & Clarke, 2006; Diehn et al., 2009), and CICs may naturally acquire invasive properties, e.g. by undergoing EMT. CICs may therefore be largely identical to **metastasis-initiating cells (MICs)** (Mani et al., 2008; Polyak & Weinberg, 2009). In PrCa, the nature of CIC/CSCs and their association with EMT (Dunning et al., 2011) is debated. While it is widely accepted that PrCa contains a functional stem compartment, the molecular characteristics of CSCs remains unclear. It is not even established if these stem cells are of luminal or basal phenotype (Maitland et al., 2011). According to this uncertainty, there is a lack of appropriate and accepted models that address the biological relevance of CSC populations experimentally. The most relevant information may be derived from mouse models, while a role for stem cells in cell lines is even more debated. Some mouse models point to a rare luminal cell type (Wang et al., 2009b), while others describe molecular profiles more consistent with a basal and/or mesenchymal phenotype (Frith et al., 2010a; Giannoni et al., 2010; Kong et al., 2010), which is consistent with observations in the breast cancer field. Some models, such as tumor spheroid ("prostaspheres") cultures and non-adherent growth conditions, promote CSC properties and result in enhanced self-reproduction potential (Rybak et al., 2011; Watanabe & Takagi, 2008). This technique is now routinely used to enrich CSCs from mouse models (Liao et al., 2010a; Liao et al., 2010b) and human cell lines alike. Isolation of CSC populations from primary tumors (Guzman-Ramirez et al., 2009) and xenografts by serial passage of spheroids (Patrawala et al., 2006; Tang et al., 2007) or FACS reproducibly result in tumorigenic cancer-initiating cells. Their properties are similar to those generated by treatment with arsenic (Tokar et al., 2010a; Tokar et al., 2010b). The ultimate test for CSC characteristics is the inoculation of a limiting number of cells subcutaneously or into the mouse prostate, resulting in formation of tumors – although there are not as many studies compared e.g. to breast cancer CSCs (Al-Hajj et al., 2003; Dontu et al., 2005). It has been criticized that such assays may be an oversimplification and could simply select for the most tumorigenic cell populations. These may or may not coincide with CSC populations. The continuous debate indicates that also here, a lack of appropriate models (and biological understanding) limit the progress of drug discovery. Nude mouse models

(NOD/SCID) commonly used for inoculation experiments are far from fully representing the complexity of human malignancies. Generally, these models critically lack immune cells and lymphocyte-related cytokine/chemokine secretion. Furthermore, in xenografts, human cancer cells become rapidly associated with mouse fibroblasts. Even co-inoculation of cancer cells with human fibroblasts typically results in their rapid, effective replacement with mouse mesenchymal cells. Cell-cell interaction of human tumor cells with human stromal cells can therefore not be investigated. This poses a particular problem to the investigation of molecular pathways such as c-Met/HGF signaling (Tu et al., 2010; Yap & de Bono, 2010), in which the ligand is typically secreted by the stromal cells, while the receptor is expressed exclusively on the epithelial cancer cells. This represents a notorious problem for the validation of inhibitors and diagnostic tools alike (Knudsen & Vande Woude, 2008; Knudsen et al., 2009). Alternatively, it may be recommended to explore such pathways by mouse cells, accepting species-to-species differences. This will nevertheless assure that receptor-ligand interactions are fully functional. Tissue recombination approaches may also be very informative. The roles of non-genetic heterogeneity in clonal selection, and the various CIC concepts do not have to be mutually exclusive; both aspects may contribute to tumor cell resistance and failure of therapy.

3. *In vitro* models for prostate cancer

3.1 Two-dimensional monolayer culture: Cell lines and primary cells
Conventional 2D monolayer cell culture in combination with models like wound healing assays and transwell migration assays (Boyden chambers) have traditionally been the most straightforward and simplistic model systems for PrCa in vitro. This is due to the uncomplicated cell culture on plastic surfaces under controlled, and highly artificial environment. In vitro cell culture systems can be classified into two types: 1) cell lines, which have an unlimited proliferation capacity; 2) primary cell cultures directly established from human tissues. Cell lines are widely used in every aspect of cancer research and clearly represent the most common models. Cell lines have the big technical advantage of infinite reproducible quality (Rhim, 2000). Their growth properties and phenotypes are essentially dictated by the genetic background, which is largely defined by the genetic background of the original tumor. Therefore, different cell lines may show strong inconsistencies or contradictions that can be attributed to differences in the genetic wiring. These may nevertheless be representative of different stages and aspects of PrCa progression or differentiation (van Bokhoven et al., 2003b; Yu et al., 2009). The spectrum of mutations found in breast cancer cell lines was shown to be largely overlapping with primary cancers (Lin et al., 2007; Wood et al., 2006; Wood et al., 2007), although no such studies were performed for PrCa. If not single lines, at least panels of multiple PrCa lines may therefore be relevant for many experimental approaches. One problem with PrCa lines is the poor representation of the basal versus luminal phenotype that is characteristic for normal prostate versus PrCa tissues. Most PrCa cell lines are routinely cultured in media with 5 – 20% bovine calf serum, which strongly promotes the luminal phenotype. This is characterized by expression of the cytokeratins CK8, CK18, AR, and androgen-dependent genes. In contrast, most non-transformed, normal and immortalized prostate-epithelial lines are cultured in serum-free media. This strongly promotes the basal phenotype (Litvinov et al., 2006b; Uzgare et al., 2004), characterized by lack of AR expression and keratins CK5, CK6, CK7 and CK14. Luminal cell lines will stop proliferating in serum-free media, while

basal cell lines may adapt to serum-containing conditions, but still fail to undergo a luminal differentiation or start expressing AR. Therefore, it is questionable if basal-type primary cells and non-transformed prostate lines (RWPE-1, PWR-1E, or EP156T) are good models for clinical aspects of prostate cancers (Kogan et al., 2006; Tokar et al., 2005), as the luminal compartment is typically lost in malignant PrCa's (Litvinov et al., 2006b). Furthermore, the immortalization of primary prostate-epithelial cells with tumor-virus oncogenes (SV40 T-antigen, HPV-16 E6 and E7) typically results in rapid tumorigenic conversion. In contrast, the use of recombinant human telomerase has been demonstrated as far less compromising (Kogan et al., 2006; Kogan-Sakin et al., 2009). The resulting hTERT-immortalized cell lines retain much of their original differentiation potential, and do not accumulate additional genetic alterations.

Only an estimated 30 PrCa cell lines have been described, which were derived from clinical prostate cancer patients. However, only a small set of these cell lines has been widely used in cancer research. This also means that a large number of findings and scientific publications is based on a very small number of models. In particular, the three spontaneously established cell lines, PC-3, DU-145 and LNCaP, represent by far the most commonly used cell culture models (Sobel & Sadar, 2005a; Sobel & Sadar, 2005b), with close to 10.000 publications altogether. The first PrCa cell lines PC-3 (Kaighn et al., 1978; Kaighn et al., 1979) and DU-145 (Mickey et al., 1977; Stone et al., 1978) were established in 1978 and are still widely used. Both PC-3 and DU-145 have been cited in over 3000 publications. PC-3 cells were isolated from a human PrCa bone metastasis and have a very high metastatic potential (Kaighn et al., 1979), a property that has resulted in a large number of xenograft studies based on PC-3 cells inoculated typically into SCID nude mice. These xenografts are characterized by robust growth and rapid tumor formation. However, PC-3 cells are androgen-insensitive and lack expression of the AR protein. Loss of AR expression in PC-3 cells is likely related to epigenetic silencing of the AR locus. PC-3 cells may therefore represent a genuine subpopulation PrCa cells with naturally absent AR expression, characterized by very high cancer-initiating capacity possibly related to CSC. Interestingly, despite the lack of AR expression, PC-3 cells are capable of undergoing near complete acinar morphogenesis upon embedding in laminin-rich ECM (Matrigel). This argues for the substantial differentiation potential of PC-3 cells and in favor of their biological relevance (Härmä et al., 2010). Despite continuous ex-vivo culture on plastic dishes for over three decades, PC-3 cells have retained an amazing potential for epithelial maturation. Re-expression of AR in PC-3 cells can either suppress or slightly promote cell proliferation, depending on which promoter drives the expression of the AR protein (Altuwaijri et al., 2007; Litvinov et al., 2006a; Yuan et al., 1993). Additionally, PC-3 cells retain the co-activator profiles required for fully functional androgen signaling (Litvinov et al., 2006a). Nevertheless, such experimental strategies have to be taken carefully as they potentially contradict the genuine biological properties of a cell line.

Similar to PC-3, DU-145 cell were derived from a brain metastasis of human PrCa (Stone et al., 1978). Like PC-3, these cells are androgen-insensitive and lack expression of AR protein due to epigenetic silencing of the AR promoter by CpG island methylation that has shut off the expression (Chlenski et al., 2001; Yu et al., 2009). DU-145 cells show a similar, strong differentiation potential analogous to PC-3 cells when embedded in Matrigel. In both cases, a significant capacity for epithelial maturation has been retained for three decades of ex vivo culture. Stable transfection of functional human AR into DU-145 cells results in cells with reduced proliferation rate. When DU-145/AR cells are treated with testosterone, proliferation rate and other properties are restored, implying that AR can still function as a regulator of proliferation of DU-145-AR cells (Scaccianoce et al., 2003). Taken together, both PC-3 and DU-145 cells represent interesting models, despite the lack of AR expression - although we lack a complete understanding of their biology and relevance for clinical PrCa. The LNCaP cell line followed in 1980 (Horoszewicz et al., 1980; Horoszewicz et al., 1983) and has since resulted in over 5000 peer-reviewed publications alone. The LNCaP cell line was isolated from a lymph node metastasis, and contains a gain-of-function mutation commonly found in many clinical CRPCs (T877A). LNCaP cells are therefore a genuine and relevant model for CRPC (Yang et al., 2005). Down-regulation of AR in LNCaP cells by siRNA inhibits cell growth and increases the level of apoptosis (Compagno et al., 2007; Eder et al., 2000; Yang et al., 2005; Yang et al., 2005). This is suggesting that LNCaP are addicted to oncogenic variants of AR which act as a key survival factor; a characteristic or CRPC.

Newer cell line models have only been added to this small collection during the late 1990's. These cell lines are typically derived from xenograft models, such as the 22rV1 and CWR-r1 lines which are both derivatives of the CWR22 xenograft (Sramkoski et al., 1999). Similarly, the PC346 panel of cell lines was derived from a human xenograft and has been developed into a comprehensive series of derivative cell lines that mimic many aspects of progression to CRPC (Marques et al., 2006; Marques et al., 2010; Vlietstra et al., 1998) and resistance against anti-androgens. The PC-310 and PC-82 cell lines represent similar models (Jongsma et al., 2000). Another panel of more recently developed and functionally relevant PrCa cell lines (MDA-PCa-2a , MDA-PCa-2b) was established from bone metastases of a single patient in 1999 (Navone et al., 1997; Zhao et al., 1999). Similarly, the DuCaP (Lee et al., 2003; Lee et al., 2001) and VCaP (Korenchuk et al., 2001) cell lines were established from soft tissue and bone metastases, respectively, of the same CRPC patient in 1999. DuCaP and VCaP currently represent the only relevant models for ETS fusion factor positive PrCa. VCaP and DuCaP are also the only PrCa cell lines that harbor a wild type, but amplified and overexpressed AR gene, a hallmark of CRPC. Both VCaP and DuCaP cells have been successfully used for xenograft models, mimicking cancer-stromal cell associations and stem-cell biology (Cooper et al., 2003; Pfeiffer et al., 2011). A specialty of DuCaP cells is their dependency on co-existing mouse fibroblasts, which represent a carry-over from the growth of these cells in xenografts. However, the dependency of DuCaP cells on the mouse stromal counterpart can be broken, resulting in a morphologically very different phenotype.

Although additional PrCa cell lines are also available, detailed studies have revealed that many of these are in fact derivatives of the other cell lines or even non-prostatic lines (Sobel & Sadar, 2005a; Sobel & Sadar, 2005b; van Bokhoven et al., 2003b).

The few bona fide cell lines, almost all derived from metastases, do not span the complete range of PrCa phenotypes, and are not fully representative of primary PrCa. It is therefore not surprising that until very recently, the lack of a variety in PrCa cell lines has probably contributed to the failure of most small molecule inhibitors against CRPC in clinical trials. A few cell lines derived from benign prostate hyperplasia have also been established (Chu et al., 2009; Cunha et al., 2003). It cannot be excluded that long-term culture changes the biological properties of a cell line, a problem that is confounded by the mismatch-repair deficiency observed in many cell lines. Therefore, primary cultures of malignant prostatic cells and their normal epithelial counterparts would be in principle preferable (Peehl, 2005) to cell lines. As the interest in "personalized medicine" is rising, well defined primary material from clinically interesting cases would be expected to provide an excellent opportunity to follow up specific questions experimentally. Primary cell cultures from clinical tissue specimens indeed offer a number of biological advantages, and are often considered to better reflect the characteristics of the original tissues. However, primary cultures are usually derived from primary adenocarcinomas, unlike PrCa cell lines that have been typically generated from metastases of CRPCs (Maroni et al., 2004; Peehl, 2005). These may therefore represent biologically different entities. Furthermore, primary cell cultures present significant technical difficulties because of the limited access, restricted lifespan and requirements for specific culture techniques. Thus, only very few studies have made use of series of primary prostate cancer cells for experimentation (Eaton et al., 2010; Guzman-Ramirez et al., 2009). At the same time, the intrinsic heterogeneity of primary tissues poses many challenges, and a relatively large number of clinical samples will have to be processed. The isolation of primary cell material from samples is notoriously difficult. In practical experience, isolation and even short-term cultivation will fail in the majority of cases. Unrestricted access to primary clinical material is critical to overcome these many limitations, but may also pose a logistic problem. The availability of dedicated and experienced personnel at the clinical site to systematically collect, process and store such material is mandatory. The clinical partners also have to properly address and document questions concerning tumor grading and staging, therapy response etc., patient relapse and survival. These represent invaluable data for bringing tumor cell behavior into the correct and clinically relevant context.

Normal human prostate epithelial cells and even primary PrCa cells often undergo approximately 10 - 30 population doublings, before they become senescent (Peehl & Feldman, 2004; Sandhu et al., 2000). This could point to the possibility that immortalization is not necessarily a prerequisite for PrCa growth in vivo, and may represent a good explanation for the difficulties in generating PrCa lines in the past. Despite these difficulties, analyses of tumor suppressor activity, gene expression and cytogenetics in primary cultures have unraveled many critical changes that are important for PrCa progression. Challenges that remain to be addressed before tapping the full capacity of primary cell culture as a reliable model system include standardized and greatly improved isolation methods, the unequivocal characterization of cancer- and normal epithelial stem cells, and the successful induction and maintenance of a differentiated androgen-responsive phenotype (Miki & Rhim, 2008; Peehl, 2005). The isolation of cancer- or normal associated fibroblasts is a different issue and usually considerably less complex.

3.2 Organotypic 3D culture models

In monolayer culture of PrCa lines, cells lose important and biologically very relevant properties like differentiation, cellular polarization, cell-cell communication and extra cellular matrix (ECM) contacts. Simultaneously, wound healing, inflammation, and hyper-proliferation are artificially promoted – which is the main reason why 2D monolayer cell culture only poorly represents tumor cell biology *in vivo*. Accordingly, the most effective small molecule inhibitors and chemotherapeutic drugs in 2D monolayer settings primarily target cell proliferation and mitosis. Other interesting drugs that may affect differentiation-related pathways or small cell populations instead of the rapidly promoting tumor bulk, are likely to go undetected in cell-based screens using monolayer cultures. Such drug candidates may be connected to cell-cell interaction, maturation, EMT and cancer stem cell turnover - aspects that that incompletely recapitulated in 2D monolayer culture. In the pre-clinical phase of drug discovery, this bias results in an unnecessary low predictive value of many in vitro experiments.

The culture of glandular epithelial cancer cells in a certain tumor microenvironment consisting of purified ECM, such as collagen, hydrogels or Matrigel, was established over two decades ago (Streuli et al., 1991; Weaver et al., 1995; Weaver et al., 1996), and initially based mainly on breast cancer models. Matrigel represents a reconstituted, laminin-rich basement membrane, which supports cell polarization, cell-cell- and cell-matrix interaction, and promotes re-expression of differentiation markers even in transformed lines (Bissell & Radisky, 2001; Streuli et al., 1995). Glandular epithelial cancer cells rapidly adapt to different microenvironments and can dynamically switch between alternative pathways that regulate proliferation, differentiation and survival. When embedded in an ECM like Matrigel or collagen, normal prostate epithelial cells differentiate into hollow polarized spheroids, characteristic for functional, glandular epithelial cells (Simian et al., 2001; Xue et al., 2001a; Xue et al., 2001b). They also develop a pronounced motility and rapidly re-populate the available space by branching and acinar morphogenesis. Similar to normal epithelial cells, PrCa cells can also move and invade the surrounding Matrigel, although their mode of migration is phenotypically different from the formation of collective, multicellular sheets or tubes of cells observed in normal cells (Fig. 2)(Friedl & Wolf, 2008). The phenotype of cancer invasion strongly depends not only on the cells, but also on the composition and density of the ECM, and can vary from amoeboid blebbing, mesenchymal fibroblast-like motility and multicellular streaming or chain migration (Friedl & Wolf, 2010). 3D models of tumor-cell invasion are thought to properly represent many aspects of cellular dynamics inside actual tumors, as the cells can utilize a comparable mode for sliding and squiggling through the mesh of the ECM (Fig. 3)(Wolf & Friedl, 2006; Wolf et al., 2007). Invasion in 3D is assisted by proteolytic processes and proteases (Friedl & Wolf, 2009; Wolf & Friedl, 2009) and soluble factors (Gaggioli et al., 2007). Furthermore, cell motility and invasion is also controlled by intrinsic physiological factors, such as re-organization of the cytoskeleton (Medjkane et al., 2009; Sanz-Moreno et al., 2008). The potential to undergo an EMT and to acquire mesenchymal migration modes is a critical aspect that is thought to contribute to PrCa invasion (Acevedo et al., 2007; Chu et al., 2009; Sequeira et al., 2008). Despite the need for 3D scaffolds, the most widely used cell culture models for tumor cell invasion are still comparably artificial assays such as transwell invasion assays (Boyden chambers), and wound healing/scratch wound migration assays. However, tumor cell migration in these models still occurs in essentially two dimensions. Any representative 3D invasion model that mimics motility inside the tumor microenvironment represents a significant improvement (Brekhman & Neufeld, 2009). Furthermore, 3D matrices more faithfully recapitulate genuine invasive pro-processes such as invadopodia formation (Harper et al., 2010; Wolf & Friedl, 2009), and embryonal, developmental processes that may be relevant also for cancers such as aspects that may be branching morphogenesis (Andrew & Ewald, 2010; Xue et al., 2001a; Xue et al., 2001b). The development of drug resistance also profits from appropriate 3D cell culture models. Drug resistance appears to be concomitant with increased cell motility and trans-differentiation features like EMT (Gupta et al., 2009; Kalluri & Weinberg, 2009; Reiman et al., 2010) also in PrCa (Armstrong et al., 2011; Giannoni et al., 2010; Kong et al., 2010). EMT has been intensely discussed as a key mechanism for future therapeutic options (Dunning et al., 2011) in PrCa. EMT and stem cell properties go together with metastatic potential (Chang et al., 2011; Li & Tang, 2011; Ling et al., 2011; Liu et al., 2011) and link EMT with the problematic of distant metastases. Also CTCs have been found to display properties of EMT, invasiveness and stem cell characteristics (Armstrong et al., 2011). To cover these morphologic and dynamic aspects properly, requires the combination of appropriate biologically relevant scaffolds that mimic the tumor microenvironment, with appropriate cell lines (or primary cells) that show invasive properties. This could be counterbalanced by their variable differentiation potential, as epithelial maturation counteracts cell motility. Using such improved models, the screening for novel anti-cancer drugs can eventually enter a new phase. Researchers should increasingly utilize well characterized 3D organotypic model systems to explore the effects of drugs and targets in multicellular organoids. Appropriate models should also be cost effective and must provide sufficient throughput for high content screening.

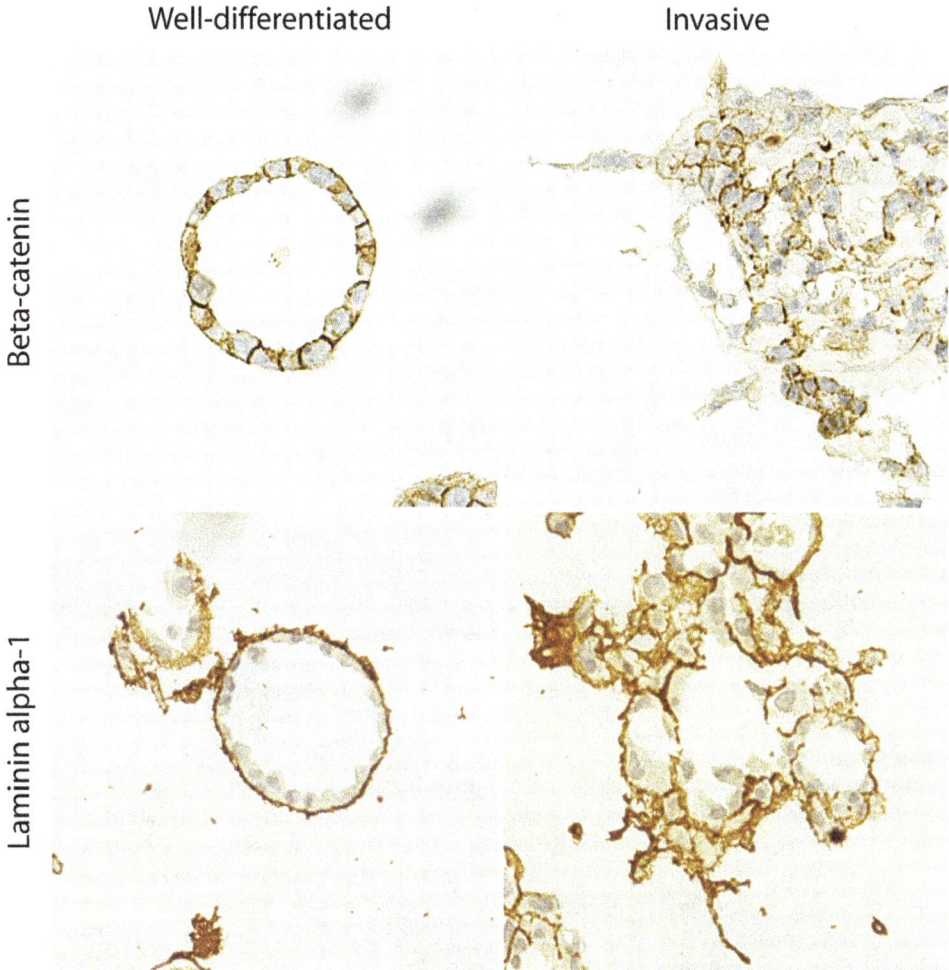

Fig. 2. Prostate adenocarcinoma cells in 3D laminin-rich microenvironment. Some PrCa cells bear the ability to differentiate into multicellular acinar structures with strong cell-cell and cell-ECM contacts (illustrated here with beta-catenin and laminin alpha-1 immunostainings). Invasive PrCa cells move by actively degrading the surrounding lrECM and tend to be less restricted by cellular contacts.

Monolayer   Prostaspheres   Embedded 3D

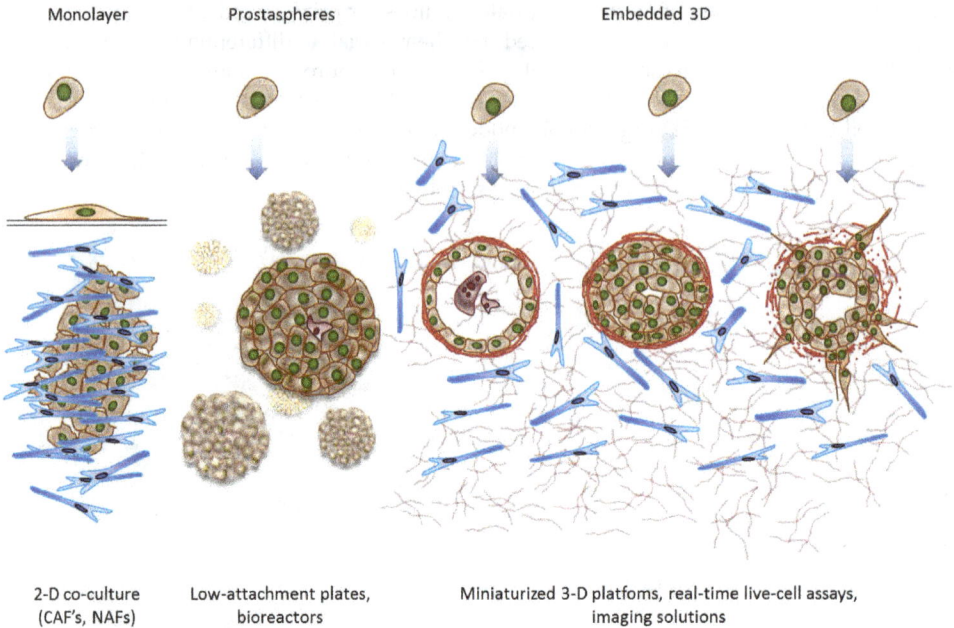

2-D co-culture   Low-attachment plates,   Miniaturized 3-D platfoms, real-time live-cell assays,
(CAF's, NAFs)   bioreactors   imaging solutions

Fig. 3. An overview of three different in vitro models for PrCa: 2-D monolayer co-culture, low-attachment culture of prostaspheres, and organotypic 3-D culture.

In the pre-clinical phase of drug discovery, the question of drug response & resistance is routinely addressed by tumor xenograft models, mainly utilizing classic tumor cell lines and nude mouse models. While in vivo models may well overcome many of the shortcomings of 2D cell culture, they are time consuming, expensive, and require ethical considerations and permissions. Nude mouse models possess no immune system, and poorly mimic the critical aspects of inflammation, tumor microenvironment, human endocrine specialities and morphology, and often fail to mimic tumor metastasis. Xenograft models only allow remote sensing, followed by post-experimental histology. With few exceptions (in vivo imaging), animal experimentation gives no direct mechanistic insights into dynamic interactions between different cell types within a tumor at the cellular level. Monitoring inducible changes in real time is a key problem, potentially addressed in the future by tissue slices (Sonnenberg et al., 2008; van der Kuip et al., 2006). Until tissue slices may become firmly established, other models could represent a valid alternative. Therefore, 2D and xenograft experiments can be readily complemented by organotypic assays. These methods, which are still in development in PrCa, generate highly valuable functional data for drug discovery. Validated 3D models may also help to reduce animal experimentation and associated cost (3R strategy: "Replacement, Refinement and Reduction of Animals in Research"). Political pressure from the European Commission to reduce animal experimentation in Europe could further contribute to a wider acceptance of organotypic models in drug discovery. Advanced and well-characterized 3D models may give important clues for lead prioritization and allow significantly cutting the need for animal experiments, - for example if compounds successful identified in 2D screens are completely ineffective in subsequent 3D organotypic assays.

Generally, 3D cell aggregates (spheroids, prostaspheres, etc.) tend to show considerably higher drug resistance compared to 2D cultures. Such comparisons may result in a vastly different dose-response curve, ideally closer to the expected in vivo data. However, to firmly establish organotypic models and to validate their relevance in the pre-clinical phase of drug discovery, systematic side-by-side comparisons between in vivo and in vitro models would be required. These efforts are currently starting.

The biological relevance of functional screens conducted in 3D organotypic cultures strongly depends on information that can be concluded from associated assays. In routine cell-based screens, mostly indirect assays measuring overall cell viability and proliferation are used. Less frequent is the use of measurements based on biomarkers (e.g. Ki67; antibody stainings, immune fluorescence) or morphological parameters (imaging). These options are central for 3D organotypic cultures; the most important parameters for evaluating drug responses will be based on multicellular morphology. To functionally validate 3D organotypic models in cancer biology, high content microscopy based on morphological features will have to be combined with automated image analysis tools (Han et al., 2009; Han et al., 2010). This combination will allow real-time monitoring of dynamic changes in spheroid morphology as a readout. Automated image analysis of 3D cultures relies on measuring morphological parameters such as size, shape, differentiation, density, surface structures and invasive properties of spheroids. Consistent morphological changes in response to perturbants (small molecule inhibitors, siRNAs, stress conditions) can then be statistically evaluated and quantified. Apoptosis and cell proliferation can also be readily evaluated based on live-cell staining with reactive dyes. These processes are difficult to automate, and represent the key bottlenecks to overcome for larger scale screens. The use of GFP-tagged cell lines (combined with luciferase) represents a widely established tool that can be utilized in both in vivo and in vitro, organotypic settings. The same tagged cells can be used for in vivo and microscopic imaging, and could facilitate the much needed side-by-side comparisons of organotypic models with mouse models. Novel assays to monitor specific mechanistic changes will become important to quantify critical aspects of pharmacology and to evaluate acute drug responses. The field of live-cell assay development, including reactive dyes and reporter constructs, is a key aspect of HCS in the pharmaceutical industry but has yet to make the move into 3D models. There is a lack of informative assays for monitoring the activity of key pathways such as NF-κB, AKT, PI3K or Wnt in living cells. Such assays would also enable researchers to monitor cellular heterogeneity, e.g. in response to drug therapy. Single cell analysis, ideally based on live-cell assays, is already a powerful tool in many aspects of biology. This could also allow researchers to identify and monitor putative stem cell populations, and quantify their dynamics in anti-cancer treatments. Imaging is also critical to make sense of the dynamics of co-culture experimentation which will be discussed later.

3.3 Non-adherent 3D culture of prostaspheres and bioreactors

Early studies by Kinbara et al (Kinbara et al., 1996) demonstrated that prostate epithelial cells, isolated from different lobes of the adult rodent prostate, exhibited stem cell like features, including an enormous proliferative potential and the potential for re-programmed epithelial differentiation. Regenerative capacity, attributed to only a small population of pluripotent progenitor epithelial cells, is rapidly lost when the cells are placed in monolayer culture or embedded in Matrigel. However, "stemness" can be strongly promoted and maintained by non-adherent cell culture, e.g. as spheroids. The first such approaches were described as "liquid overlay" technology, which prohibits successful cell attachment. Cells are then forced to adhere to themselves to overcome the lack of critical survival signals provided by cell and matrix adhesion, and to avoid anoikis or apoptosis. Low-attachment technologies have been introduced multiple times, e.g. by Poly-HEMA coated plastic plates. Placing prostate epithelial cells in non-adherent culture e.g. on a layer of hydrogel has a similar effect, resulting in the formation of spheroids or "prostaspheres" (Fig. 3)(Sauer et al., 1997; Sauer et al., 1998; Wartenberg et al., 1998). Such spheroids undergo a dynamic process of de-differentiation and reproducibly acquire properties of stem- and precursor cells (Patrawala et al., 2007; Pfeiffer & Schalken, 2010; Tang et al., 2007). Spheroid culture represents one of the oldest in vitro cell culture technologies and was pioneered already over 40 years ago by Sutherland et al (Sutherland et al., 1971; Sutherland et al., 1977).

Prostaspheres can be easily generated from most PrCa cell lines (Rajasekhar et al., 2011; Rybak et al., 2011), and serially passaged. Prostaspheres exhibit increased expression of putative stem cell markers, and represent 3D clusters of tumor cells derived from one or several cell clones that develop into multicellular globes of fairly large size. Spheroids often contain different subpopulations of cells that can be quiescent, hypoxic and necrotic and display a spatial geometry which provides a number of practical experimental advantages over adherent cell culture (Freyer & Sutherland, 1980; Kostarelos et al., 2004; Sutherland, 1988). To date, prostaspheres (and mammospheres, the equivalent in breast cancer cells) represent a widely used tool to study the processes of self-renewal, differentiation and cancer stem cell research (Lang et al., 2009). An intriguing recent application is the combination of spheroid culture to enrich for human prostate progenitor cells rat urogenital sinus mesenchymal cells. Inoculation of the formed chimeric prostate tissue under the renal capsule of nude mice (Hu et al., 2011) leads to tumor masses with human functionality, indicated by expression of PSA and hormone-dependent PrCa lesions. This represents an elegant system for the experimental recapitulation of carcinogenesis.

Another classic application for prostaspheres is within bioreactors (Ingram et al., 2010). These provide a low-turbulence environment which promotes the formation of very large and complex spheroids. A bioreactor is typically rotated or stirred, to provide a gentle mixing of fresh and spent nutrients without inducing excessive shear forces that may damage the structures. Bioreactors are also an ideal tool to generate co-culture spheroids, e.g. with stromal and epithelial/tumor cells (Yates et al., 2007a; Yates et al., 2007b), or to promote the self-renewal potential and stem cell characteristics (Frith et al., 2010b). Bioreactor research could be instrumental in helping scientists to prepare better models for cancerous tissues, and is expected to facilitate drug and peptide development. Improved characterization of these models and comparisons to other alternatives would be important also in this case.

3.4 Co-culture models for the investigation of tumor-stroma interactions

In a tumor, fibroblasts, smooth muscle cells, endothelial cells and leukocytes, interact physically or via the secretion of paracrine signalling molecules with tumor cells. These cell types make up the main components of the breast tumor microenvironment (Bissell & Radisky, 2001; Polyak et al., 2009; Radisky et al., 2002; Shipitsin et al., 2007). The situation in PrCa has also been explored in detail (Cunha et al., 2003; Cunha et al., 2004). Stromal cells secrete a variety of growth factors like FGF-2, FGF-7, and FGF-10 (Chambers et al., 2011), insulin-like growth factor (IGF), epidermal growth factor (EGF), and a panel of chemokines

(Kogan-Sakin et al., 2009). FGFs like FGF-10, which signals through the FGFR1 receptor, play a particularly critical role in regulating PrCa cell morphology and invasive properties (Abate-Shen & Shen, 2007; Chambers et al., 2011). Dysregulated FGF-10 expression has been observed in advanced PrCa and suggests the FGF-10/FGFR1 axis as a potential therapeutic target in treating both hormone-sensitive or CRPC (Memarzadeh et al., 2007). Exposure to paracrine growth factors like FGF-10 and FGF-7 may be critical for the initiation of oncogenic transformation (Fata et al., 2007). Additional secreted factors including chemokines like CCL2 act as key factors for PrCa invasion and bone metastasis (Li et al., 2009; Loberg et al., 2006a). These and others like IL-6 are thought to support differentiation and stimulate cancer cell growth (Culig et al., 1995; Malinowska et al., 2009). A tumor is clearly the product of intricate cross-talk between the epithelial and stromal cells; with the secretion of cytokines and chemokines as the common language. Identification of these environmental, paracrine cues which induce important changes in cell fate during development, has caused a fundamental re-evaluation of the process of tumorigenesis.

In vitro co-culture systems could also provide better models to address the interaction of epithelial AR functions in cell proliferation and metastasis (Fig. 3). For example, the immortalized human prostate stromal cell line WPMY-1 expresses functional AR and secretes paracrine growth factors (Webber et al., 1999), with an impact on the morphology and proliferation of the epithelial counterpart. Stromal AR expression promote epithelial cell invasion via paracrine secretion of growth factors, chemokines or cytokines. The stromal cells, via AR expression, can therefore modulate tumor cell proliferation and invasion (Tanner et al., 2011; Yu et al., 2011; Zhang et al., 2008). Their key effects are mediated e.g. by estrogen receptor signaling or the ERK kinase family, but also secreted high-molecular weight glycoproteins like endoglin (Romero et al., 2011). Expression of eccrine factors is mediated by TGF beta, another key factor and signaling pathway that massively affects the tumor-stroma interaction (Chambers et al., 2011; Pu et al., 2009). TGF beta dependent mechanisms play a key role in regulating paracrine stromal signals, and strongly affect epithelial cell adhesion via adhesion/cytoskeleton interactions. These and many other reports indicate a fundamental role for the stroma and stroma-derived secreted factors in maintaining adult prostate epithelial tissue morphology and integrity.

Simple, modular and reproducible 3D co-culture systems might allow researchers to further address the interdependence of tumor and stromal cells in straightforward settings. These systems would ideally allow the analysis of morphological features and epithelial differentiation/maturation. Optimal systems should also be standardized and miniaturized to facilitate the use of imaging and automated image analysis tools, and provide a higher experimental throughput. Such advanced, reproducible 3D co-culture models could then be utilized to systematically explore the importance of molecular signalling pathways AR, PI3K/AKT, and c-MET on heterogeneous co-culture and tissue formation. For example, stable stromal-tumor co-cultures are expected to be more resistant to anti-androgens or c-MET inhibitors than the isolated counterparts (Maeda et al., 2006; Tu et al., 2010), but this has not been properly investigated across multiple model systems. Which molecular and cell-cell interactions determine the response? Can resistance to anti-cancer therapeutics, e.g. androgen independence, be generated more readily in co-culture than by isolated mono-cultures, or even better in xenografts; and which molecular changes can be identified in resistant populations arising? What are the differences between human and mouse fibroblasts in terms of heterogeneity and response to anti-cancer therapeutics (Kiskowski et al., 2011)? For such fundamental questions, the use of 3D co-culture settings could represent a critical "missing link" between reductionist cell culture models and more complex xenograft experiments or even GEMMs.

4. Conclusions

The heterogeneous nature of PrCa has made it difficult to understand the factors involved in the onset and progression of the disease. Advanced in vitro experimental systems should ideally try to recapitulate, as closely as possible, the 3D organization of tumors and mimic aspects of cellular heterogeneity and tumor-host cell interactions within the tumor microenvironment. Other important aspects are cell motility, the dynamics of clonal selection and tumor cell heterogeneity generated during chemotherapy. To provide a more comprehensive, biologically relevant context to investigate these processes experimentally, an ideal situation would be to combine in vitro models (2D, 3D and co-culture), transgenic mouse models (GEMMs), and xenografts into a bigger picture. A maximum of information can be generated by the systematic comparison of multiple models. The tissue architecture and heterogeneity formed by these various model systems may be vastly different, but the ultimate standard will be to relate these morphologies to the human clinical pathology and histology. Although the role of pathologists has not been featured prominently in this review, it remains one of the key aspects for cancer biology and the drug discovery process as a whole.

5. References

Abate-Shen, C., Banach-Petrosky W. A., Sun X., Economides K. D., Desai N., Gregg J. P. et al. (2003). Nkx3.1; pten mutant mice develop invasive prostate adenocarcinoma and lymph node metastases. *Cancer Res, 63*, 3886-3890.

Abate-Shen, C. & Shen M. M. (2007). FGF signaling in prostate tumorigenesis--new insights into epithelial-stromal interactions. *Cancer Cell, 12*, 495-497.

Abou-Kheir, W. G., Hynes P. G., Martin P. L., Pierce R. & Kelly K. (2010). Characterizing the contribution of stem/progenitor cells to tumorigenesis in the pten-/-TP53-/- prostate cancer model. *Stem Cells, 28*, 2129-2140.

Acevedo, V. D., Gangula R. D., Freeman K. W., Li R., Zhang Y., Wang F. et al. (2007). Inducible FGFR-1 activation leads to irreversible prostate adenocarcinoma and an epithelial-to-mesenchymal transition. *Cancer Cell, 12*, 559-571.

Agarwal, N., Hutson T. E., Vogelzang N. J. & Sonpavde G. (2010). Abiraterone acetate: A promising drug for the treatment of castration-resistant prostate cancer. *Future Oncol, 6*, 665-679.

Al-Hajj, M., Wicha M. S., Benito-Hernandez A., Morrison S. J. & Clarke M. F. (2003). Prospective identification of tumorigenic breast cancer cells. *Proc Natl Acad Sci U S A, 100*, 3983-3988.

Alimonti, A., Nardella C., Chen Z., Clohessy J. G., Carracedo A., Trotman L. C. et al. (2010). A novel type of cellular senescence that can be enhanced in mouse models and human tumor xenografts to suppress prostate tumorigenesis. *J Clin Invest, 120*, 681-693.

Altuwaijri, S., Wu C. C., Niu Y. J., Mizokami A., Chang H. C. & Chang C. (2007). Expression of human AR cDNA driven by its own promoter results in mild promotion, but not suppression, of growth in human prostate cancer PC-3 cells. *Asian J Androl, 9*, 181-188.

Andrew, D. J. & Ewald A. J. (2010). Morphogenesis of epithelial tubes: Insights into tube formation, elongation, and elaboration. *Dev Biol, 341*, 34-55.

Armstrong, A. J., Marengo M. S., Oltean S., Kemeny G., Bitting R. L., Turnbull J. D. et al. (2011). Circulating tumor cells from patients with advanced prostate and breast cancer display both epithelial and mesenchymal markers. *Mol Cancer Res, .*

Attard, G., Clark J., Ambroisine L., Fisher G., Kovacs G., Flohr P. et al. (2008). Duplication of the fusion of TMPRSS2 to ERG sequences identifies fatal human prostate cancer. *Oncogene, 27*, 253-263.

Attard, G., de Bono J. S., Clark J. & Cooper C. S. (2010). Studies of TMPRSS2-ERG gene fusions in diagnostic trans-rectal prostate biopsies. *Clin Cancer Res, 16*, 1340; author reply 1340.

Attard, G., Reid A. H., A'Hern R., Parker C., Oommen N. B., Folkerd E. et al. (2009a). Selective inhibition of CYP17 with abiraterone acetate is highly active in the treatment of castration-resistant prostate cancer. *J Clin Oncol, 27*, 3742-3748.

Attard, G., Reid A. H., Olmos D. & de Bono J. S. (2009b). Antitumor activity with CYP17 blockade indicates that castration-resistant prostate cancer frequently remains hormone driven. *Cancer Res, 69*, 4937-4940.

Attard, G., Richards J. & de Bono J. S. (2011). New strategies in metastatic prostate cancer: Targeting the AR signaling pathway. *Clin Cancer Res, 17*, 1649-1657.

Attard, G., Swennenhuis J. F., Olmos D., Reid A. H., Vickers E., A'Hern R. et al. (2009). Characterization of ERG, AR and PTEN gene status in circulating tumor cells from patients with castration-resistant prostate cancer. *Cancer Res, 69*, 2912-2918.

Banach-Petrosky, W., Jessen W. J., Ouyang X., Gao H., Rao J., Quinn J. et al. (2007). Prolonged exposure to reduced levels of androgen accelerates prostate cancer progression in Nkx3.1; pten mutant mice. *Cancer Res, 67*, 9089-9096.

Bello-DeOcampo, D., Kleinman H. K., Deocampo N. D. & Webber M. M. (2001). Laminin-1 and alpha6beta1 integrin regulate acinar morphogenesis of normal and malignant human prostate epithelial cells. *Prostate, 46*, 142-153.

Bissell, M. J. & Radisky D. (2001). Putting tumours in context. *Nat Rev Cancer, 1*, 46-54.

Bjorkman, M., Iljin K., Halonen P., Sara H., Kaivanto E., Nees M. et al. (2008). Defining the molecular action of HDAC inhibitors and synergism with androgen deprivation in ERG-positive prostate cancer. *Int J Cancer, 123*, 2774-2781.

Blando, J. M., Carbajal S., Abel E., Beltran L., Conti C., Fischer S. et al. (2011). Cooperation between Stat3 and akt signaling leads to prostate tumor development in transgenic mice. *Neoplasia, 13*, 254-265.

Boormans, J. L., Korsten H., Ziel-van der Made A. C., van Leenders G. J., Verhagen P. C. & Trapman J. (2010). E17K substitution in AKT1 in prostate cancer. *Br J Cancer, 102*, 1491-1494.

Brekhman, V. & Neufeld G. (2009). A novel asymmetric 3D in-vitro assay for the study of tumor cell invasion. *BMC Cancer, 9*, 415.

Brenner, J. C., Ateeq B., Li Y., Yocum A. K., Cao Q., Asangani I. A. et al. (2011). Mechanistic rationale for inhibition of poly(ADP-ribose) polymerase in ETS gene fusion-positive prostate cancer. *Cancer Cell*, 19, 664-678.

Brock, A., Chang H. & Huang S. (2009). Non-genetic heterogencity--a mutation-independent driving force for the somatic evolution of tumours. *Nat Rev Genet*, 10, 336-342.

Cai, C., Wang H., Xu Y., Chen S. & Balk S. P. (2009). Reactivation of AR-regulated TMPRSS2:ERG gene expression in castration-resistant prostate cancer. *Cancer Res*, 69, 6027-6032.

Carver, B. S., Tran J., Chen Z., Carracedo-Perez A., Alimonti A., Nardella C. et al. (2009a). ETS rearrangements and prostate cancer initiation. *Nature*, 457, E1; discussion E2-3.

Carver, B. S., Tran J., Gopalan A., Chen Z., Shaikh S., Carracedo A. et al. (2009b). Aberrant ERG expression cooperates with loss of PTEN to promote cancer progression in the prostate. *Nat Genet*, 41, 619-624.

Chambers, K. F., Pearson J. F., Aziz N., O'Toole P., Garrod D. & Lang S. H. (2011). Stroma regulates increased epithelial lateral cell adhesion in 3D culture: A role for actin/cadherin dynamics. *PLoS One*, 6, e18796.

Chang, H. H., Chen B. Y., Wu C. Y., Tsao Z. J., Chen Y. Y., Chang C. P. et al. (2011). Hedgehog overexpression leads to the formation of prostate cancer stem cells with metastatic property irrespective of AR expression in the mouse model. *J Biomed Sci*, 18, 6.

Chen, Y., Clegg N. J. & Scher H. I. (2009). Anti-androgens and androgen-depleting therapies in prostate cancer: New agents for an established target. *Lancet Oncol*, 10, 981-991.

Chlenski, A., Nakashiro K., Ketels K. V., Korovaitseva G. I. & Oyasu R. (2001). AR expression in androgen-independent prostate cancer cell lines. *Prostate*, 47, 66-75.

Chu, J. H., Yu S., Hayward S. W. & Chan F. L. (2009). Development of a three-dimensional culture model of prostatic epithelial cells and its use for the study of epithelial-mesenchymal transition and inhibition of PI3K pathway in prostate cancer. *Prostate*, 69, 428-442.

Clegg, N. J., Couto S. S., Wongvipat J., Hieronymus H., Carver B. S., Taylor B. S. et al. (2011). MYC cooperates with AKT in prostate tumorigenesis and alters sensitivity to mTOR inhibitors. *PLoS One*, 6, e17449.

Compagno, D., Merle C., Morin A., Gilbert C., Mathieu J. R., Bozec A. et al. (2007). SIRNA-directed in vivo silencing of AR inhibits the growth of castration-resistant prostate carcinomas. *PLoS One*, 2, e1006.

Cooper, C. R., Chay C. H., Gendernalik J. D., Lee H. L., Bhatia J., Taichman R. S. et al. (2003). Stromal factors involved in prostate carcinoma metastasis to bone. *Cancer*, 97, 739-747.

Couto, S. S., Cao M., Duarte P. C., Banach-Petrosky W., Wang S., Romanienko P. et al. (2009). Simultaneous haploinsufficiency of pten and Trp53 tumor suppressor genes accelerates tumorigenesis in a mouse model of prostate cancer. *Differentiation*, 77, 103-111.

Culig, Z., Hobisch A., Cronauer M. V., Radmayr C., Trapman J., Hittmair A. et al. (1995). AR activation in prostatic tumor cell lines by insulin-like growth factor-I, keratinocyte growth factor and epidermal growth factor. *Eur Urol*, 27 Suppl 2, 45-47.

Cunha, G. R., Hayward S. W., Wang Y. Z. & Ricke W. A. (2003). Role of the stromal microenvironment in carcinogenesis of the prostate. *Int J Cancer*, 107, 1-10.

Cunha, G. R., Ricke W., Thomson A., Marker P. C., Risbridger G., Hayward S. W. et al. (2004). Hormonal, cellular, and molecular regulation of normal and neoplastic prostatic development. *J Steroid Biochem Mol Biol, 92,* 221-236.

Dahut, W. L. & Madan R. A. (2010). Revisiting the ultimate target of treatment for prostate cancer. *Lancet, 375,* 1409-1410.

Danila, D. C., Fleisher M. & Scher H. I. (2011). Circulating tumor cells as biomarkers in prostate cancer. *Clin Cancer Res, 17,* 3903-3912.

Danila, D. C., Morris M. J., de Bono J. S., Ryan C. J., Denmeade S. R., Smith M. R. et al. (2010). Phase II multicenter study of abiraterone acetate plus prednisone therapy in patients with docetaxel-treated castration-resistant prostate cancer. *J Clin Oncol, 28,* 1496-1501.

de Bono, J. S., Logothetis C. J., Molina A., Fizazi K., North S., Chu L. et al. (2011). Abiraterone and increased survival in metastatic prostate cancer. *N Engl J Med, 364,* 1995-2005.

Debnath, J. & Brugge J. S. (2005). Modelling glandular epithelial cancers in three-dimensional cultures. *Nat Rev Cancer, 5,* 675-688.

Debnath, J., Muthuswamy S. K. & Brugge J. S. (2003). Morphogenesis and oncogenesis of MCF-10A mammary epithelial acini grown in three-dimensional basement membrane cultures. *Methods, 30,* 256-268.

Diehn, M., Cho R. W. & Clarke M. F. (2009). Therapeutic implications of the cancer stem cell hypothesis. *Semin Radiat Oncol, 19,* 78-86.

Diehn, M. & Clarke M. F. (2006). Cancer stem cells and radiotherapy: New insights into tumor radioresistance. *J Natl Cancer Inst, 98,* 1755-1757.

Dontu, G., Liu S. & Wicha M. S. (2005). Stem cells in mammary development and carcinogenesis: Implications for prevention and treatment. *Stem Cell Rev, 1,* 207-213.

Dubrovska, A., Kim S., Salamone R. J., Walker J. R., Maira S. M., Garcia-Echeverria C. et al. (2009). The role of PTEN/Akt/PI3K signaling in the maintenance and viability of prostate cancer stem-like cell populations. *Proc Natl Acad Sci U S A, 106,* 268-273.

Dunning, N. L., Laversin S. A., Miles A. K. & Rees R. C. (2011). Immunotherapy of prostate cancer: Should we be targeting stem cells and EMT? *Cancer Immunol Immunother, 60,* 1181-1193.

Eaton, C. L., Colombel M., van der Pluijm G., Cecchini M., Wetterwald A., Lippitt J. et al. (2010). Evaluation of the frequency of putative prostate cancer stem cells in primary and metastatic prostate cancer. *Prostate, 70,* 875-882.

Eder, I. E., Culig Z., Ramoner R., Thurnher M., Putz T., Nessler-Menardi C. et al. (2000). Inhibition of LncaP prostate cancer cells by means of AR antisense oligonucleotides. *Cancer Gene Ther, 7,* 997-1007.

Fata, J. E., Mori H., Ewald A. J., Zhang H., Yao E., Werb Z. et al. (2007). The MAPK(ERK-1,2) pathway integrates distinct and antagonistic signals from TGFalpha and FGF7 in morphogenesis of mouse mammary epithelium. *Dev Biol, 306,* 193-207.

Feldman, B. J. & Feldman D. (2001). The development of androgen-independent prostate cancer. *Nat Rev Cancer, 1,* 34-45.

Figg, W. D., Woo S., Zhu W., Chen X., Ajiboye A. S., Steinberg S. M. et al. (2010). A phase I clinical study of high dose ketoconazole plus weekly docetaxel for metastatic CRPC. *J Urol, 183,* 2219-2226.

Freyer, J. P. & Sutherland R. M. (1980). Selective dissociation and characterization of cells from different regions of multicell tumor spheroids. *Cancer Res,* 40, 3956-3965.

Friedl, P. & Wolf K. (2010). Plasticity of cell migration: A multiscale tuning model. *J Cell Biol,* 188, 11-19.

Friedl, P. & Wolf K. (2009). Proteolytic interstitial cell migration: A five-step process. *Cancer Metastasis Rev,* 28, 129-135.

Friedl, P. & Wolf K. (2008). Tube travel: The role of proteases in individual and collective cancer cell invasion. *Cancer Res,* 68, 7247-7249.

Frith, J. E., Thomson B. & Genever P. G. (2010a). Dynamic three-dimensional culture methods enhance mesenchymal stem cell properties and increase therapeutic potential. *Tissue Eng Part C Methods,* 16, 735-749.

Frith, J. E., Thomson B. & Genever P. G. (2010b). Dynamic three-dimensional culture methods enhance mesenchymal stem cell properties and increase therapeutic potential. *Tissue Eng Part C Methods,* 16, 735-749.

Gaggioli, C., Hooper S., Hidalgo-Carcedo C., Grosse R., Marshall J. F., Harrington K. et al. (2007). Fibroblast-led collective invasion of carcinoma cells with differing roles for RhoGTPases in leading and following cells. *Nat Cell Biol,* 9, 1392-1400.

Gao, H., Ouyang X., Banach-Petrosky W. A., Shen M. M. & Abate-Shen C. (2006). Emergence of androgen independence at early stages of prostate cancer progression in Nkx3.1; pten mice. *Cancer Res,* 66, 7929-7933.

Giannoni, E., Bianchini F., Masieri L., Serni S., Torre E., Calorini L. et al. (2010). Reciprocal activation of prostate cancer cells and cancer-associated fibroblasts stimulates epithelial-mesenchymal transition and cancer stemness. *Cancer Res,* 70, 6945-6956.

Gupta, P. B., Chaffer C. L. & Weinberg R. A. (2009). Cancer stem cells: Mirage or reality? *Nat Med,* 15, 1010-1012.

Gupta, S., Iljin K., Sara H., Mpindi J. P., Mirtti T., Vainio P. et al. (2010). FZD4 as a mediator of ERG oncogene-induced WNT signaling and epithelial-to-mesenchymal transition in human prostate cancer cells. *Cancer Res,* .

Guzman-Ramirez, N., Voller M., Wetterwald A., Germann M., Cross N. A., Rentsch C. A. et al. (2009). In vitro propagation and characterization of neoplastic stem/progenitor-like cells from human prostate cancer tissue. *Prostate,* 69, 1683-1693.

Han, J., Chang H., Fontenay G., Wang N. J., Gray J. W. & Parvin B. (2009). Morphometric subtyping for a panel of breast cancer cell lines. *Proc IEEE Int Symp Biomed Imaging,* 6, 791-794.

Han, J., Chang H., Giricz O., Lee G. Y., Baehner F. L., Gray J. W. et al. (2010). Molecular predictors of 3D morphogenesis by breast cancer cell lines in 3D culture. *PLoS Comput Biol,* 6, e1000684.

Härmä, V., Virtanen J., Mäkelä R., Happonen A., Mpindi J. P., Knuuttila M. et al. (2010). A comprehensive panel of three-dimensional models for studies of prostate cancer growth, invasion and drug responses. *PLoS One,* 5, e10431.

Harper, K., Arsenault D., Boulay-Jean S., Lauzier A., Lucien F. & Dubois C. M. (2010). Autotaxin promotes cancer invasion via the lysophosphatidic acid receptor 4: Participation of the cyclic AMP/EPAC/Rac1 signaling pathway in invadopodia formation. *Cancer Res,* 70, 4634-4643.

Havens, A. M., Pedersen E. A., Shiozawa Y., Ying C., Jung Y., Sun Y. et al. (2008). An in vivo mouse model for human prostate cancer metastasis. *Neoplasia*, 10, 371-380.

Hensley, P. J. & Kyprianou N. (2011). Modeling prostate cancer in mice: Limitations and opportunities. *J Androl*, .

Hermans, K. G., Boormans J. L., Gasi D., van Leenders G. J., Jenster G., Verhagen P. C. et al. (2009). Overexpression of prostate-specific TMPRSS2(exon 0)-ERG fusion transcripts corresponds with favorable prognosis of prostate cancer. *Clin Cancer Res*, 15, 6398-6403.

Hermans, K. G., Bressers A. A., van der Korput H. A., Dits N. F., Jenster G. & Trapman J. (2008a). Two unique novel prostate-specific and androgen-regulated fusion partners of ETV4 in prostate cancer. *Cancer Res*, 68, 3094-3098.

Hermans, K. G., van der Korput H. A., van Marion R., van de Wijngaart D. J., Ziel-van der Made A., Dits N. F. et al. (2008b). Truncated ETV1, fused to novel tissue-specific genes, and full-length ETV1 in prostate cancer. *Cancer Res*, 68, 7541-7549.

Horoszewicz, J. S., Leong S. S., Chu T. M., Wajsman Z. L., Friedman M., Papsidero L. et al. (1980). The LNCaP cell line--a new model for studies on human prostatic carcinoma. *Prog Clin Biol Res*, 37, 115-132.

Horoszewicz, J. S., Leong S. S., Kawinski E., Karr J. P., Rosenthal H., Chu T. M. et al. (1983). LNCaP model of human prostatic carcinoma. *Cancer Res*, 43, 1809-1818.

Hu, W. Y., Shi G. B., Lam H. M., Hu D. P., Ho S. M., Madueke I. C. et al. (2011). Estrogen-initiated transformation of prostate epithelium derived from normal human prostate stem-progenitor cells. *Endocrinology*, 152, 2150-2163.

Hu, Y., Dobi A., Sreenath T., Cook C., Tadase A. Y., Ravindranath L. et al. (2008). Delineation of TMPRSS2-ERG splice variants in prostate cancer. *Clin Cancer Res*, 14, 4719-4725.

Ingram, M., Techy G. B., Ward B. R., Imam S. A., Atkinson R., Ho H. et al. (2010). Tissue engineered tumor models. *Biotech Histochem*, 85, 213-229.

Jeet, V., Russell P. J. & Khatri A. (2010). Modeling prostate cancer: A perspective on transgenic mouse models. *Cancer Metastasis Rev*, 29, 123-142.

Jenster, G., Trapman J. & Brinkmann A. O. (1993). Nuclear import of the human AR. *Biochem J*, 293 (Pt 3), 761-768.

Jhavar, S., Reid A., Clark J., Kote-Jarai Z., Christmas T., Thompson A. et al. (2008). Detection of TMPRSS2-ERG translocations in human prostate cancer by expression profiling using GeneChip human exon 1.0 ST arrays. *J Mol Diagn*, 10, 50-57.

Jiao, J., Wang S., Qiao R., Vivanco I., Watson P. A., Sawyers C. L. et al. (2007). Murine cell lines derived from pten null prostate cancer show the critical role of PTEN in hormone refractory prostate cancer development. *Cancer Res*, 67, 6083-6091.

Jongsma, J., Oomen M. H., Noordzij M. A., Van Weerden W. M., Martens G. J., van der Kwast T. H. et al. (2000). Androgen deprivation of the PC-310 [correction of prohormone convertase-310] human prostate cancer model system induces neuroendocrine differentiation. *Cancer Res*, 60, 741-748.

Kaighn, M. E., Lechner J. F., Narayan K. S. & Jones L. W. (1978). Prostate carcinoma: Tissue culture cell lines. *Natl Cancer Inst Monogr*, (49), 17-21.

Kaighn, M. E., Narayan K. S., Ohnuki Y., Lechner J. F. & Jones L. W. (1979). Establishment and characterization of a human prostatic carcinoma cell line (PC-3). *Invest Urol, 17,* 16-23.

Kalluri, R. & Weinberg R. A. (2009). The basics of epithelial-mesenchymal transition. *J Clin Invest,* 119, 1420-1428.

Karnoub, A. E., Dash A. B., Vo A. P., Sullivan A., Brooks M. W., Bell G. W. et al. (2007). Mesenchymal stem cells within tumour stroma promote breast cancer metastasis. *Nature,* 449, 557-563.

Kim, M. J., Bhatia-Gaur R., Banach-Petrosky W. A., Desai N., Wang Y., Hayward S. W. et al. (2002). Nkx3.1 mutant mice recapitulate early stages of prostate carcinogenesis. *Cancer Res,* 62, 2999-3004.

Kinbara, H., Cunha G. R., Boutin E., Hayashi N. & Kawamura J. (1996). Evidence of stem cells in the adult prostatic epithelium based upon responsiveness to mesenchymal inductors. *Prostate,* 29, 107-116.

King, J. C., Xu J., Wongvipat J., Hieronymus H., Carver B. S., Leung D. H. et al. (2009). Cooperativity of TMPRSS2-ERG with PI3-kinase pathway activation in prostate oncogenesis. *Nat Genet,* 41, 524-526.

Kiskowski, M. A., Jackson R. S.,2nd, Banerjee J., Li X., Kang M., Iturregui J. M. et al. (2011). Role for stromal heterogeneity in prostate tumorigenesis. *Cancer Res,* 71, 3459-3470.

Knudsen, B. S. & Vande Woude G. (2008). Showering c-MET-dependent cancers with drugs. *Curr Opin Genet Dev,* 18, 87-96.

Knudsen, B. S., Zhao P., Resau J., Cottingham S., Gherardi E., Xu E. et al. (2009). A novel multipurpose monoclonal antibody for evaluating human c-met expression in preclinical and clinical settings. *Appl Immunohistochem Mol Morphol,* 17, 57-67.

Kogan, I., Goldfinger N., Milyavsky M., Cohen M., Shats I., Dobler G. et al. (2006). hTERT-immortalized prostate epithelial and stromal-derived cells: An authentic in vitro model for differentiation and carcinogenesis. *Cancer Res,* 66, 3531-3540.

Kogan-Sakin, I., Cohen M., Paland N., Madar S., Solomon H., Molchadsky A. et al. (2009). Prostate stromal cells produce CXCL-1, CXCL-2, CXCL-3 and IL-8 in response to epithelia-secreted IL-1. *Carcinogenesis,* 30, 698-705.

Koivisto, P., Kononen J., Palmberg C., Tammela T., Hyytinen E., Isola J. et al. (1997). AR gene amplification: A possible molecular mechanism for androgen deprivation therapy failure in prostate cancer. *Cancer Res,* 57, 314-319.

Koivisto, P. A., Schleutker J., Helin H., Ehren-van Eekelen C., Kallioniemi O. P. & Trapman J. (1999). AR gene alterations and chromosomal gains and losses in prostate carcinomas appearing during finasteride treatment for benign prostatic hyperplasia. *Clin Cancer Res,* 5, 3578-3582.

Kong, D., Banerjee S., Ahmad A., Li Y., Wang Z., Sethi S. et al. (2010). Epithelial to mesenchymal transition is mechanistically linked with stem cell signatures in prostate cancer cells. *PLoS One,* 5, e12445.

Korenchuk, S., Lehr J. E., MClean L., Lee Y. G., Whitney S., Vessella R. et al. (2001). VCaP, a cell-based model system of human prostate cancer. *In Vivo,* 15, 163-168.

Korkaya, H., Paulson A., Charafe-Jauffret E., Ginestier C., Brown M., Dutcher J. et al. (2009). Regulation of mammary stem/progenitor cells by PTEN/Akt/beta-catenin signaling. *PLoS Biol,* 7, e1000121.

Korsten, H., Ziel-van der Made A., Ma X., van der Kwast T. & Trapman J. (2009). Accumulating progenitor cells in the luminal epithelial cell layer are candidate tumor initiating cells in a pten knockout mouse prostate cancer model. *PLoS One*, 4, e5662.

Kostarelos, K., Emfietzoglou D., Papakostas A., Yang W. H., Ballangrud A. & Sgouros G. (2004). Binding and interstitial penetration of liposomes within avascular tumor spheroids. *Int J Cancer*, 112, 713-721.

Lang, S. H., Frame F. M. & Collins A. T. (2009). Prostate cancer stem cells. *J Pathol*, 217, 299-306.

Lang, S. H., Sharrard R. M., Stark M., Villette J. M. & Maitland N. J. (2001). Prostate epithelial cell lines form spheroids with evidence of glandular differentiation in three-dimensional matrigel cultures. *Br J Cancer*, 85, 590-599.

Laxman, B., Morris D. S., Yu J., Siddiqui J., Cao J., Mehra R. et al. (2008). A first-generation multiplex biomarker analysis of urine for the early detection of prostate cancer. *Cancer Res*, 68, 645-649.

Lee, H. L., Pienta K. J., Kim W. J. & Cooper C. R. (2003). The effect of bone-associated growth factors and cytokines on the growth of prostate cancer cells derived from soft tissue versus bone metastases in vitro. *Int J Oncol*, 22, 921-926.

Lee, Y. G., Korenchuk S., Lehr J., Whitney S., Vessela R. & Pienta K. J. (2001). Establishment and characterization of a new human prostatic cancer cell line: DuCaP. *In Vivo*, 15, 157-162.

Li, H. & Tang D. G. (2011). Prostate cancer stem cells and their potential roles in metastasis. *J Surg Oncol*, 103, 558-562.

Li, X., Loberg R., Liao J., Ying C., Snyder L. A., Pienta K. J. et al. (2009). A destructive cascade mediated by CCL2 facilitates prostate cancer growth in bone. *Cancer Res*, 69, 1685-1692.

Liao, C. P., Adisetiyo H., Liang M. & Roy-Burman P. (2010a). Cancer stem cells and microenvironment in prostate cancer progression. *Horm Cancer*, 1, 297-305.

Liao, C. P., Adisetiyo H., Liang M. & Roy-Burman P. (2010b). Cancer-associated fibroblasts enhance the gland-forming capability of prostate cancer stem cells. *Cancer Res*, 70, 7294-7303.

Liao, C. P., Liang M., Cohen M. B., Flesken-Nikitin A., Jeong J. H., Nikitin A. Y. et al. (2010c). Mouse prostate cancer cell lines established from primary and post-castration recurrent tumors. *Horm Cancer*, 1, 44-54.

Lin, J., Gan C. M., Zhang X., Jones S., Sjoblom T., Wood L. D. et al. (2007). A multidimensional analysis of genes mutated in breast and colorectal cancers. *Genome Res*, 17, 1304-1318.

Ling, P. M., Cheung S. W., Tay D. K. & Ellis-Behnke R. G. (2011). Using self-assembled nanomaterials to inhibit the formation of metastatic cancer stem cell colonies in vitro. *Cell Transplant*, 20, 127-131.

Litvinov, I. V., Antony L., Dalrymple S. L., Becker R., Cheng L. & Isaacs J. T. (2006a). PC3, but not DU145, human prostate cancer cells retain the coregulators required for tumor suppressor ability of AR. *Prostate*, 66, 1329-1338.

Litvinov, I. V., Vander Griend D. J., Xu Y., Antony L., Dalrymple S. L. & Isaacs J. T. (2006b). Low-calcium serum-free defined medium selects for growth of normal prostatic epithelial stem cells. *Cancer Res,* 66, 8598-8607.

Liu, C., Kelnar K., Liu B., Chen X., Calhoun-Davis T., Li H. et al. (2011). The microRNA miR-34a inhibits prostate cancer stem cells and metastasis by directly repressing CD44. *Nat Med,* 17, 211-215.

Loberg, R. D., Day L. L., Harwood J., Ying C., St John L. N., Giles R. et al. (2006a). CCL2 is a potent regulator of prostate cancer cell migration and proliferation. *Neoplasia,* 8, 578-586.

Loberg, R. D., St John L. N., Day L. L., Neeley C. K. & Pienta K. J. (2006b). Development of the VCaP androgen-independent model of prostate cancer. *Urol Oncol,* 24, 161-168.

Loberg, R. D., Tantivejkul K., Craig M., Neeley C. K. & Pienta K. J. (2007). PAR1-mediated RhoA activation facilitates CCL2-induced chemotaxis in PC-3 cells. *J Cell Biochem,* 101, 1292-1300.

Maeda, A., Nakashiro K., Hara S., Sasaki T., Miwa Y., Tanji N. et al. (2006). Inactivation of AR activates HGF/c-met system in human prostatic carcinoma cells. *Biochem Biophys Res Commun,* 347, 1158-1165.

Mailleux, A. A., Overholtzer M. & Brugge J. S. (2008). Lumen formation during mammary epithelial morphogenesis: Insights from in vitro and in vivo models. *Cell Cycle,* 7, 57-62.

Maitland, N. J., Frame F. M., Polson E. S., Lewis J. L. & Collins A. T. (2011). Prostate cancer stem cells: Do they have a basal or luminal phenotype? *Horm Cancer,* 2, 47-61.

Malinowska, K., Neuwirt H., Cavarretta I. T., Bektic J., Steiner H., Dietrich H. et al. (2009). Interleukin-6 stimulation of growth of prostate cancer in vitro and in vivo through activation of the AR. *Endocr Relat Cancer,* 16, 155-169.

Mani, S. A., Guo W., Liao M. J., Eaton E. N., Ayyanan A., Zhou A. Y. et al. (2008). The epithelial-mesenchymal transition generates cells with properties of stem cells. *Cell,* 133, 704-715.

Mao, X., Shaw G., James S. Y., Purkis P., Kudahetti S. C., Tsigani T. et al. (2008). Detection of TMPRSS2:ERG fusion gene in circulating prostate cancer cells. *Asian J Androl,* 10, 467-473.

Maroni, P. D., Koul S., Meacham R. B. & Koul H. K. (2004). Mitogen activated protein kinase signal transduction pathways in the prostate. *Cell Commun Signal,* 2, 5.

Marques, R. B., Dits N. F., Erkens-Schulze S., van Weerden W. M. & Jenster G. (2010). Bypass mechanisms of the AR pathway in therapy-resistant prostate cancer cell models. *PLoS One,* 5, e13500.

Marques, R. B., van Weerden W. M., Erkens-Schulze S., de Ridder C. M., Bangma C. H., Trapman J. et al. (2006). The human PC346 xenograft and cell line panel: A model system for prostate cancer progression. *Eur Urol,* 49, 245-257.

Marusyk, A. & Polyak K. (2010). Tumor heterogeneity: Causes and consequences. *Biochim Biophys Acta,* 1805, 105-117.

Massard, C. & Fizazi K. (2011). Targeting continued AR signaling in prostate cancer. *Clin Cancer Res,* 17, 3876-3883.

Medjkane, S., Perez-Sanchez C., Gaggioli C., Sahai E. & Treisman R. (2009). Myocardin-related transcription factors and SRF are required for cytoskeletal dynamics and experimental metastasis. *Nat Cell Biol*, 11, 257-268.

Mehrian-Shai, R., Chen C. D., Shi T., Horvath S., Nelson S. F., Reichardt J. K. et al. (2007). Insulin growth factor-binding protein 2 is a candidate biomarker for PTEN status and PI3K/Akt pathway activation in glioblastoma and prostate cancer. *Proc Natl Acad Sci U S A*, 104, 5563-5568.

Memarzadeh, S., Xin L., Mulholland D. J., Mansukhani A., Wu H., Teitell M. A. et al. (2007). Enhanced paracrine FGF10 expression promotes formation of multifocal prostate adenocarcinoma and an increase in epithelial AR. *Cancer Cell*, 12, 572-585.

Mertz, K. D., Setlur S. R., Dhanasekaran S. M., Demichelis F., Perner S., Tomlins S. et al. (2007). Molecular characterization of TMPRSS2-ERG gene fusion in the NCI-H660 prostate cancer cell line: A new perspective for an old model. *Neoplasia*, 9, 200-206.

Mickey, D. D., Stone K. R., Wunderli H., Mickey G. H., Vollmer R. T. & Paulson D. F. (1977). Heterotransplantation of a human prostatic adenocarcinoma cell line in nude mice. *Cancer Res*, 37, 4049-4058.

Miki, J. & Rhim J. S. (2008). Prostate cell cultures as in vitro models for the study of normal stem cells and cancer stem cells. *Prostate Cancer Prostatic Dis*, 11, 32-39.

Mohamed, A. A., Tan S. H., Sun C., Shaheduzzaman S., Hu Y., Petrovics G. et al. (2011). ERG oncogene modulates prostaglandin signaling in prostate cancer cells. *Cancer Biol Ther*, 11, 410-417.

Molina, A. & Belldegrun A. (2011). Novel therapeutic strategies for CRPC: Inhibition of persistent androgen production and AR mediated signaling. *J Urol*, 185, 787-794.

Mosquera, J. M., Perner S., Genega E. M., Sanda M., Hofer M. D., Mertz K. D. et al. (2008). Characterization of TMPRSS2-ERG fusion high-grade prostatic intraepithelial neoplasia and potential clinical implications. *Clin Cancer Res*, 14, 3380-3385.

Mulholland, D. J., Xin L., Morim A., Lawson D., Witte O. & Wu H. (2009). Lin-sca-1+CD49fhigh stem/progenitors are tumor-initiating cells in the pten-null prostate cancer model. *Cancer Res*, 69, 8555-8562.

Navone, N. M., Olive M., Ozen M., Davis R., Troncoso P., Tu S. M. et al. (1997). Establishment of two human prostate cancer cell lines derived from a single bone metastasis. *Clin Cancer Res*, 3, 2493-2500.

Ouyang, X., DeWeese T. L., Nelson W. G. & Abate-Shen C. (2005). Loss-of-function of Nkx3.1 promotes increased oxidative damage in prostate carcinogenesis. *Cancer Res*, 65, 6773-6779.

Park, S. I., Kim S. J., McCauley L. K. & Gallick G. E. (2010). Pre-clinical mouse models of human prostate cancer and their utility in drug discovery. *Curr Protoc Pharmacol*, 51, 14.15-14.15.27.

Patrawala, L., Calhoun T., Schneider-Broussard R., Li H., Bhatia B., Tang S. et al. (2006). Highly purified CD44+ prostate cancer cells from xenograft human tumors are enriched in tumorigenic and metastatic progenitor cells. *Oncogene*, 25, 1696-1708.

Patrawala, L., Calhoun-Davis T., Schneider-Broussard R. & Tang D. G. (2007). Hierarchical organization of prostate cancer cells in xenograft tumors: The CD44+alpha2beta1+ cell population is enriched in tumor-initiating cells. *Cancer Res*, 67, 6796-6805.

Peehl, D. M. (2005). Primary cell cultures as models of prostate cancer development. *Endocr Relat Cancer,* 12, 19-47.

Peehl, D. M. & Feldman D. (2004). Interaction of nuclear receptor ligands with the vitamin D signaling pathway in prostate cancer. *J Steroid Biochem Mol Biol,* 92, 307-315.

Peehl, D. M., Seto E., Hsu J. Y. & Feldman D. (2002). Preclinical activity of ketoconazole in combination with calcitriol or the vitamin D analogue EB 1089 in prostate cancer cells. *J Urol,* 168, 1583-1588.

Perner, S., Mosquera J. M., Demichelis F., Hofer M. D., Paris P. L., Simko J. et al. (2007). TMPRSS2-ERG fusion prostate cancer: An early molecular event associated with invasion. *Am J Surg Pathol,* 31, 882-888.

Pfeiffer, M. J. & Schalken J. A. (2010). Stem cell characteristics in prostate cancer cell lines. *Eur Urol,* 57, 246-254.

Pfeiffer, M. J., Smit F. P., Sedelaar J. P. & Schalken J. A. (2011). Steroidogenic enzymes and stem cell markers are up-regulated during androgen deprivation in prostate cancer. *Mol Med.*

Pisters, L. L., Troncoso P., Zhau H. E., Li W., von Eschenbach A. C. & Chung L. W. (1995). C-met proto-oncogene expression in benign and malignant human prostate tissues. *J Urol,* 154, 293-298.

Polyak, K., Haviv I. & Campbell I. G. (2009). Co-evolution of tumor cells and their microenvironment. *Trends Genet,* 25, 30-38.

Polyak, K. & Weinberg R. A. (2009). Transitions between epithelial and mesenchymal states: Acquisition of malignant and stem cell traits. *Nat Rev Cancer,* 9, 265-273.

Pu, H., Collazo J., Jones E., Gayheart D., Sakamoto S., Vogt A. et al. (2009). Dysfunctional transforming growth factor-beta receptor II accelerates prostate tumorigenesis in the TRAMP mouse model. *Cancer Res,* 69, 7366-7374.

Radisky, D., Muschler J. & Bissell M. J. (2002). Order and disorder: The role of ECM in epithelial cancer. *Cancer Invest,* 20, 139-153.

Rajasekhar, V. K., Studer L., Gerald W., Socci N. D. & Scher H. I. (2011). Tumour-initiating stem-like cells in human prostate cancer exhibit increased NF-kappaB signalling. *Nat Commun,* 2, 162.

Reiman, J. M., Knutson K. L. & Radisky D. C. (2010). Immune promotion of epithelial-mesenchymal transition and generation of breast cancer stem cells. *Cancer Res,* 70, 3005-3008.

Rhim, J. S. (2000). Development of human cell lines from multiple organs. *Ann N Y Acad Sci,* 919, 16-25.

Romero, D., O'Neill C., Terzic A., Contois L., Young K., Conley B. A. et al. (2011). Endoglin regulates cancer-stromal cell interactions in prostate tumors. *Cancer Res,* 71, 3482-3493.

Ryan, C. J., Smith M. R., Fong L., Rosenberg J. E., Kantoff P., Raynaud F. et al. (2010). Phase I clinical trial of the CYP17 inhibitor abiraterone acetate demonstrating clinical activity in patients with castration-resistant prostate cancer who received prior ketoconazole therapy. *J Clin Oncol,* 28, 1481-1488.

Rybak, A. P., He L., Kapoor A., Cutz J. C. & Tang D. (2011). Characterization of sphere-propagating cells with stem-like properties from DU145 prostate cancer cells. *Biochim Biophys Acta,* 1813, 683-694.

Samuels, Y., Wang Z., Bardelli A., Silliman N., Ptak J., Szabo S. et al. (2004). High frequency of mutations of the PIK3CA gene in human cancers. *Science*, 304, 554.

Sandhu, C., Peehl D. M. & Slingerland J. (2000). p16INK4A mediates cyclin dependent kinase 4 and 6 inhibition in senescent prostatic epithelial cells. *Cancer Res*, 60, 2616-2622.

Sanz-Moreno, V., Gadea G., Ahn J., Paterson H., Marra P., Pinner S. et al. (2008). Rac activation and inactivation control plasticity of tumor cell movement. *Cell*, 135, 510-523.

Saramaki, O. R., Harjula A. E., Martikainen P. M., Vessella R. L., Tammela T. L. & Visakorpi T. (2008). TMPRSS2:ERG fusion identifies a subgroup of prostate cancers with a favorable prognosis. *Clin Cancer Res*, 14, 3395-3400.

Sarker, D., Reid A. H., Yap T. A. & de Bono J. S. (2009). Targeting the PI3K/AKT pathway for the treatment of prostate cancer. *Clin Cancer Res*, 15, 4799-4805.

Sauer, H., Diedershagen H., Hescheler J. & Wartenberg M. (1997). Calcium-dependence of hydrogen peroxide-induced c-fos expression and growth stimulation of multicellular prostate tumor spheroids. *FEBS Lett*, 419, 201-205.

Sauer, H., Ritgen J., Hescheler J. & Wartenberg M. (1998). Hypotonic Ca2+ signaling and volume regulation in proliferating and quiescent cells from multicellular spheroids. *J Cell Physiol*, 175, 129-140.

Sawyers, C. L. (2007). Where lies the blame for resistance--tumor or host? *Nat Med*, 13, 1144-1145.

Scaccianoce, E., Festuccia C., Dondi D., Guerini V., Bologna M., Motta M. et al. (2003). Characterization of prostate cancer DU145 cells expressing the recombinant AR. *Oncol Res*, 14, 101-112.

Scher, H. I., Beer T. M., Higano C. S., Anand A., Taplin M. E., Efstathiou E. et al. (2010). Antitumour activity of MDV3100 in castration-resistant prostate cancer: A phase 1-2 study. *Lancet*, 375, 1437-1446.

Scher, H. I. & Sawyers C. L. (2005). Biology of progressive, castration-resistant prostate cancer: Directed therapies targeting the androgen-receptor signaling axis. *J Clin Oncol*, 23, 8253-8261.

Sequeira, L., Dubyk C. W., Riesenberger T. A., Cooper C. R. & van Golen K. L. (2008). Rho GTPases in PC-3 prostate cancer cell morphology, invasion and tumor cell diapedesis. *Clin Exp Metastasis*, 25, 569-579.

Shackleton, M., Quintana E., Fearon E. R. & Morrison S. J. (2009). Heterogeneity in cancer: Cancer stem cells versus clonal evolution. *Cell*, 138, 822-829.

Shah, S. & Ryan C. (2010). Abiraterone acetate for CRPC. *Expert Opin Investig Drugs*, 19, 563-570.

Sharifi, N. (2010). New agents and strategies for the hormonal treatment of castration-resistant prostate cancer. *Expert Opin Investig Drugs*, .

Shen, M. M. & Abate-Shen C. (2007). Pten inactivation and the emergence of androgen-independent prostate cancer. *Cancer Res*, 67, 6535-6538.

Shipitsin, M., Campbell L. L., Argani P., Weremowicz S., Bloushtain-Qimron N., Yao J. et al. (2007). Molecular definition of breast tumor heterogeneity. *Cancer Cell*, 11, 259-273.

Simian, M., Hirai Y., Navre M., Werb Z., Lochter A. & Bissell M. J. (2001). The interplay of matrix metalloproteinases, morphogens and growth factors is necessary for branching of mammary epithelial cells. *Development*, 128, 3117-3131.

Sobel, R. E. & Sadar M. D. (2005a). Cell lines used in prostate cancer research: A compendium of old and new lines--part 1. *J Urol*, 173, 342-359.

Sobel, R. E. & Sadar M. D. (2005b). Cell lines used in prostate cancer research: A compendium of old and new lines--part 2. *J Urol*, 173, 360-372.

Song, H., Zhang B., Watson M. A., Humphrey P. A., Lim H. & Milbrandt J. (2009). Loss of Nkx3.1 leads to the activation of discrete downstream target genes during prostate tumorigenesis. *Oncogene*, 28, 3307-3319.

Sonnenberg, M., van der Kuip H., Haubeis S., Fritz P., Schroth W., Friedel G. et al. (2008). Highly variable response to cytotoxic chemotherapy in carcinoma-associated fibroblasts (CAFs) from lung and breast. *BMC Cancer*, 8, 364.

Squire, J. A. (2009). TMPRSS2-ERG and PTEN loss in prostate cancer. *Nat Genet*, 41, 509-510.

Sramkoski, R. M., Pretlow T. G.,2nd, Giaconia J. M., Pretlow T. P., Schwartz S., Sy M. S. et al. (1999). A new human prostate carcinoma cell line, 22Rv1. *In Vitro Cell Dev Biol Anim*, 35, 403-409.

Stone, K. R., Mickey D. D., Wunderli H., Mickey G. H. & Paulson D. F. (1978). Isolation of a human prostate carcinoma cell line (DU 145). *Int J Cancer*, 21, 274-281.

Streuli, C. H., Bailey N. & Bissell M. J. (1991). Control of mammary epithelial differentiation: Basement membrane induces tissue-specific gene expression in the absence of cell-cell interaction and morphological polarity. *J Cell Biol*, 115, 1383-1395.

Streuli, C. H., Schmidhauser C., Bailey N., Yurchenco P., Skubitz A. P., Roskelley C. et al. (1995). Laminin mediates tissue-specific gene expression in mammary epithelia. *J Cell Biol*, 129, 591-603.

Sun, C., Dobi A., Mohamed A., Li H., Thangapazham R. L., Furusato B. et al. (2008). TMPRSS2-ERG fusion, a common genomic alteration in prostate cancer activates C-MYC and abrogates prostate epithelial differentiation. *Oncogene*, 27, 5348-5353.

Sutherland, R. M. (1988). Cell and environment interactions in tumor microregions: The multicell spheroid model. *Science*, 240, 177-184.

Sutherland, R. M., MacDonald H. R. & Howell R. L. (1977). Multicellular spheroids: A new model target for in vitro studies of immunity to solid tumor allografts. *J Natl Cancer Inst*, 58, 1849-1853.

Sutherland, R. M., McCredie J. A. & Inch W. R. (1971). Growth of multicell spheroids in tissue culture as a model of nodular carcinomas. *J Natl Cancer Inst*, 46, 113-120.

Szabo, R., Rasmussen A. L., Moyer A. B., Kosa P., Schafer J. M., Molinolo A. A. et al. (2011). c-met-induced epithelial carcinogenesis is initiated by the serine protease matriptase. *Oncogene*.

Takahashi, S., Watanabe T., Okada M., Inoue K., Ueda T., Takada I. et al. (2011). Noncanonical wnt signaling mediates androgen-dependent tumor growth in a mouse model of prostate cancer. *Proc Natl Acad Sci U S A*, 108, 4938-4943.

Tang, D. G., Patrawala L., Calhoun T., Bhatia B., Choy G., Schneider-Broussard R. et al. (2007). Prostate cancer stem/progenitor cells: Identification, characterization, and implications. *Mol Carcinog*, 46, 1-14.

Tanner, M. J., Welliver R. C.,Jr, Chen M., Shtutman M., Godoy A., Smith G. et al. (2011). Effects of AR and androgen on gene expression in prostate stromal fibroblasts and paracrine signaling to prostate cancer cells. *PLoS One,* 6, e16027.

Taylor, B. S., Schultz N., Hieronymus H., Gopalan A., Xiao Y., Carver B. S. et al. (2010). Integrative genomic profiling of human prostate cancer. *Cancer Cell,* 18, 11-22.

Tokar, E. J., Ancrile B. B., Cunha G. R. & Webber M. M. (2005). Stem/progenitor and intermediate cell types and the origin of human prostate cancer. *Differentiation,* 73, 463-473.

Tokar, E. J., Diwan B. A. & Waalkes M. P. (2010a). Arsenic exposure transforms human epithelial stem/progenitor cells into a cancer stem-like phenotype. *Environ Health Perspect,* 118, 108-115.

Tokar, E. J., Qu W., Liu J., Liu W., Webber M. M., Phang J. M. et al. (2010b). Arsenic-specific stem cell selection during malignant transformation. *J Natl Cancer Inst,* 102, 638-649.

Tomlins, S. A., Bjartell A., Chinnaiyan A. M., Jenster G., Nam R. K., Rubin M. A. et al. (2009). ETS gene fusions in prostate cancer: From discovery to daily clinical practice. *Eur Urol,* 56, 275-286.

Tomlins, S. A., Laxman B., Dhanasekaran S. M., Helgeson B. E., Cao X., Morris D. S. et al. (2007). Distinct classes of chromosomal rearrangements create oncogenic ETS gene fusions in prostate cancer. *Nature,* 448, 595-599.

Tomlins, S. A., Laxman B., Varambally S., Cao X., Yu J., Helgeson B. E. et al. (2008). Role of the TMPRSS2-ERG gene fusion in prostate cancer. *Neoplasia,* 10, 177-188.

Tomlins, S. A., Mehra R., Rhodes D. R., Smith L. R., Roulston D., Helgeson B. E. et al. (2006). TMPRSS2:ETV4 gene fusions define a third molecular subtype of prostate cancer. *Cancer Res,* 66, 3396-3400.

Tomlins, S. A., Rhodes D. R., Perner S., Dhanasekaran S. M., Mehra R., Sun X. W. et al. (2005). Recurrent fusion of TMPRSS2 and ETS transcription factor genes in prostate cancer. *Science,* 310, 644-648.

Tran, C., Ouk S., Clegg N. J., Chen Y., Watson P. A., Arora V. et al. (2009). Development of a second-generation antiandrogen for treatment of advanced prostate cancer. *Science,* 324, 787-790.

Tu, W. H., Zhu C., Clark C., Christensen J. G. & Sun Z. (2010). Efficacy of c-met inhibitor for advanced prostate cancer. *BMC Cancer,* 10, 556.

Uzgare, A. R., Xu Y. & Isaacs J. T. (2004). In vitro culturing and characteristics of transit amplifying epithelial cells from human prostate tissue. *J Cell Biochem,* 91, 196-205.

van Bokhoven, A., Caires A., Maria M. D., Schulte A. P., Lucia M. S., Nordeen S. K. et al. (2003a). Spectral karyotype (SKY) analysis of human prostate carcinoma cell lines. *Prostate,* 57, 226-244.

van Bokhoven, A., Varella-Garcia M., Korch C., Johannes W. U., Smith E. E., Miller H. L. et al. (2003b). Molecular characterization of human prostate carcinoma cell lines. *Prostate,* 57, 205-225.

van de Wijngaart, D. J., Molier M., Lusher S. J., Hersmus R., Jenster G., Trapman J. et al. (2010). Systematic structure-function analysis of AR Leu701 mutants explains the properties of the prostate cancer mutant L701H. *J Biol Chem,* 285, 5097-5105.

van der Kuip, H., Murdter T. E., Sonnenberg M., McClellan M., Gutzeit S., Gerteis A. et al. (2006). Short term culture of breast cancer tissues to study the activity of the anticancer drug taxol in an intact tumor environment. *BMC Cancer*, 6, 86.

van der Pluijm, G. (2011). Epithelial plasticity, cancer stem cells and bone metastasis formation. *Bone*, 48, 37-43.

van Golen, K. L., Ying C., Sequeira L., Dubyk C. W., Reisenberger T., Chinnaiyan A. M. et al. (2008). CCL2 induces prostate cancer transendothelial cell migration via activation of the small GTPase rac. *J Cell Biochem*, 104, 1587-1597.

van Weerden, W. M., Bangma C. & de Wit R. (2009). Human xenograft models as useful tools to assess the potential of novel therapeutics in prostate cancer. *Br J Cancer*, 100, 13-18.

Verhagen, P. C., van Duijn P. W., Hermans K. G., Looijenga L. H., van Gurp R. J., Stoop H. et al. (2006). The PTEN gene in locally progressive prostate cancer is preferentially inactivated by bi-allelic gene deletion. *J Pathol*, 208, 699-707.

Visakorpi, T., Hyytinen E., Koivisto P., Tanner M., Keinanen R., Palmberg C. et al. (1995). In vivo amplification of the AR gene and progression of human prostate cancer. *Nat Genet*, 9, 401-406.

Vlietstra, R. J., van Alewijk D. C., Hermans K. G., van Steenbrugge G. J. & Trapman J. (1998). Frequent inactivation of PTEN in prostate cancer cell lines and xenografts. *Cancer Res*, 58, 2720-2723.

Wang, F. (2011). Modeling human prostate cancer in genetically engineered mice. *Prog Mol Biol Transl Sci*, 100, 1-49.

Wang, Q., Li W., Zhang Y., Yuan X., Xu K., Yu J. et al. (2009a). AR regulates a distinct transcription program in androgen-independent prostate cancer. *Cell*, 138, 245-256.

Wang, X., Kruithof-de Julio M., Economides K. D., Walker D., Yu H., Halili M. V. et al. (2009b). A luminal epithelial stem cell that is a cell of origin for prostate cancer. *Nature*, 461, 495-500.

Wang, Z. A. & Shen M. M. (2011). Revisiting the concept of cancer stem cells in prostate cancer. *Oncogene*, 30, 1261-1271.

Wartenberg, M., Hescheler J., Acker H., Diedershagen H. & Sauer H. (1998). Doxorubicin distribution in multicellular prostate cancer spheroids evaluated by confocal laser scanning microscopy and the "optical probe technique". *Cytometry*, 31, 137-145.

Watanabe, M. & Takagi A. (2008). Biological behavior of prostate cancer cells in 3D culture systems. *Yakugaku Zasshi*, 128, 37-44.

Weaver, V. M., Fischer A. H., Peterson O. W. & Bissell M. J. (1996). The importance of the microenvironment in breast cancer progression: Recapitulation of mammary tumorigenesis using a unique human mammary epithelial cell model and a three-dimensional culture assay. *Biochem Cell Biol*, 74, 833-851.

Weaver, V. M., Howlett A. R., Langton-Webster B., Petersen O. W. & Bissell M. J. (1995). The development of a functionally relevant cell culture model of progressive human breast cancer. *Semin Cancer Biol*, 6, 175-184.

Weaver, V. M., Lelievre S., Lakins J. N., Chrenek M. A., Jones J. C., Giancotti F. et al. (2002). Beta4 integrin-dependent formation of polarized three-dimensional architecture confers resistance to apoptosis in normal and malignant mammary epithelium. *Cancer Cell*, 2, 205-216.

Webber, M. M., Trakul N., Thraves P. S., Bello-DeOcampo D., Chu W. W., Storto P. D. et al. (1999). A human prostatic stromal myofibroblast cell line WPMY-1: A model for stromal-epithelial interactions in prostatic neoplasia. *Carcinogenesis*, 20, 1185-1192.

Weinberg, R. A. (2008). Coevolution in the tumor microenvironment. *Nat Genet*, 40, 494-495.

Wolf, K. & Friedl P. (2009). Mapping proteolytic cancer cell-ECM interfaces. *Clin Exp Metastasis*, 26, 289-298.

Wolf, K. & Friedl P. (2006). Molecular mechanisms of cancer cell invasion and plasticity. *Br J Dermatol*, 154 Suppl 1, 11-15.

Wolf, K., Wu Y. I., Liu Y., Geiger J., Tam E., Overall C. et al. (2007). Multi-step pericellular proteolysis controls the transition from individual to collective cancer cell invasion. *Nat Cell Biol*, 9, 893-904.

Wood, L. D., Calhoun E. S., Silliman N., Ptak J., Szabo S., Powell S. M. et al. (2006). Somatic mutations of GUCY2F, EPHA3, and NTRK3 in human cancers. *Hum Mutat*, 27, 1060-1061.

Wood, L. D., Parsons D. W., Jones S., Lin J., Sjoblom T., Leary R. J. et al. (2007). The genomic landscapes of human breast and colorectal cancers. *Science*.

Xue, Y., Smedts F., Ruijter E. T., Debruyne F. M., de la Rosette J. J. & Schalken J. A. (2001a). Branching activity in the human prostate: A closer look at the structure of small glandular buds. *Eur Urol*, 39, 222-231.

Xue, Y., Sonke G., Schoots C., Schalken J., Verhofstad A., de la Rosette J. et al. (2001b). Proliferative activity and branching morphogenesis in the human prostate: A closer look at pre- and postnatal prostate growth. *Prostate*, 49, 132-139.

Yang, Q., Fung K. M., Day W. V., Kropp B. P. & Lin H. K. (2005). AR signaling is required for androgen-sensitive human prostate cancer cell proliferation and survival. *Cancer Cell Int*, 5, 8.

Yap, T. A. & de Bono J. S. (2010). Targeting the HGF/c-met axis: State of play. *Mol Cancer Ther*, 9, 1077-1079.

Yates, C., Shepard C. R., Papworth G., Dash A., Beer Stolz D., Tannenbaum S. et al. (2007a). Novel three-dimensional organotypic liver bioreactor to directly visualize early events in metastatic progression. *Adv Cancer Res*, 97, 225-246.

Yates, C. C., Shepard C. R., Stolz D. B. & Wells A. (2007b). Co-culturing human prostate carcinoma cells with hepatocytes leads to increased expression of E-cadherin. *Br J Cancer*, 96, 1246-1252.

Yu, J., Yu J., Mani R. S., Cao Q., Brenner C. J., Cao X. et al. (2010). An integrated network of AR, polycomb, and TMPRSS2-ERG gene fusions in prostate cancer progression. *Cancer Cell*, 17, 443-454.

Yu, L., Wang C. Y., Shi J., Miao L., Du X., Mayer D. et al. (2011). Estrogens promote invasion of prostate cancer cells in a paracrine manner through up-regulation of matrix metalloproteinase 2 in prostatic stromal cells. *Endocrinology*, 152, 773-781.

Yu, S. Q., Lai K. P., Xia S. J., Chang H. C., Chang C. & Yeh S. (2009). The diverse and contrasting effects of using human prostate cancer cell lines to study AR roles in prostate cancer. *Asian J Androl*, 11, 39-48.

Yuan, S., Trachtenberg J., Mills G. B., Brown T. J., Xu F. & Keating A. (1993). Androgen-induced inhibition of cell proliferation in an androgen-insensitive prostate cancer cell line (PC-3) transfected with a human AR complementary DNA. *Cancer Res*, 53, 1304-1311.

Zhang, S., Pavlovitz B., Tull J., Wang Y., Deng F. M. & Fuller C. (2010). Detection of TMPRSS2 gene deletions and translocations in carcinoma, intraepithelial neoplasia, and normal epithelium of the prostate by direct fluorescence in situ hybridization. *Diagn Mol Pathol*, 19, 151-156.

Zhang, Z., Duan L., Du X., Ma H., Park I., Lee C. et al. (2008). The proliferative effect of estradiol on human prostate stromal cells is mediated through activation of ERK. *Prostate*, 68, 508-516.

Zhao, X. Y., Boyle B., Krishnan A. V., Navone N. M., Peehl D. M. & Feldman D. (1999). Two mutations identified in the AR of the new human prostate cancer cell line MDA PCa 2a. *J Urol*, 162, 2192-2199.

Zong, Y., Xin L., Goldstein A. S., Lawson D. A., Teitell M. A. & Witte O. N. (2009). ETS family transcription factors collaborate with alternative signaling pathways to induce carcinoma from adult murine prostate cells. *Proc Natl Acad Sci U S A*, 106, 12465-12470.

Part 3

Signaling Pathways

5

Signalling Pathways and Gene Expression Profiles in Prostate Cancer

Sophia Marsella-Hatziieremia, Pamela McCall and Joanne Edwards
University of Glasgow
UK

1. Introduction

In general, cancer, encompassing prostate cancer (PCa), is a disease that utilises signalling pathways to progress through the uncontrolled proliferation of cancerous cells. Although the mechanisms of how the cells evade intrinsic or extrinsic signals of death and keep on dividing is not completely understood, there is a plethora of evidence that point to certain signalling molecules that are crucial conveyors of the fine tuning that slightly differs in cancer in comparison to control states. The present chapter provides a detailed description of the key regulators of PCa cell life and unveils their closely communicating proteins that aid in the fine tuning of the cancerous state.

2. Androgen receptor (AR) signalling

A major insight into the potential role of androgens in PCa came almost 70 years ago, from the observation that castration of patients with metastatic PCa resulted in a marked reduction in the levels of prostate specific antigen (PSA), a PCa serum acid phosphatase marker (Huggins and Hodges, 1941). In the same study, injection of androgens in some PCa patients resulted in significant increase of PSA. This clearly demonstrated the androgen dependency of PCa. The treatment of PCa has been based on inhibition of the synthesis or action of the ligand (testosterone and its active metabolite 5-diydrotestosterone (5-DHT)) on the androgen receptor (AR). In addition, there are numerous evidence that demonstrate the involvement of AR in PCa progression especially castration-recurrent PCa, despite the absence of circulating testicular androgens.

As activation of the AR is associated with induction of proliferation and apoptosis in PCa cells, manipulation of androgen-AR relationship such as non steroidal AR antagonists such as bicalutamide and flutamide in conjunction with chemical or surgical castration is the main therapeutic option available to patients with locally advanced or metastatic cancer. However, the AR has been demonstrated to be activated even in castrate conditions, independent of testicular androgens. Mechanisms known to be involved with AR transactivation are: increased expression of receptor which allows its activation even in low levels of andrenal androgens, mutation of AR, non canonical variants of AR, modified expression or activity of AR coregulators and cross talk with other pathways regulating survival, cell death and proliferation of PCa cells. Usually a combination of these mechanisms occur simultaneously to provide PCa cells with an increase in the expression of genes that regulate proliferation and apoptosis.

Numerous studies, initiated almost a decade ago, are dedicated in unravelling androgen regulated gene expression in both normal and tumorgenic prostate cells (please refer to review for complete references; Dehm and Tindall, 2006). The majority of large scale studies have been performed in LNCaP cells based on their AR-sensitive properties. The number of genes regulated by the function of androgens through the AR was recently estimated to be between 10,570 and 23,448 polyadenylated RNAs, however this number is set to grow if microRNAs are included (Dehm and Tindall, 2006). Furthermore, a recent study utilising a microarray analysis of androgen related genes in the cell line LNCaP has demonstrated that a large number of genes falling under the regulation of androgens are still of unknown function (Ngan et al., 2009). The genes regulated by AR regulate functions of the prostate cell related to cell proliferation, cell cycle, survival, death, lipid and steroid metabolism, protein products resulting from gene fusions and microRNAs.

AR signalling that regulates cell proliferation and apoptosis usually arises from cross-talk of the pathway with other pathways that are known to regulate these functions. For example, the insulin like growth factor-1 (IGF-1) pathway falls under the numerous genes affected by the AR-pathway (Schayek et al., 2010). Some of the SMAD and ID proteins involved in the transforming growth factor-beta (TGFβ) pathway are also regulated. Androgens negatively regulate the expression of SMAD1, 3, 6 and 7, while ID3 expression is markedly increased (Ngan et al., 2009). Some of the forkhead box (FOX) family of transcription factors which are important in cell survival are differentially regulated by AR activity (Takayama et al., 2008). Furthermore some of the FOX genes can influence AR expression and activity itself. For example, FOXP1 has been shown to negatively regulate AR expression (Takayama et al., 2008). Cyclin D, cdc6 and genes such as UBEC2 are some of the genes regulated by the androgenic signalling that control cell cycle checkpoints of PCa cells. In addition, the AR signalling can regulate PCa cells apoptosis by regulation of anti-apoptotic molecules such as FLIP (Gao et al., 2005; Raclaw et al., 2008).

Androgens also control the lipid and steroid metabolic pathways that are important in providing energy to cells undergoing proliferation. Sterol regulatory element-binding proteins (SREBPs), which are responsible for activation of numerous enzymes involved in cholesterol processes such as HMG-CoA, acyl CoA:cholesterol acyltransferase (ACAT) are regulated by AR (Locke et al., 2008; Leon et al., 2010).

Recently, reports are exploring the impact of AR signalling in the formation of fusion protein arrangements. Androgenic signalling has demonstrated the ability to promote interactions of genomic regions and DNA breaks (Lin et al., 2009).

MicroRNA profiling in the parental hormone naive cell line LNCaP in comparison to castrate resistant LNCaP- derived cell line has identified 17 differentially expressed miRNAs between the two cells lines (deVere White et al., 2009). In the same study, miR-125b was shown to be highly expressed in AR expressing cell lines such as CWR22R, PC-346C, LNCaP, cds1 and cds2 cells when in AR negative cell lines (DU145, PC3, pRNS-1-1 and RWPE-1) its expression was diminished. These findings suggest that miR-125b may be related to prostatic tumorigenesis and androgen independent (AI) growth, and the AR may regulate the expression of this miRNA in CaP cells. That notion is further supported by the altered expression of miR-125b upon anti-androgen treatment (deVere White et al., 2009).

There are numerous evidence demonstrating the ability of PCa cells to respond to lower levels of androgens due to overexpression of AR protein (Chen et al., 2008). The AR is upregulated in most CRPCs, of which only 10–20% exhibit amplification of the AR gene

(Edwards et al., 2003), indicating that increased AR expression in CRPC may result from factors other than gene amplification such as increased transcription from endogenous promoters or from stabilisation of mRNA (Lammond and Tindall, 2010; Shiota et al., 2011).

Depletion of androgens during PCa treatment can lead to structural and functional changes of AR in the PCa cells in order to adjust and survive in the hormone depleted environment (Pienta et al., 2006). Somatic mutations in the ligand binding pocket of the ligand binding domain (LBD) of AR are a common feature amongst castrate resistant and metastatic prostate tumours, with more than 50% of tumors presented with this type of mutations. AR mutations can alter the binding specificity of AR. For example, the missense mutation of threonine to alanine at amino acid 877 (T877A) leads to an increase in the type of ligands that can bind AR; with estrogens and progesterone having a similar binding affinity as androgens in this instance (Montgomery et al., 2001; Han et al., 2005). Recently seven more variants have been discovered to be over-expressed in castrate resistant PCa (CRPC). Two of these, AR-V1 and AR-V7 that were studied in full detail, were shown to possess premature termination codons. High expressions of both variants correlated with poor prognosis of patients at CRPC (Hu et al., 2009). The splicing variant AR23, that was recently detected in a patient with metastatic CRPC has impaired nuclear localisation and increases androgen signalling only in the presence of endogenous wild-type AR (Jagla et al., 2007). Furthermore this variant has the ability to regulate other signalling pathways such as increasing the transcriptional activity of nuclear factor kappa B (NFκB) and decreasing the activity of activator protein-1 (AP-1). The presence of AR variants have been investigated in CRPC cell lines also. AR3, AR4 and AR5 variants were identified in C-821, CWR-R1 and CWR22Rv1 cell lines, with AR3 being the most abundant variant in these cell lines. AR3 showed both cytoplasmic and nuclear localisation of AR, however, AR3 function, activity and expression was not affected by the presence of androgens or anti-androgens demonstrating the androgen independence of PCa cells in CRPC state. Furthermore, the same study has pinpointed Akt-1 through a microarray analysis, as the key difference between the AR and AR3 signalling pathway to drive growth of CRPC cells (Guo et al. 2009). Another AR mutation has been identified in the CRPC cell line CWR22Rv1 that was absent in the parental hormone naive mimicking cell line CWR22. This mutation resulted in the generation of AR protein fragments; one characterised by a duplication of exon 3 of AR leading to AR[ex3dup] protein with molecular weight of 114kDa, and a second protein ARΔLBD with a truncated ligand binding domain and a lower molecular weight of 75-80kDa (Dehm et al. 2008). Both variants have distinct roles in the hormone naive and CRPC states; AR[ex3dup] protein affects the growth of hormone naive cells while ARΔLBD protein affects the growth of castrate resistant cells (Tepper et al., 2002).

3. Heat shock proteins

Heat shock proteins (Hsps) are a superfamily of proteins produced in cells in response to environmental stresses and in particular heat. It is now well established that Hsp70 and Hsp90 are bound to the AR when it is held in its inactive form in the cytoplasm. The function of the Hsps is to stabilise the receptor and protect it from protelytic degradation. However when androgens bind to the AR, Hsp 70 and 90 dissociate, allowing the AR to form homodimers and transolcate to the nucleus. The first evidence that Hsps were involved in PCa was obtained almost two decades ago from the direct interaction of the Hsp members Hsp90, Hsp70 and Hsp56 with AR (Veldscholte et al., 1992). Furthermore, this interaction has been recently verified in a heterologous AR expression system in the 293HEK cell line. This recapitulates AR SHR activity in PCa cells that identified these Hsps as putative AR-binding proteins in the cytosolic extracts using the ICAT method (Jasavala et al., 2007).

Hsps have been implicated in apoptosis and survival of PCa cells as well as response to chemotherapeutic treatment. The role of Hsps in these cell processes differs depending on the Hsp member involved. The anti-apoptotic role of Hsp70 in PCa, which is known to bind to the AR in the inactive state, was demonstrated *in vitro* by direct transfection of adenoviral Ad.asHsp70 in PCa cells such as PC-3 and DU145 cells. The result was impressive, leading to cell death of tumorigenic cells within three to five days post-transfection (Nylandsted et al., 2000). Increase of Hsp27 and Hsp72 have also been implicated in resistance to apoptotic signals *in vitro* (Gibbons et al., 2000; Garrido et al., 2003). Hsp27 modulates apoptosis through prevention of the apoptosome formation and activation of caspases through direct sequestration of cytochrome c released from the mitochondria into the cytosol or cytochrome c–mediated caspase activation by sequestering both pro-caspase-3 and cytochrome c (Bruye et al., 2000, Paul et al., 2000). Also, Hsp27 at high levels may prevent the caspase-8 activation of the pro-apoptotic Bid protein, a member Bcl-2 family (Concannon et al., 2000). Results from a tissue microarray study on changes in Hsp27 protein expression in 232 specimens from hormone naive and posthormone-treated cancers showed that Hsp27 expression was low or absent in untreated human PCas but increased 4 weeks after beginning androgen-ablation to become uniformly highly expressed in AI tumors (Rocchi et al., 2004). The same group has evaluated the functional relevance of Hsp27 changes in AI progression providing a mechanism by which castration-induced changes in Hsp27 expression serves as an upstream regulator of Stat3 activity (Rocchi et al., 2005). The correlation of the expression of Hsp27, Hsp70 and Hsp90 has also been evaluated in relation to clinicopathological outcomes in patients undergoing radical prostatectomy (Kurashami et al., 2007). Only Hsp27 expression is significantly associated with pathological stage, Gleason score, surgical margin status, lymph node metastasis and tumor volume as well as cell proliferative activity.

4. Src expression

The Src family encompasses nine non-receptor protein kinases: Src, Fyn, Yes, Blk, Yrk, Fgr, Hck, Lck and Lyn with similar structural features. Numerous *in vitro* studies have shown the significance of Src in the development of PCa and its progression to a hormone-independent state (Slack et al., 2001; Recchia et al., 2003; Nam et al., 2005). In addition, the clinical association between Src family kinase (SFK) activity and PCa patient survival suggests that SFK activity is up-regulated in a subgroup of CRPC patients (Tatarov et al., 2009). Furthermore, the same study suggested that an increase in SFK activity in CRPC patients may result in higher likelihood of metastatic disease, which could potentially contribute to the reduction in survival.

Extensive cross-talk and co-regulation are two features of the SFK member action. Moreover, the Src proline-rich sequences of AR have the affinity for SH3 domain of Src, so that the resulting complexes release Src intramolecular constrains activating the tyrosine kinase. Androgen stimulation acts as a trigger for the AR-Src complex formation, which is followed by activation of Src/Raf-1/Erk-2 pathway and, as a result, increases in PCa cell proliferation. Application of androgen antagonists, expression of Src lacking SH3 domain and treatment with Src inhibitor prevented androgen stimulated S-phase entry (Migliaccio et al., 2000). A significant correlation between AR and Src activation in human prostate tumours has been found with proposed tyrosine Y534 as a Src-specific phosphorylation site. Introduction of a dominant negative mutant of Src kinase prevents AR activation and its translocation to the nucleus (Lee et al., 2001). These findings suggest that androgen deprivation therapy may result in Src activation by growth factors, which can then stimulate AR activity as a potential hormone escape mechanism (Guo et al., 2006). Epidermal growth factor (EGF) acting through epidermal growth factor receptor (EGFR) has been shown to activate Src in PCa cells, experiencing acute androgen withdrawal by triggering AR-Src complex formation. Resulting DNA synthesis and cytoskeletal changes were abrogated by treatment with androgen antagonists, suggesting that the relationship between AR and Src play an important role in PCa cells biology (Migliaccio et al., 2005; Hitosugi et al., 2007). Androgen independent growth and cell migration stimulated by Interleukin-8 (IL-8) signalling may involve transactivation of AR by Src as application of Src inhibitors and AR antagonists significantly inhibited these biological processes (Lee et al., 2004). Interaction between IGF system and steroid receptor signalling is thought to play an important role in prostatic carcinogenesis, although the precise mechanism of action is not completely understood (129;130). Androgens have been shown to up-regulate IGF-1R expression and IGF-1-induced Src/MAPK signalling in AR-positive prostate cancer cells (Pandini et al., 2005). Activation of oestrogen receptor β (ERβ), known to form complexes with Src and AR in prostate cancer cells, can result in similar effect on IGF-1R expression and activation (Pandini et al., 2007).

SFK members are involved in the regulation of focal adhesions, thus playing a key role in the regulation of cell motility, migration and invasion. Activation of guanosine phosphate binding protein coupled receptors (GPCRs) results in complex formation between Src and FAK in focal adhesions, whereas Lyn is thought to inhibit these cellular functions by acting as an intermediary between NEP and p85 subunit of PI3-K, preventing association of PI3-K and FAK (Sumitomo et al., 2000). Src is thought to be the main factor in tyrosine phosphorylation of ezrin, an adaptor protein which is implicated in invasion, migration and is important for the development of metastatic PCa (Curto and McClutchey, 2004). Application of Src inhibitor PP2 reduced ezrin phosphorylation and decreased invasive capacity of androgen stimulated PCa cells (Chuan et al., 2006). Growth factors released into the bone microenvironment, including transforming growth factor β (TGFβ), fibroblast growth factor (FGF), IGF, and platelet derived growth factor (PDGF) stimulate Src-mediated osteoclast activity, leading to further bone destruction and release of biologically active substances from the bone matrix, stimulating the proliferation and migration of tumour cells (Araujo and Logothetis, 2009; Edwards, 2010).

5. PI3K signalling

Several key components of the PI3K/Akt cascade have been implemented in prostate carcinogenesis and castration resistance. PI3K inhibition has been studied *in vitro* for some time and evidence of its key role in carcinogenesis continue to emerge. Genetic analysis of high Gleason grade PCas revealed 3% of patients had PIK3CA mutation and 13% had PIK3CA amplification (Sun et al., 2009). Up regulation of PI3K signalling may also be due to overexpression of receptor tyrosine kinases (RTKs) which have been previously reported to be overexpressed in prostate tumours and cell lines (Grasso et al., 1997; Yeh et al., 1999; Barlett et al., 2005). PI3K has shown to be an important signalling molecule and key survival factor involved in PCa proliferation and invasion. Studies have reported that treatment of LNCaP, PC-3 and DU145 with PI3K pharmacological inhibitor, LY294002, potently suppresses the invasive properties in each of these cell lines and restoration of the PTEN gene to highly invasive prostate cancer PC-3 cells or expression of a dominant negative version of Akt also significantly inhibits invasion and down regulates protein expression of urokinase type plasminogen activator (uPA) and matrix metalloproteinase (MMP)-9, markers for cell invasion. Increased levels of PI3K (p110) and regulatory (p85) and Akt were also observed in these cell lines (Shukla et al., 2007).

A somatic mutation in AKT1 (E17K) has been detected in numerous cancers including prostate (Bleeker et al., 2008; Boorman et al., 2010). The E17K substitution leads to a PI3K independent activation of AKT1. In PCa, AKT1 mutation was reported to have a prevalence of just 1.4% and the mutation seemed to be associated with favourable clinical outcome and was not associated with a specific tumour growth pattern (Boormans et al., 2010). Overexpression of Akt in PCa is hypothesised to be due to defective PTEN gene as discussed below. Prostate tumours are reported to have significantly higher Akt expression than BPH (Liao et al., 2003), and only 10% of well-differentiated prostate tumours strongly express pAkt compared to 92% of poorly differentiated tumours (Malik et al., 2002; Ayala et al., 2004). Additionally, in hormone-naive tumours Akt1 and Akt2 expression has been associated with shorter time to biochemical relapse; and amplification was observed in castrate resistant tumours (Kirkegaard et al., 2010). In addition phosphorylation of Akt increases with the development of castrate resistant disease and is associated with reduced disease specific survival (McCall et al. 2008; Edwards et al., 2006). Loss of PTEN has been associated with advanced prostate cancer (Gray et al., 1998) and loss of PTEN expression is associated with increased risk of recurrence in human tumours (McMennin et al., 1999, McCall et al., 2008).

PCa cell lines that have been cultured from metastatic sites such as the lymph nodes (LNCaP) or brain metastasis (PC3) have highly active PI3K/Akt signalling and PTEN deletion (Davies et al., 1999; Murillo et al., 2001) The magnitude of loss of function of PTEN is best described in both localised and metastatic PCas and includes homozygous deletions, loss of heterozygosity (LOH) and inactivating mutations (Sarker et al., 2009). The reported frequency and mode of inactivation at different stages of PCa varies. Homozygous deletions of PTEN have been detected in up to 15% of locally confined PCa and up to 30% in metastatic cases (Verhagen et al., 2006; Yoshimoto et al., 2007). Heterozygous loss has been reported in 13% of locally confined prostate cancers and up to 39% in metastatic cases (Samuels et al., 2004; Verhagen et al., 2006; Yoshimoto et al., 2007). PTEN mutation has been associated with 5-27% of localised and 30-60% of metastatic prostate tumours (Feiloter et al., 1998; Suzuki et al., 1998) In addition, loss of PTEN expression is associated with disease progression and increased risk of recurrence (Fenci et al., 2002) although substantial heterogeneity has been observed between different metastatic sites within the same patients (Suzuki et al., 1998).

Many oncoproteins and tumor suppressors intersect in the PI3K cascade, regulating cellular functions at the interface of signal transduction and classical metabolic regulation. This careful balance is altered in human cancer by a variety of activating and inactivating mechanisms that target both Akt and interrelated proteins. Numerous studies have suggested that PI3K signalling enhances its oncogenic signal through interaction with other signalling networks such as the transcription factor Nuclear factor Kappa B (NFκB) (Romashkova and Makarov, 1999). Recent reports suggest that suppression of NFκB activity by inhibitory kappa B (IκB) superepressor induces a strong and selective resistance to PI3K or Akt induced oncogenic transformation which suggests an essential role for NFκB in the transforming mechanisms induced by this signalling cascade (Bai et al., 2009).

6. NFκB signalling

NFκB has been shown to be constitutively activated in PCa cells. Evidence on the direct involvement of NFκB in the regulation of angiogenesis and metastasis of PCa cells have already been obtained. Suppression of NFκB activity in human PCa cells by inhibitory kappa B alpha (IκBα) mutation transfection inhibits their tumorigenic and metastatic properties in nude mice by suppressing angiogenesis and invasion. In the same experiments, IκBαM transfection-blocked NFκB activity was associated with downregulation of several angiogenic genes such as vascular endothelial growth factor (VEGF), interleukin 8 (IL-8) and matrix metalloprotease-9 (MMP-9) in cultured cells and in cells implanted into the prostate gland of nude mice. The decreased expression of VEGF, IL-8 and MMP-9 *in vivo* directly correlated with decreased neovascularization and production of lymph node metastasis. In addition, direct clinical correlations of the expression levels the angiogenic genes, including VEGF, basic fibroblast growth factor (Bfgf), IL-8 and MMP-2 and MMP-9 with the metastatic potential of PCa cells has already been established (Huang et al., 2002;Andela et al., 2003).

The association between steroid hormone receptor expression and NFκB activation has been of substantial interest in prostate cancer. Prominent constitutive NFκB has been observed in the prostate cancer cell lines PC-3 and DU-145 which lack AR expression however, only very low levels of NFκB were seen in the AR positive cell line LNCaP (Suh et al., 2002). Moreover, a markedly higher NFκB activity in an androgen independent prostate cancer xenograft model than in its androgen dependent counterpart (Chen et al., 2002). Here NFκB activated expression of AR regulated gene PSA. This data may suggest that either the presence of AR actually inhibits NFκB activity in prostate cancer or alternatively that constitutive activation of NFκB may correlate with AR loss, which in turn may contribute to compensatory cellular changes, allowing cell survival and growth in the absence of AR activation.

NFκB has been implicated with PCa progression via two mechanisms, promotion of metastases via MMP-9 expression or promotion of androgen independence via an as yet unknown mechanism. It was suggested that the absence of PTEN might contribute to constitutive activation of NFκB induced by PI3K/Akt pathway. However no direct correlation has been observed in prostate cancer cell lines.

7. Bcl-2 signalling

Bcl-2 family plays a central role in the mitochondrial pathway of apoptosis by regulation of the integrity of the outer membranes of mitochondria. Members of this family have different role in apoptosis; Bcl-2, Bcl-xL, Bcl-w, A1, and Mcl-1 members are considered as anti-apoptotic molecules while Bax, Bak, and Bok have pro-apoptotic functions and Bad, Bim, Bid, Puma, and Noxa control the activation of pro-apoptotic proteins.

In PCa, Bcl-2 expression is correlated with a higher Gleason score and pT category and is lower in localized PCa compared with HRPC change to CRPC (McDonnell et al., 1992; Apakama et al., 1992; Bubendorf et al., 1996). It has been reported that high expression of Bcl-2 may enable the PCa cells to survive in an androgen-deprived environment, and to confer resistance to anti-androgen therapy (McDonnell et al., 1992). On the other hand, Bak and Bax expression is significantly higher in localized PCa than in HRPC. In addition, decreased Bax expression is associated with an increased pre-operative PSA level in localized PCa and early disease progression in HRPC (Yoshino et al., 2006). These findings suggest that differential regulation of anti-apoptotic Bcl-2 protein and pro-apoptotic proteins may be involved with the processes controlling the development of HRPC as well as disease progression in PCa (Yoshino et al., 2006). *In vitro*, Bax and Bcl-X overexpression resulted in apoptotic cell death in PCa cells such as PC3 and DU145, which are known to offer resistance to a variety of chemical proapoptotic agents as well as LNCaP cells (Marcelli et al., 2000; Li et al., 2001; Castilla et al., 2006). Bcl-X expression is observed in all tumours and was generally stronger in high grade primary tumors (grade 8 to 10) and metastases compared with PIN and low grade neoplasms (P < 0.0001) (Krajewska M et al., 1996; Castilla et al., 2006). On the other hand, a recent study in a 58 patient cohort of PCa patients aith matched tissue from androgen-dependent to CRPC tumours, showed that there was a trend with improved overall survival in patients with increased Bad expression at diagnosis.

In addition, there were trends towards a decrease in Bad and Bax expression with disease progression (Teo et al., 2007). These results might signify that Bad expression may represent a possible positive prognostic marker and useful therapeutic target in HRPC management in the future.

8. IL-6R/STAT3

The IL-6R/gp130/JAK/STAT3 pathway is also implicated in the development of PCa. It is known that circulating levels of IL-6 in sera of patients with CRPC are elevated in comparison to hormone naive patients (Hobisch et al., 1998; Drachenberg et al., 1999). The initial hypothesis of cross-talk between IL-6 and the AR, by measuring the effects of IL-6 on AR transcriptional activity, was investigated in two cell lines, DU-145 which transiently expresses the AR and LNCaP which contains a promiscuous mutated AR. In both cell lines IL-6 activated the AR in a ligand-independent and synergistic manner with low concentrations of a synthetic androgen (methyltrienolone) (Hobisch et al., 1998). Later, Yang et al (2003) was to demonstrate that IL-6, enhanced AR transactivation via IL-6R/STAT3 pathway. Lee et al (2004) observed that androgen sensitive LNCaP cells in the presence of IL-6 were protected from apoptosis when deprived of androgen. However, the anti-apoptotic activity of IL-6 was prevented by the expression of a dominant-negative STAT3 mutant, STAT3F. Furthermore, androgen deprivation induced LNCaP cell death which was antagonized by ectopic expression of a constitutively active STAT3 (Lee et al., 2004). DeMiguel et al (2002) has demonstrated that constitutive activation of STAT3 is associated with increased cell growth and prolonged survival in androgen sensitive LNCaP cells. The study was extended to involve *in vivo* work using both intact and castrated nude male mice. Activation of STAT3 resulted in an increase in tumour growth in both groups of mice. This study shows that STAT3 can enhance the growth of hormone sensitive tumour even in low circulating androgen conditions *in vivo*. More *in vivo* work demonstrated that constitutive activation of STAT3 was found in 82% of human prostate tumours as compared with matched adjacent non-tumour prostate tissue in radical prostatectomy samples (Edwards et al., 2005). Furthermore higher levels of STAT3 activation correlated with a more aggressive tumour or a higher Gleason score. In addition to this, three prostate cancer cell lines, DU145, PC3 and LNCaP cells were examined all of which displayed constitutive activation of STAT3, though substantially lower levels of STAT3 activation was observed in hormone sensitive LNCaP cells. This further supports the fact that STAT3 activation is involved in the progression of prostate cancer. The fact that activated STAT3 is found in tumour and not around its normal margins of prostatectomy samples was further supported by Barton et al (2004). In addition they also showed that directly inhibiting STAT3 either using antisense STAT3 oligonucleotides or by transfecting cells with a dominant negative (DN) STAT3 plasmid, resulted in apoptosis. Cell lines used were NRP-154 and DU145 and apoptosis was seen in both lines when inhibition of STAT3 was performed. From these data the authors conclude that STAT3 specific inhibitors could be used in treating CRPC. Similar conclusions were drawn by (Tam et al, 2007) who reported that cytoplasmic pSTAT3[Tyr 705] expression is associated with time to death from hormone relapse and disease specific survival of the prostate cancer patients that develop castrate resistant disease.

9. Mitogen activated protein (MAP) kinase pathway

Alterations to members of the Raf/MAP kinase pathway have been linked with the progression of several solid tumours including prostate cancer (Weinstein-Oppenheimer et al., 2000). Most solid tumours demonstrate a link between Ras mutation and MAP Kinase activation (Edwards et al., 2004). Mutated Ras has been linked with increased levels of activated MAP Kinase and the development of androgen-independent growth in LNCaP cells (Bakin et al., 2003; Edwards et al., 2004). Activated MAP Kinase and MEK are also differentially expressed during the progression of prostate cancer in a transgenic mouse model (Uzgare et al., 2003-as referenced in Edwards et al., 2004). Raf and MEK are known to be expressed in both non-metastatic and metastatic prostate cancer cells (Weinstein-Oppenheimer et al., 2000; Fu et al., 2003). Increased MAP Kinase activity is known to be elevated in androgen insensitive cell-lines and in clinical CRPC (Abreu-Martin et al., 1999; Gioeli et al., 1999). Recently increasing levels of Raf-1 and/or MAPK correlated with a more rapid biochemical relapse and rapid decline into CRPC, thus negatively impacting on survival time (Mukherjee et al., 2011). Intriguingly, the constitutively active form of MAP Kinase also induces Raf-1 activation in cell-line studies, forming the positive feedback loop required for chronic autocrine stimulation (Allessandrini et al., 1997; Weinstein-Oppenheimer et al., 2000). MAP Kinase has also been demonstrated to increase transcription of androgen-dependent genes, independently of androgens, via either direct or indirect phosphorylation of the AR (Abreu-Martin et al., 1999; Bakin et al., 2003; Franco et al., 2003). MAP Kinase is known to activate the AR N terminal domain (NTD) by phosphorylation of the serine 515 site independently of androgen (Yeh et al. 1999; Rochette-Egly, 2003). Inhibition of MAP Kinase in cell-line studies is known to abrogate IL-6 and PKA activation of the AR, suggesting a crucial role in the convergence of both pathways towards the AR NTD (Ueda et al., 2002). Hydroxyflutamide has been shown to activate the Raf/MAP Kinase pathway independently stimulating cell proliferation, possibly via a member of the EGFR receptor family (Lee et al., 2002). Activation of the pathway has therefore been linked with the pathogenesis of the androgen-withdrawal syndrome, by stimulating androgen-independent cell growth in response to antiandrogens. Data has also revealed increased activation of the MAP Kinase pathway in prostate cancer in patients with tumour progression (Gioeli et al., 1999; Lee et al. 2002). Taken together, the MAP Kinase pathway appears to play a crucial role in cross-talking with the AR-signalling pathway, modulating its response to ligands. It may also function as a surrogate for ligand-activation during androgen withdrawal, resulting in the progression to CRPC.

10. Human epidermal growth factor receptor (her) signalling

The Human Epidermal Growth Factor Receptor (HER) family consists of 4 transmembrane glycoprotein receptor molecules and their variants; Epidermal Growth Factor Receptor (EGFR also known as HER1 and ErbB1), HER2 (ErbB2), HER3 (ErbB3) and HER4 (ErbB4). The HER family members are all differentially expressed in malignant compared to benign prostatic tissue. Great variability of EGFR has been reported amongst studies, with 17-100% detactable levels observed (Di Lorenzo et al., 2002) which has been attributed mainly in PCa disease heterogeneity amongst tissue specimens and variation in IHC technique procedures (Hernes et al., 2004). EGFR overexpression both at the protein and transcript level has been reported in metastatic PCa in numerous studies (Kumar et al., 1996, Kim et al., 1999). Furthermore, the expression of EGFR variant EGFRvII has only been detected in PCa cells and not in benign prostate tissue. In addition EGFRvII expression is greater in CRPC samples compared to hormone naive tissue (Olepade and Oleopa, 2001). Contradictory is also the expression of HER2 in studies in patient tissue; some studies have noted greater expression of HER2 in PCa than benign tissue (Hernes et al., 2004; Okegawa et al., 2006) while others demonstrated no significant difference between the two states (Mellon et al., 1992). In general, HER2 expression in PCa is lower than other tumor types (Edwards, 2003). Furthermore, HER2 gene amplification is not a feature of the transition of hormone naive PCa to CRPC (Bartlett et al., 2005). HER3 is consistently expressed in PCa tissue, however, only nuclear expression and not cytoplasmic is significantly different from benign tissue (Koumakpayi et al., 2006). On the other hand, HER4 is expressed at low levels in PCa tissue and its expression in CRPC samples may offer up to 2 years survival (Hernes et al., 2004). This is contradictory to HER1-3 expression which is associated with worse prognosis. Heregulins are highly expressed in benign prostate tissue compared to malignant (prostatectomy derived PCa) (Lyne et al., 1998). This may indicate that HRGs may act as tumor suppressors and its loss might signify an early stage in PCa oncogenesis.

HER role in prostate carcinogenesis relies in cross-talk interactions with other pathways. EGFR member can cross-talk with the signalling pathways of P13K/Akt, MAP kinase and PKC to increase growth, modulate cell cycle progression, cell motility and angiogenesis of CaP oncogenesis (Mimeault et al., 2003). Overexpression of the EGFR-HER2 heterodimer in comparison to other HER dimers is considered an alternative mechanism of HER-induced carcinogenesis (Xia et al., 1999). EGFR activity has been implicated in hormone escape. EGFR signalling has been shown to activate AR in the absence of adrogenic stimulation (Mimeault, 2003). Cross-talk between HER2 and AR pathways is also apparent (Mellinghoff et al., 2004; Yeh et al., 1999). HER2 and HER3 expression, stimulated by HRG, have also been shown to increase AR transactivation and tumour proliferation in a recurrent CaP cell line in the absence of androgen (Gregory et al., 2005). Overexpression of HER2 has been shown to be induced by low androgen environments *in vitro* and *in vivo* (Berger et al., 2006). Androgen independent AR transactivation can be induced by spontaneous HER2 homodimerisation in the presence of extreme overexpression of HER2 (Wen et al., 2000). *In vitro*, the Q646C constitutively active HER4 mutant inhibits formation of colonies in DU-145 and PC-3 CaP cell lines suggesting that the HER4 signalling is coupled to PCa cell growth arrest and tumor suppression (Williams et al., 2003).

11. Fibroblast growth factor (FGF) receptor signalling

FGF functions are mediated through high ligand-specific affinity receptor signalling. FGF receptor overexpression has been evident in malignant PCa biopsies of patients. In particular, FGFR1 and FGFR4 receptor expression at protein and transcript level are significantly upregulated compared to benign prostates (Sahadevan et al., 2007). Furthermore, FGFR1 is involved in PCa initiation (Acevedo et al., 2007) and promotes tumour progression (Feng et al. 1997). Transgenic models that express constitutively active FGFR-1 in the prostate epithelium develop hyperplasia and PIN (Wang et al. 2002, 2004a) and increased expression accelerates the appearance of this phenotype (Jin et al. 2003; Kwabi-Addo et al., 2004). The role of FGFR2 in prostate cancer is dependent on the expression of its specific isoform (Kwabi-Addo et al., 2001). More specifically, increased expression of FGFR2IIIc isoform and not of FGFR2IIIb was observed in only in a subset of PCa tissue compared to normal epithelial cells. No significant change in the levels of FGFR3 expression and cellular localisation is observed in both benign prostatic hyperplasia (BPH) and PCa tissue (Gowardhan et al., 2005). Increased FGFR4 expression and the germline FGFR4 Gly388Arg polymorphism is associated with adverse survival of patients with PCa (Wang et al. 2004; Gowardhan et al., 2005; Murphy et al., 2010). Moreover, the presence of the FGFR4 GlyArg388 polymorphism is correlated with the occurrence of pelvic lymph node metastasis and PSA recurrence in men undergoing radical prostatectomy. Expression of the FGFR-4 Arg388 in immortalized PCa epithelial cells results in increased cell motility and invasion and upregulation of the urokinase-type plasminogen activator receptor (uPAR), which is known to promote invasion and metastasis (Sidenius & Blasi, 2003; Kwabi-Addo et al., 2004).

In PCa, upregulation of some ligands of the FGF system has also been reported; FGF1, FGF2, FGF6, FGF8, FGF10 and FGF17 mainly used as autocrine or paracrine factors for PCa cells (Heer et al., 2004; Kwabi et al., 2004). FGF1 is known to be expressed in more than 80% of PCa (Dorkins et al., 1999) and be increased in PIN. FGF1 was shown to induce the expression of matrix metalloproteinase MT1-MMP which is also overexpressed in PIN and invasive cancers and might provide a link to the role of FGF1 in the progression of PCa (Udayakumar et al., 2004). FGF2 expression is altered during the progression of PCa; evidence shows that paracrine stromal expression can be observed during early stages of PCa which eventually switches to autocrine expression by epithelial cells (Dorkin et al., 1999; Girri and Ittmann, 2001). FGF1 and FGF2 regulate angiogenesis. In particular, expression of FGF2 in PCa cells and stromal cells can induce tumour vasculature formation (Powers et al., 2000; Kwabi-Addo et al., 2004). FGF6 is expressed by normal prostatic basal cells in extremely small amounts, and expression in basal cells is markedly increased in PIN lesions. The acquisition of FGF6 expression by the prostate cancers implies but does not prove that it may play a role in cancer cell proliferation or perhaps in other aspects of tumor progression (Ropiquet et al., 2000). The role of FGF7 still remains unclear although it was one of the first factors shown to regulate AR transcription in PCa cells, along with EGF and IGF-I (Culig et al.,1994). Recent evidence support the role of paracrine mesenchymal FGF10 in driving tumourgenesis as enhanced expression of mesenchymal FGF10 was sufficient for histologic transformation of the adjacent prostate epithelium in CB.17$^{SCID/SCID}$ mice (Memarzadeh et al., 2007). FGFs play an important role in all stages of bone formation. Thus, it is not surprising that some FGF members have been linked with bone metastasis of PCa. FGF8 secreted by cancer cells regulates osteoblast differentiation by enhancing osteoprogenitor cell proliferation and their osteogenic capacity (Valta et al., 2006). Moreover, FGF8 in particular is expressed highly in PCa bone metastasis and was recently shown to increase the growth of intratibial PC3 tumors in nude mice used as an experimental model for PCa bone metastasis (Valta et al., 2008). FGF8 can also induce FGF17 expression which has also been associated with bone metastasis (Heer et al., 2004).

12. Insulin growth factor receptor (igfr) signalling

The insulin-like growth factor (IGF) system, is composed of the receptors IGFR-IR, IGFR-IIR, insulin receptor (IR), numerous atypical receptors, two ligands (IGF-I and IGF-II), and six binding proteins (IGFBP-1 to -6) (Nakae et al., 2001). Involvement of the IGF system in the progression of hormone naïve PCa to CRPC and metastasis of PCa tumour has had a long standing role, and along with androgens and EGF, IGFs represent another important class of mitogens in PCa. Early *in vitro* work has shown that treatment with IGF-I and IGF-II can increase the proliferation of PCa DU145 cells (Connolly and Rose, 1994). However, in LNCaP cells, IGF-I alone was unable to increase cell growth in growth factor free conditions, revealing the need of IGF signalling for co-operation with other factors in order to promote tumour cell growth (Ngo et al., 2003). Although most of the members of the IGF system are expressed in PCa patients the results from numerous studies are fairly contradictory. Studies on the IGF-I serum levels and PCa risk have shown mixed results with some studies showing a positive correlation while others showing no or inverse correlation. Furthermore similar associations were produced for IGFBP3 and PCa. A large study from the Cancer Research UK Epidemiology Unit in 2007 examining 630 specimens from PCa patients at diagnosis and 630 matched control samples, did not identify a strong correlation between serum IGF-I neither IGFBP3 and PCa risk and only a small increase in risk was noted for advanced stage disease.

Significant interactions of IGF-I have been reported with AR, depicting a significant involvement of this pathway in CRPC. *In vitro* experiments in M12AR cells showed that IGF-I enhances nuclear translocation of AR in the absence of any androgenic signal and this effect can be inversed by an IGF-IR inhibitory antibody (Wu et al., 2006). *In vitro* studies have demonstrated that IGF-1R downstream signalling via MAPK pathway may promote proliferation of prostate cancer cells whereas involvement of PI3K-AKT pathway is required to inhibit apoptosis (Genningens et al., 2006).

IGF-I plays an important role in PCa bone metastasis. IGF-I can cross-talk with the NFκB pathway by direct upregulation of RANK ligand and osteoblasts and binding to RANK. Activation of NFκB leads to osteoclast synthesis and osteoprotegerin (OPG) thus driving bone formation and resorption (Fizzazi et al., 2003).

13. Conclusion

The signalling pathways involved in the initiation and progression of PCa are complex and require further investigation. However in this chapter we have attempted to elucidate which receptors (HER, FGFR and IGFR) and intracellular signalling pathways play major roles in prostate cancer. In addtion, we also demonstrate that the AR has a central role to play in both hormone naïve and castrate resistant disease, and it is only by unravelling the interactions between cell surface receptors, intracellular signalling and steroid receptors that we are going to move forward with a targeted personalised approach to treatment of PCa.

14. References

Abreu-Martin, M.T., Chari, A., Palladino, A.A., et al. (1999) Mitogen-activated protein kinase kinase kinase 1 activates androgen receptor-dependent transcription and apoptosis in prostate cancer. *Mol Cell Biol*, Vol.19, pp. 5143– 5154.

Acevedo, V.D., Gangula, R.D., Freeman, K.W., et al. (2007) Inducible FGFR-1 activation leads to irreversible prostate adenocarcinoma and an epithelial-to-mesenchymal transition. *Cancer Cell*, Vol.12, pp.559–571.

Alessandrini, A., Chiaur, D.S., Pagano, M. (1997) Regulation of the cyclindependent kinase inhibitor p27 by degradation and phosphorylation. *Leukemia*, Vol.11, pp.342 – 345.

Andela, V.B., Gordon, A.H., Zotalis, G., et al. (2003) NF kappa B: A pivotal transcription factor in prostate cancer metastasis to bone. *Clinical Orthopaedics and Related Research*, Vol.415, pp.S75-S85.

Apakama, I., Robinson, M.C., Walter, N.M., et al. (1996) Bcl-2 overexpression combined with p53 protein accumulation correlates with hormone-refractory prostate cancer. *Br J Cancer*, Vol.74, pp.1258–62.

Araujo, J., Logothetis, C. (2009) Targeting Src signaling in metastatic bone disease. *Int J Cancer*, Vol.124, pp.1-6.

Ayala, G., Thompson, T., Yang, G., et al. (2004) High Levels of Phosphorylated Form of Akt-1 in Prostate Cancer and Non-Neoplastic 208 Prostate Tissues Are Strong Predictors of Biochemical Recurrence. *Clin Cancer Res*, Vol. 10, pp. 6572-6578.

Bai, D., Ueno, L., Vogt, P.K. (2009) Akt-mediated regulation of NFkappaB and the essentialness of NFkappaB for the oncogenicity of PI3K and Akt. *Int J Cancer*, Vol. 125, pp.2863-2870.

Bakin, R.E., Gioeli, D., Sikes, R.A., et al. (2003) Constitutive activation of the Ras/mitogen-activated protein kinase signaling pathway promotes androgen hypersensitivity in LNCaP prostate cancer cells. *Cancer Res*, Vol.63, pp.1981– 1989.

Bartlett, J.M., Brawley, D., Grigor, K., et al. (2005) Type I receptor tyrosine kinases are associated with hormone escape in prostate cancer. *J Pathol*, Vol. 205, pp.522-529.

Barton BE, Karras JG, Murphy TF, et al. (2004) Signal transducer and activator of transcription 3 (STAT3) activation in prostate cancer: direct STAT3 inhibition induces apoptosis in prostate cancer lines. Mol Cancer Ther 3: 11 - 20

Bleeker, F.E., Felicioni, L., Buttitta, F., et al. (2008) AKT1(E17K) in human solid tumours. Oncogene 2008.

Boormans JL, Korsten H, Ziel-van der Made AC, et al. (2010) E17K substitution in AKT1 in prostate cancer. BrJ Cancer, Vol. 102, pp.1491-1494.

Bruey, J.M., Paul, C., Fromentin, A., et al. (2000) Differential regulation of HSP27 oligomerization in tumor cells grown in vitro and in vivo. Oncogene, Vol. 19, pp. 4855–4863.

Bubendorf, L., Sauter, G., Moch, H., et al. (1996) Prognostic significance of Bcl-2 in clinically localized prostate cancer. Am J Pathol, Vol.148, pp.1557–1565.

Castilla, C., Congregado, B., Chinchón, D., et al. (2006) Bcl-xL is overexpressed in hormone-resistant prostate cancer and promotes survival of LNCaP cells via interaction with proapoptotic Bak. Endocrinology, Vol.147, pp.4960-7.

Chen, Y., Sawyers, C.L., Sche,r H.I. (2008) Targeting the androgen receptor pathway in prostate cancer. Curr Opin Pharmacol, Vol. 8, pp. 440-448.

Chen, C.D., Sawyers, C.L.(2002) NF-kappa B activates prostate-specific antigen expression and is upregulated in androgen-independent prostate cancer. Mol Cell Biol, Vol.22, pp. 2862-2870.

Chuan, Y.C., Pang, S.T., Cedazo-Minguez, A, et al. (2006) Androgen induction of prostate cancer cell invasion is mediated by ezrin. J Biol Chem, Vol.281, pp.29938-29948.

Concannon, C.G, Orrenius, S., Samali, A. (2000) Hsp27 inhibits cytochrome c-mediated caspase activation by sequestering both pro-caspase-3 and cytochrome c. Gene Expr, Vol. 9, pp.195–201.

Connolly JM, Rose DP. (1994) Regulation of DU145 human prostate cancer cell proliferation by insulin-like growth factors and its interaction with the epidermal growth factor autocrine loop. Prostate, Vol.24, pp.167-175.

Culig, Z., Hobisch, A., Cronauer, M.V. (1994) Androgen receptor activation in prostatic tumor cell lines by insulin-like growth factor-I, keratinocyte growth factor, and epidermal growth factor. Cancer Res, Vol. 54, pp. 5474-5478.

Curto, M., McClatchey, A.I. (2004) Ezrin...a metastatic detERMinant? Cancer Cell, Vol. 5, pp. 113-114.

Davies, M.A., Koul, D., Dhesi, H., et al. (1999) Regulation of Akt/PKB activity, cellular growth, and apoptosis in prostate carcinoma cells by MMAC/PTEN. Cancer Res, Vol.59, pp.2551-2556.

Dehm, S.M., Tindall, D.J.(2006) Molecular regulation of androgen action in prostate cancer. J Cell Biochem, Vol.99, pp.333-44.

Dehm, S.M., Schmidt, L.J., Heemers, H.V. (2008) Splicing of a novel androgen receptor exon generates a constitutively active androgen receptor that mediates prostate cancer therapy resistance. Cancer Res, Vol. 68, pp. 5469-5477.

DeMiguel, F., Lee, S.O., Lou, W., et al. (2002) Stat3 enhances the growth of LNCaP human prostate cancer cells in intact and castrated male nude mice. Prostate, Vol.52, pp.123-129.

DeVere White, R.W., Vinall, R.L., Tepper, C.G., et al. (2009) MicroRNAs and their potential for translation in prostate cancer. *Urol Oncol*, Vol.27, pp.307-311.

Di Lorenzo, G., Tortora, G., D'Armiento, F.P. (2002) Expression of epidermal growth factor receptor correlates with disease relapse and progression to androgen-independence in human prostate cancer. *Clin Cancer Res*, Vol. 8, pp. 3438-3444.

Dorkin, T.J., Robinson, M.C., Marsh, C., et al. (1999) aFGF immunoreactivity in prostate cancer and its colocalization with bFGF and FGF8. *Journal of Pathology*, Vol.189, pp. 564-569.

Drachenberg, D.E., Elgamal, A.A., Rowbotham, R., et al. (1999) Circulating levels of interleukin-6 in patients with hormone refractory prostate cancer. *Prostate*, Vol.41, pp.127 - 133.

Edwards, J. (2010) Src kinase inhibitors: an emerging therapeutic treatment option for prostate cancer. Expert *Opin Investig Drugs*, Vol.19, pp.605-614.

Edwards, J., Traynor, P., Munro, A.., et al. (2006) The role of HER1-HER4 and EGFRvIII in hormone-refractory prostate cancer. *Clin.Cancer Res*, Vol.12, pp.123-130.

Edwards, J. and Bartlett, J.M.S. (2005) The androgen receptor and signal-transduction pathways in hormone-refractory prostate cancer. Part 2: Androgen-receptor cofactors and bypass pathways. *BJU Int*, Vol.95, pp.1327-1335.

Edwards, J., Krishna, N.S., Mukherjee, R., et al. (2004) The role of c-Jun and c-Fos expression in androgen-independent prostate cancer. J Pathol, Vol.204, pp.153 - 158.

Edwards, J., Krishna, N.S., Grigor, K.M., et al. (2003) Androgen receptor gene amplification and protein expression in hormone refractory prostate cancer. *Br.J Cancer*, Vol.89, pp.552-556.

Feilotter, H.E., Nagai, M.A., Boag, A.H., et al. (1998) Analysis of PTEN and the 10q23 region in primary prostate carcinomas. *Oncogene*, Vol. 16, pp.1743-1748.

Fenci, I., Woenckhaus, J. (2002) The tumour suppressor PTEN and the cell cycle inhibitor p27(KIP1) in prostate carcinoma and prostatic intraepithelial neoplasia (PIN) - An immunohistochemical study. *British Journal of Cancer*, Vol. 86, pp.S79-S80.

Fizazi, K., Yang, J., Peleg, S. et al. (2003) Prostate cancer cells-osteoblast interaction shifts expression of growth/survival-related genes in prostate cancer and reduces expression of osteoprotegerin in osteoblasts. *Clin.Cancer Res*, Vol. 9, pp.2587-2597.

Franco, O.E., Onishi, T., Yamakawa, K., et al. (2003) Mitogen-activated protein kinase pathway is involved in androgen-independent PSA gene expression in LNCaP cells. *Prostate*, Vol.56, pp.319 - 325.

Gao, S., Lee, P., Wang, et al. (2005) The Androgen Receptor Directly Targets the Cellular Fas/FasL-Associated Death Domain Protein-Like Inhibitory Protein Gene to Promote the Androgen-Independent Growth of Prostate Cancer Cells. *Mol Endocrinol*, 19, pp.1792-1802.

Garrido, C., Schmitt, E., Cande, C., et al. (2003) HSP27 and HSP70: potentially oncogenic apoptosis inhibitors. Cell Cycle, Vol.2, pp.579-584.

Gennigens, C., Menetrier-Caux, C., Droz, J.P. (2006) Insulin-Like Growth Factor (IGF) family and prostate cancer. *Crit Rev Oncol Hematol*, Vol.58, pp.124-145.

Gibbons, N.B., Watson, R.W., Coffey, R.N., et al. (2000) Heat-shock proteins inhibit induction of prostate cancer cell apoptosis.*Prostate*, Vol.45, pp.58-65.

Gioeli, D., Mandell, J.W., Petroni, G.R., et al. (1999) Activation of mitogen-activated protein kinase associated with prostate cancer progression. *Cancer Res*, Vol.59, pp.279 – 284.

Giri, D. & Ittmann, M. (2001) Interleukin-8 is a paracrine inducer of fibroblast growth factor 2, a stromal and epithelial growth factor in benign prostatic hyperplasia. Am J Pathol, Vol.159, pp. 139–147.

Gowardhan, B., Douglas, D.A.,Mathers, M.E., et al. Evaluation of the fibroblast growth factor system as a potential target for therapy in human prostate cancer. Br J Cancer 2005;92:320-327.

Grasso, A.W., Wen, D., Miller, C.M., et al. (1997) ErbB kinases and NDF signaling in human prostate cancer cells. *Oncogene*, Vol.15, pp.2705-2716.

Gray, I.C., Stewart, L.M., Phillips, et al. (1998) Mutation and expression analysis of the putative prostate tumoursuppressor gene PTEN. *Br J Cancer*, Vol.78, pp.300.

Guo, Z., Dai, B., Jiang, T., et al. (2006) Regulation of androgen receptor activity by tyrosine phosphorylation. *Cancer Cell*, Vol.10, pp.309-319.

Guo, Z., Yang, X., Sun, F. (2009)A novel androgen receptor splice variant is up-regulated during prostate cancer progression and promotes androgen depletion-resistant growth. *Cancer Res*, Vol. 69, pp. 2305-13.

Han, G., Buchanan, G., Ittmann, M. (2005) Mutation of the androgen receptor causes oncogenic transformation of the prostate. *Proc Natl Acad Sci U S A*, Vol. 25, pp. 1151-6.

Heer, R., Douglas, D., Mathers, M.E., et al. (2004) Fibroblast growth factor 17 is over-expressed in human prostate cancer. *J Pathol*, Vol.204, pp.578–586.

Hitosugi, T., Sasaki, K., Sato, M., et al. (2007) Epidermal growth factor directs sex-specific steroid signaling through Src activation. *J Biol Chem*, Vol.282, pp.10697-10706.

Hernes, E., Fosså, S.D., Berner, A. (2004) Expression of the epidermal growth factor receptor family in prostate carcinoma before and during androgen-independence. *Br J Cancer*, Vol. 90, pp. 449-454.

Hobisch A, Eder IE, Putz T, et al. (1998) Interleukin-6 regulates prostate-specific protein expression in prostate carcinoma cells by activation of the androgen receptor. *Cancer Res*, Vol.58, pp.4640– 4645.

Hu, R., Dunn, T.A., Wei, S. (2009) Ligand-independent androgen receptor variants derived from splicing of cryptic exons signify hormone-refractory prostate cancer. *Cancer Res*, Vol. 69, pp.16-22.

Huang, S.Y., Pettaway, C.A., Uehara, H., et al. (2001) Blockade of NFkappa B activity in human prostate cancer cells is associated with suppression of angiogenesis, invasion, and metastasis. *Oncogene*, Vol.20, pp.4188-4197.

Huggins, C. & Hodges, C.V. (1971) Studies on prostatic cancer: I. The effect of castration, of estrogen and of androgen injection on serum phosphatases in metastatic carcinoma of the prostate. *Cancer Research*, Vol.1, pp.293-297.

Jagla, M., Fève, M., Kessler, P. (2007) A splicing variant of the androgen receptor detected in a metastatic prostate cancer exhibits exclusively cytoplasmic actions.*Endocrinology*, Vol. 148, pp. 4334-4343.

Jasavala, R., Martinez, H., Thumar, J., et al. (2007) Identification of putative androgen receptor interaction protein modules: cytoskeleton and endosomes modulate androgen receptor signaling in prostate cancer cells. *Mol Cell Proteomics*. Vol.6, pp.252-271.

Kim, H.G., Kassis, J., Souto, J.C. (1999) EGF receptor signaling in prostate morphogenesis and tumorigenesis. *Histol Histopathol*, Vol. 14, pp. 1175-82.

Koumakpayi, I.H., Diallo, J.S., Le Page, C. (2006)Expression and nuclear localization of ErbB3 in prostate cancer. *Clin Cancer Res*, Vol. 12, pp.2730-2737.

Kirkegaard, T., Witton, C.J., Edwards, J., et al. (2010) Molecular alterations in AKT1, AKT2 and AKT3 detected in breast and prostate cancer by FISH. *Histopathology*, Vol., pp.

Krajewska, M., Krajewski, S., Epstein, J.I., et al. (1996) Immunohistochemical analysis of bcl-2, bax, bcl-X, and mcl-1 expression in prostate cancers. *Am J Pathol*, Vol.148, pp.1567–1576.

Kumar, A., Goel, A.S., Hill, T.M. (1996) Expression of human glandular kallikrein, hK2, in mammalian cells. *Cancer Res*, Vol. 56, pp. 5397-5402.

Kurahashi, T., Miyake, H., Hara, I., et al. (2001) Expression of major heat shock proteins in prostate cancer: correlation with clinicopathological outcomes in patients undergoing radical prostatectomy. *J Urol*, Vol. 177, pp.757-761.

Kwabi-Addo, B., Ropiquet, F., Giri, D., et al. (2001) Alternative splicing of fibroblast growth factor receptors in human prostate cancer. *Prostate*, Vol.46, pp.163-172.

Kwabi-Addo, B., Ozen, M., Ittmann, M. (2004) The role of fibroblast growth factors and their receptors in prostate cancer. *Endocr Relat Cancer*, Vol.11, pp.709–24.

Lammont, K.R., Tindall, D.J. (2010) Androgen regulation of gene expression *Adv Cancer Res*, Vol. 107, pp.137-162.

Lee, L.F., Guan, J., Qiu, Y., et al. (2001) Neuropeptide-induced androgen independence in prostate cancer cells: roles of nonreceptor tyrosine kinases Etk/Bmx, Src, and focal adhesion kinase. *Mol Cell Biol*, Vol.21, pp.8385-8397.

Lee, L.F., Louie, M.C., Desai, S.J., et al. (2004) Interleukin-8 confers androgen-independent growth and migration of LNCaP: differential effects of tyrosine kinases Src and FAK. *Oncogene*, Vol.23, pp.2197-2205.

Lee, S.O., Lou, W., Johnson, C.S., et al. (2004) Interleukin-6 protects LNCaP cells from apoptosis induced by androgen deprivation through the Stat3 pathway. *Prostate*, Vol.60, pp.178 – 186.

Le Page, C., Koumakpayi, I.H., Alam-Fahmy, M., et al. (2006) Expression and localisation of Akt-1, Akt-2 and Akt-3 correlate with clinical outcome of prostate cancer patients. *Br J Cancer*, Vol.94, pp. 1906-1912.

Leon, C.G., Locke, J.A., Adomat, H.H., et al. (2010) Alterations in cholesterol regulation contribute to the production of intratumoral androgens during progression to castration-resistant prostate cancer in a mouse xenograft model. *Prostate*, Vol.70, pp.390-400.

Li, X., Marani, M., Mannucci, R., et al. (2001) Overexpression of BCL-XL underlies the molecular basis for resistance to staurosporine-induced apoptosis in PC-3 cells. *Cancer Res*, Vol.61, pp.1699–1706.

Liao, Y., Grobholz, R., Abel, U., et al. (2003) Increase of AKT/PKB expression correlates with gleason pattern in human prostate cancer. *Int J Cancer*, Vol.107, pp.676-680.

Lin, B., Wang, J., Hong, X., et al. (2009) Integrated expression profiling and ChIP-seq analyses of the growth inhibition response program of the androgen receptor. PLoS One, Vol.4, pp.e6589.

Locke, J.A., Wasan, K.M., Nelson, C.C., et al. (2008) Androgenmediated cholesterol metabolismin LNCaPand PC-3 cell lines is regulated through two different isoforms of acyl-coenzyme A:cholesterol acyltransferase (ACAT). Prostate, Vol.68, pp.20–33.

Malik, S.N., Brattain, M., Ghosh, P.M., et al. (2002) Immunohistochemical demonstration of phospho-Akt in high Gleason grade prostate cancer. *Clin Cancer Res*, Vol.8, pp. 1168-1171.

Marcelli, M., Marani, M., Li, X., et al. (2000) Heterogeneous apoptotic responses of prostate cancer cell lines identify an association between sensitivity to staurosporine-induced apoptosis, expression of Bcl-2 family members, and caspase activation. *Prostate*, Vol.42, pp.260–273.

McCall, P., Gemmell, L.K., Mukherjee, R., et al. (2008) Phosphorylation of the Androgen Receptor is associated with reduced survival in hormone refractory prostate cancer patients. *Br J Cancer*, Vol.98, pp.1094-1101.

McCall, P., Witton, C.J., Nielsen, K.V., et al. (2008). Is PTEN loss associated with clinical outcome measures in human prostate cancer? *Br J Cancer*, Vol.99, pp.1296-1301.

McDonnell, T.J., Troncoso, P., Brisbay, S.M., et al. (1992) Expression of the protooncogene bcl-2 in the prostate and its association with emergence of androgen-independent prostate cancer. *Cancer Res*, Vol.52, pp.6940–6944.

McMenamin, M.E., Soung, P., Perera, S., et al. (1999) Loss of PTEN expression in paraffin-embedded primary prostate cancer correlates with high Gleason score and advanced stage. *Cancer Res*, Vol.59, pp. 4291- 4296.

Mellinghoff, I,K,, Vivanco, I,, Kwon, A. (2004) HER2/neu kinase-dependent modulation of androgen receptor function through effects on DNA binding and stability. *Cancer Cell*, Vol. 6, pp.517-527.

Mimeault, M., Pommery, N., Hénichart, J.P. (2003) New advances on prostate carcinogenesis and therapies: involvement of EGF-EGFR transduction system. *Growth Factors*, Vol. 21, pp. 1-14.

Montgomery, J.S., Price, D.K., Figg, W.D. (2001) The androgen receptor gene and its influence on the development and progression of prostate cancer. *J Pathol*, Vol.195, pp.138-46.

Memarzadeh, S., Xin, L., Mulholland, D.J., et al. (2007) Enhanced paracrine FGF10 expression promotes formation of multifocal prostate adenocarcinoma and an increase in epithelial androgen receptor. *Cancer Cell*, Vol.12, pp.572-85.

Migliaccio, A., Castoria, G., Di Domenico, M., et al. (2000) Steroid-induced androgen receptor-oestradiol receptor beta-Src complex triggers prostate cancer cell proliferation. *EMBO J*, Vol.19, pp.5406-5417.

Migliaccio, A., Di Domenico, M., Castoria, G., et al. (2005) Steroid receptor regulation of epidermal growth factor signaling through Src in breast and prostate cancer cells: steroid antagonist action. *Cancer Res*, Vol.65, pp.10585-10593.

Mukherjee, R., McGuinness, D.H., McCall, P. (2011) Upregulation of MAPK pathway is associated with survival in castrate-resistant prostate cancer. *Br J Cancer*, Vol.104, pp.1920 – 1928.

Murillo, H., Huang, H., Schmidt, L.J., et al. (2001) Role of PI3K Signaling in Survival and Progression of LNCaP Prostate Cancer Cells to the Androgen Refractory State. *Endocrinology*, Vol.142, pp.4795-4805.

Nakae, J., Kido, Y., Accili, D. (2001). Distinct and overlapping functions of insulin and IGF-I receptors. *Endocrine Rev*, Vol.22, pp.818–835.

Nam, S., Kim, D., Cheng, J.Q. (2005) Action of the Src family kinase inhibitor, dasatinib (BMS-354825), on human prostate cancer cells. *Cancer Res*, Vol. 65, pp. 9185-9189.

Ngan, S., Stronach, E.A., Photiou, A., et al. (2009) Microarray coupled to quantitative RT-PCR analysis of androgen-regulated genes in human LNCaP prostate cancer cells. *Oncogene*, Vol.28, pp.2051-2063.

Ngo, T.H., Barnard, R.J., Leung, P.S. et al. (2003) Insulin-like growth factor I (IGF-I) and IGF binding protein-1 modulate prostate cancer cell growth and apoptosis: possible mediators for the effects of diet and exercise on cancer cell survival. *Endocrinology*, Vol.144, pp.2319–2324.

Nylandsted, J., Brand, K., Jäättelä, M. (2000) Heat shock protein 70 is required for the survival of cancer cells. *Ann N Y Acad Sci*, Vol.926, pp.122-125.

Okegawa, T., Kinjo, M., Nutahara, K. (2006) Pretreatment serum level of HER2/nue as a prognostic factor in metastatic prostate cancer patients about to undergo endocrine therapy. *Int J Urol*, Vol. 13, pp. 1197-1201.

Pandini, G., Mineo, R., Frasca, F., et al. (2005) Androgens up-regulate the insulin-like growth factor-I receptor in prostate cancer cells. *Cancer Res*, Vol. 65, pp.1849-1857.

Pandini, G., Genua, M., Frasca, F., et al. (2007) 17beta-estradiol up-regulates the insulin-like growth factor receptor through a nongenotropic pathway in prostate cancer cells. *Cancer Res*, Vol.67, pp.8932-8941.

Paul, C., Manero, F., Gonin, S., et al. (2000) Hsp27 as a negative regulator of cytochrome C release. *Mol Cell Biol*, Vol.22, pp. 816–34.

Pienta, K.J., Bradley, D. (2006) Mechanisms underlying the development of androgen-independent prostate cancer. *Clin Cancer Res*, Vol. 15, pp. 1665-71.

Raclaw, K.A., Heemers, H.V., Kidd, E.M., et al. (2008) Induction of FLIP expression by androgens protects prostate cancer cells from TRAIL-mediated apoptosis. *Prostate*, Vol.68, pp.1696-706.

Recchia, I., Rucci, N., Festuccia, C. (2003) Pyrrolopyrimidine c-Src inhibitors reduce growth, adhesion, motility and invasion of prostate cancer cells in vitro. *Eur J Cancer*, Vol. 39, pp. 1927-1935.

Rocchi, P., So, A., Kojima, S., et al. (2004) Heat shock protein 27 increases after androgen ablation and plays a cytoprotective role in hormone-refractory prostate cancer. *Cancer Res*, Vol.64, pp.6595-602.

Rocchi, P., Beraldi, E., Ettinger, S., et al. (2005) Increased Hsp27 after androgen ablation facilitates androgen-independent progression in prostate cancer via signal transducers and activators of transcription 3-mediated suppression of apoptosis. *Cancer Res*, Vol.65, pp.11083-93.

Rochette-Egly, C. (2003) Nuclear receptors: integration of multiple signalling pathways through phosphorylation. *Cell Signal*, Vol.15, pp.355-366.

Romashkova, J.A., Makarov, S.S. (1999) NF-kappaB is a target of AKT in antiapoptotic PDGF signalling. *Nature*, Vol.401, pp.86-90.

Ropiquet, F., Giri, D., Kwabi-Addo, B., et al. (2000) Increased expression of fibroblast growth factor 6 in human prostatic intraepithelial neoplasia and prostate cancer. *Cancer Research*, Vol.60, pp.4245–4250.

Sahadevan, K., Darby, S., Leung, H.Y. (2007) Selective over-expression of fibroblast growth factor receptors 1 and 4 in clinical prostate cancer. *J Pathol*, Vol. 213, pp. 82-90.

Sarker, D., Reid, A.H.M., Yap, T.A., et al. (2009) Targeting the PI3K/AKT Pathway for the Treatment of Prostate Cancer. *Clin Cancer Res*, Vol.15, pp.4799-4805.

Samuels, Y., Wang, Z., Bardelli, A., et al. (2004) High frequency of mutations of the PIK3CA gene in human cancers. *Science* Vol.304, pp.554.

Schayek, H., Seti, H., Greenberg, N.M., et al. (2010) Differential regulation of insulin-like growth factor-I receptor gene expression by wild type and mutant androgen receptor in prostate cancer cells. *Mol Cell Endocrinol*, Vol.323, pp.239-45.

Shiota, M., Yokomizo, A., Naito, S. (2011) J Increased androgen receptor transcription: a cause of castration-resistant prostate cancer and a possible therapeutic target. *Mol Endocrinol*, Apr 19.

Shukla, S., MacLennan, G.T., Hartman, D.J., et al. (2007) Activation of PI3K-Akt signaling pathway promotes prostate cancer cell invasion. Int J Cancer, Vol.121, pp.1424-1432.

Sidenius, N. & Blasi, F. (2003) The urokinase plasminogen activator system in cancer: recent advances and implication for prognosis and therapy. *Cancer Metastasis Reviews*, Vol.22, pp.205–222.

Slack, J.K., Adams, R.B., Rovin, J.D, et al. (2001) Alterations in the focal adhesion kinase/Src signal transduction pathway correlate with increased migratory capacity of prostate carcinoma cells. *Oncogene*, Vol.20, pp.1152–63.

Suh, J., Payvandi, F., Edelstein, L.C., et al. (2002) Mechanisms of constitutive NF-kappaB activation in human prostate cancer cells. *Prostate*, Vol.52, pp.183-200.

Sumitomo, M., Shen, R., Walburg, M., et al. (2000) Neutral endopeptidase inhibits prostate cancer cell migration by blocking focal adhesion kinase signaling. *J Clin Invest*, Vol.106, pp.1399-1407.

Sun, X., Huang, J., Homma, T., et al. (2009) Genetic alterations in the PI3K pathway in prostate cancer. *Anticancer Res*, Vol.29, pp.1739-1743.

Suzuki, H., Freije, D., Nusskern, D.R., et al. (1998) Interfocal heterogeneity of PTEN/MMAC1 gene alterations in multiple metastatic prostate cancer tissues. *Cancer Res*, Vol.58, pp.204-209.

Tam, L., McGlynn, L.M., Traynor, P., et al. (2007) The Role of IL-6R/JAK/STAT3 Pathway in Hormone Refractory Prostate Cancer. *Br J Cancer*, Vol.97, pp.378-383.

Takayama, K., Horie-Inoue, K., Ikeda, K., et al. (2008) FOXP1 is an androgen-responsive transcription factor that negatively regulates androgen receptor signaling in prostate cancer cells. *Chem Biophys Res Commun*, Vol.374, pp.388-93.

Tatarov, O., Mitchell, T.J., Seywright, M. (2009) SRC family kinase activity is up-regulated in hormone-refractory prostate cancer. *Clin Cancer Res*, Vol. 15, pp. 3540-3549.

Tepper, C.G., Boucher, D.L., Ryan, P.E. (2002) Characterization of a novel androgen receptor mutation in a relapsed CWR22 prostate cancer xenograft and cell line. Cancer Res, Vol. 62, pp. 6606-6614.

Teo, K., Gemmell, L., Mukherjee, R. (2007) Bad expression influences time to androgen escape in prostate cancer. *BJU Int*, Vol.100, pp.691-696.

Udayakumar, T.S., Nagle, R.B., Bowden, G.T. (2004) Fibroblast growth factor-1 transcriptionally induces membrane type-1 matrix metalloproteinase expression in prostate carcinoma cell line. *Prostate*, Vol.58, pp.66-75.

Ueda, T., Bruchovsky, N., Sadar, M.D. (2002) Activation of the androgen receptor N-terminal domain by interleukin-6 via MAPK and STAT3 signal transduction pathways. *J Biol Chem*, Vol.277, pp.7076– 7085.

Valta, M.P., Hentunen, T., Qu, Q., et al. (2006) Regulation of osteoblast differentiation: a novel function for fibroblast growth factor 8. *Endocrinology*, Vol. 147, pp. 2171-2182.

Valta, M. P., Tuomela, J., Bjartell, A., et al. (2008) FGF-8 is involved in bone metastasis for prostate cancer. *Int J Cancer*, Vol. 123, pp.22-31.

Veldscholte, J., Berrevoets, C.A., Brinkmann, A.O., et al. (1992) Anti-androgens and the mutated androgen receptor of LNCaP cells: differential effects on binding affinity, heat-shock protein interaction, and transcription activation. *Biochemistry*, Vol.31, pp.2393-2399.

Verhagen, P.C., van Duijn, P.W., Hermans, K.G., et al. (2006) The PTEN gene in locally progressive prostate cancer is preferentially inactivated by bi-allelic gene deletion. *J Pathol*, Vol. 208, pp.699-707.

Wang, J., Stockton, D.W., Ittmann, M. (2004) The fibroblast growth factor receptor-4 Arg388 allele is associated with prostate cancerinitiation and progression. *Clin Cancer Res*, Vol.10, pp.6169–6178.

Wen, Y., Hu, M.C., Makino, K. (2000) HER-2/neu promotes androgen-independent survival and growth of prostate cancer cells through the Akt pathway. *Cancer Res*, Vol. 60, pp. 6841-6845.

Weinstein-Oppenheimer, C.R., Blalock, W.L., Steelman, L.S., et al. (2000) The Raf signal transduction cascade as a target for chemotherapeutic intervention in growth factor-responsive tumors. Pharmacol Ther, Vol. 88, pp.229 – 279.

Wu, J.D., Haugk, K., Woodke, L. et al. (2006) Interaction of IGF signaling and the androgen receptor in prostate cancer progression. *J. Cell Biochem*, Vol.99, pp. 392–401.

Yeh, S., Lin, H.K., Kang, H.Y. (1999) From HER2/Neu signal cascade to androgen receptor and its coactivators: a novel pathway by induction of androgen target genes through MAP kinase in prostate cancer cells. *Proc Natl Acad Sci U S A*, Vol. 96, pp. 5458-5463.

Yeh, S., Lin, H.K., Kang HY, et al. (1999) From HER2/Neu signal cascade to androgen receptor and its coactivators: a novel pathway by induction of androgen target genes through MAP kinase in prostate cancer cells. Proc Natl Acad Sci U S A, Vol.96, pp.5458-5463.

Yoshimoto, M., Cunha, I.W., Coudry, R.A., et al. (2007) FISH analysis of 107 prostate cancers shows that PTEN genomic deletion is associated with poor clinical outcome. *Br J Cancer*, Vol.97, pp.678-685.

Yoshino, T., Shiina, H., Urakami, S., et al. (2006) Bcl-2 expression as a predictive marker of hormone-refractory prostate cancer treated with taxane-based chemotherapy. *Clin Cancer Res*, Vol.12, pp.6116-6124.

6

Prostate Cancer Dephosphorylation Atlas

Carmen Veríssima Ferreira[1], Renato Milani[1], Willian Fernando Zambuzzi[2],
Thomas Martin Halder[3], Eduardo Galembeck[1] and Hiroshi Aoyama[1]
[1]University of Campinas
[2]Federal Fluminense University
[3]TopLab GmbH
[1,2]Brazil
[3]Germany

1. Introduction

The widespread nature of protein phosphorylation/dephosphorylation underscores its key role in cell metabolism. Phosphate moiety balance on proteins is regulated by protein kinases (PK) and protein phosphatases (PP), which are milestone players of eukaryotic signaling pathways. In general, signaling proteins involved in intracellular pathways are transiently active or inactive by phosphorylation and dephosphorylation mechanisms, covalently executed by PK and PP, respectively (Hooft et al. 2002; Tonks, 2005). It is accepted that the phosphorylation state of these proteins must be kept at a dynamic equilibrium in biological systems. Any deviation in this balance (generally associated with augmented PK signaling) can cause the intracellular accumulation of serine, threonine, tyrosine-phosphorylated proteins, which will cause abnormal cell proliferation and differentiation, thereby resulting in different kinds of diseases (Souza et al., 2009). Similar deviation from this equilibrium can be also induced by decreased activity of protein tyrosine phosphatases (PTP) resulting from gene mutation or gene deletion, leading to an increase in tyrosine phosphorylated proteins in cells. PPs are subdivided into two major families, with regard to their physiological substrates: protein tyrosine phosphatases and serine/threonine phosphatases. In particular, tyrosine phosphorylation of key proteins is a critical event in the regulation of intracellular signaling pathways (Aoyama et al., 2003; Gee and Mansuy, 2004; Souza et al., 2009). There is strong evidence pointing that low SHP-1 PTP activity is associated with a high proliferation rate and an increased risk of recurrence after radical prostatectomy for localized prostate cancer (Tassidis et al., 2010). Moreover, it has been proposed that specific PTPs may be related to determining the developmental stage and aggressiveness degree of prostate cancer (Chuang et al, 2010). Thus, it is reasonable to suggest that the chemical modulation of PTPs may, therefore, be a good spot for pharmacological intervention for overcoming prostate cancer, in combination with conventional cancer chemotherapeutic strategies. However, the critical bottleneck in deciphering the role of PTPs in prostate cancer biology is the identification of their physiological substrates and how their enzymatic activity is related to molecular changes in proliferation and cell death. In this chapter we shall focus on the contribution of the low molecular weight protein tyrosine phosphatase (LMWPTP), Src homology 2 (SH2) domain-containing PTP (SHP-1), cell division cycle 25 (Cdc25), acid phosphatase, phosphatase and tensin homolog (PTEN) and dual-specificity phosphatase (DUSP) for prostate carcinogenesis and describe their participation in the molecular events that lead to tumor survival and osteomimetic properties, highlighting perspectives and directions for future research that improve current knowledge on these critical signaling molecules.

2. Protein phosphatases

The ubiquitous nature of protein phosphorylation/dephosphorylation underscores its key role in cell signaling metabolism, growth and differentiation. In fact, cells respond to internal and external stimuli through integrated networks of intracellular signaling pathways that act via cascades of sequential phosphorylation or dephosphorylation reactions which are governed by the action of PK and PPs, respectively (Hooft van Huijsduijnen et al., 2002; Tonks, 2005).

PPs have been classified by structure and substrate specificity into protein serine/threonine phosphatases (PSTPs) and protein tyrosine phosphatases (PTPs) (Aoyama et al., 2003; Gee and Mansuy, 2005).

In general, PTPs control fundamental physiological processes such as cell growth and differentiation, cell cycle, metabolism, immune response and cytoskeletal function. Furthermore, interfering with the delicate balance between counteracting PTKs and PTPs is involved in the development of numerous inherited and acquired human diseases such as autoimmunity, diabetes and cancer (Alonso et al., 2004; Andersen et al., 2004; Ferreira et al., 2006; Souza et al., 2009; Zambuzzi et al., 2010; Zambuzzi et al., 2011).

2.1 PTPs classification

Up to now, 107 genes encoding PTPs have been discovered in the human genome, whereas 81 of them have been predicted to be active PTPs (Alonso et al., 2004). Classically, PTPs were divided into four classes: receptor type PTPs, non-receptor PTPs, dual specificity PTPs and low molecular weight PTPs. However, some authors have proposed an alternative way to classify this enzyme family based on the amino acid residues of their catalytic domains (Alonso et al., 2004; Bialy and Waldmann et al., 2005). In fact, comparison of the crystal structure of the PTPs that have been solved to date demonstrates that the PTPs domains are conserved in both sequence and structure. Additionally the sequences (domains) outside the catalytic domain are diverse and may regulate PTP activity and/or function (Table 1).

- Class I cysteine-based PTPs catalyze the enzymatic reaction in which an active-site cysteine group plays a central role and renders the PTP susceptible to oxidant agents that can lead to oxidation of the key cysteine and inhibition of PTP activity. This class contains the "classical" PTPs and the "dual specificity" protein phosphatases (DSPs), both evolved from a common ancestor. The "classical PTPs" members are strictly tyrosine-specific and according to their subcellular localization can be further divided into intracellular PTPs (PTP1B and SHP) and receptor-like PTPs (CD45, PTPα and PTPγ), both containing one or two catalytic domain(s) of approximately 240 amino acids. The DSPs (VH1-like enzymes) are the most diverse group in terms of substrate specificity and can be distinguished by their ability to hydrolyze pSer/pThr as well as pTyr residues and non-protein substrates, such as inositol phospholipids. The DSP family contains, amongst others, highly specialized types of phosphatases. For instance, members of this family include mitogen-activated protein kinases phosphatases (MKPs), members of the myotubularin family, RNA triphosphatases, and PTEN (phosphatase and tensin homologue deleted on chromosome 10) type phosphatase (Alonso et al., 2004; Wishart and Dixon, 2006).
- Class II cysteine-based PTPs are especially common in bacteria and enzymes of this class appear to be more ancient than class I PTPs. In humans this class is represented by an 18 kDa tyrosine-specific low M_r phosphatase (LMPTP). LMPTP is able to

dephosphorylate tyrosine kinases and their substrates but its biological functions remain unclear. The correlation between expression and activity of variants of this PTP with some human diseases, including cancer, indicates that this phosphatase may be involved in pivotal processes in cell physiology (Malentacchi et al., 2005).

- Class III cysteine-based PTPs are tyrosine/threonine specific phosphatases and probably evolved from a bacterial rhodanese-like enzyme. In humans, this class is represented by the group of Cdc 25 phosphatases: Cdc25A, Cdc25B and Cdc25C. These three cell cycle regulators act by dephosphorylation of Cdks at their inhibitory N-terminal phosphor-Thr/Tyr motifs, a reaction that is required for the activation of these kinases to drive progression of the cell cycle (Hoffman et al., 2004; Kristjansdottir and Rudolph, 2004).

- The fourth class of PTPs is represented by aspartate-based PTPs, which use a different catalytic mechanism with a key aspartic acid and dependence on a cation (Rayapureddi et al., 2003).

PTP family	Members
Class I cys-based	Receptor PTP CD45, RPTPμ, RPTPκ, RPTPρ, RPTPλ, RPTPσ, RPTPδ, RPTPα, RPTPε, RPTPγ, RPTPξ, RPTPβ, DEP1, SAP1, GLEPP, PTPS31, PCPTP, STEP, IA2 and IA2β Nonreceptor PTP PTP1B, TCPTP, PTP-MEG2, HePTP, STEP, LYP, PTP-PEST, PTP-HSCF, Typ-PTP and HD-PTP MPKs PAC-1, MKP1, MKP2, MKP3, MKP4, VH3, VH5, PYST2, MKP5, MKP7 and MK-STYX Atypical DSPs VHR, PIR1, BEDP, TMDP, MKP6, DSP20, SKRP, DSP21, MOSP, MGC1136, VHZ, FMDSP, VHX, VHY, HYVH1, VHP, Laforin, RNGTT and STYX PRLs PRL1, PRL2 and PRL3, CDC14s CDC14A, CDC14B, KAP and PTP9Q22 Slingshots SSH1, SSH2 and SSH3 PTENs PTEN, TPIP, TPTE, tensin and C-1-TEN Myotubularins MTM1, MTMR1, MTMR2, MTMR3, MTMR4, MTMR5, MTMR6, MTMR7, MTMR8, MTMR9, MTMR10, MTMR11, MTMR12, MTMR13 and MTMR14
Class II cys-based	LMWPTP
Class III cys-based	CDC25A, CDC25B and CDC25C
Class IV asp-based	EyA1, EyA2, EyA3 and EyA4

Alonso et al., 2004; Souza et al., 2009.

Table 1. Classification of protein tyrosine phosphatases based on amino acid sequences of the catalytic domains

2.2 Mechanisms of PTP catalysis

Different experimental approaches, such as X-ray crystallography, directed site mutagenesis and circular dichroism, have contributed to our understanding of catalysis and substrate recognition by PTPs. Although PTPs have conserved catalytic domains and share a common mechanism of action, substrate specificity of individual PTPs may display substantial specificity, thus resulting in these enzymes to regulate highly specialized and often fundamentally important processes.

The PTP family shares a strictly conserved active site comprising the "P-loop" residues $(H/V)C(X)_5R(S/T)$ and a conserved acidic residue (Denu et al., 1996; Fauman et al., 1996; Zhang 2003; Aoyama et al., 2003). In all structurally characterized PTPs to date, the three-dimensional structure of active-site components is also highly conserved suggesting a common catalytic mechanism. In general, the catalytic site is located in a groove at the protein surface. Its size is responsible for explaining the higher substrate selectivity of classical PTPs (Alonso et al., 2004).

In vitro studies based on model substrates, such as phenyl phosphate or *p*-nitrophenyl phosphate, have provided much of the information on the mechanistic aspects of catalysis. In particular, it is well established that the enzyme completes its action in two major steps. In the first step, the phosphoryl group from the substrate is transferred to the nucleophilic cysteine, forming a phosphoenzyme intermediate. In the second step, this intermediate is hydrolyzed, leading to the regeneration of the enzyme and the release of an inorganic phosphate (Aoyama et al., 2003; Zhang, 1997). Although this two-step mechanism is well-established, some mechanistic aspects still need to be clarified, such as regulatory and inhibitory mechanisms.

3. Protein tyrosine phosphatases and prostate cancer

3.1 LMWPTP

3.1.1 Signaling features

Chernoff and Li (1985) purified a PTP from bovine heart whose characteristics were similar to those described for the low molecular weight acid phosphatase (See item 3.4.1). This low molecular weight (about 18 kDa) protein tyrosine phosphatase (LMWPTP) shares very low sequence homology in relation to the other protein tyrosine phosphatase families, except for the consensus active site motif CX_5R, that contains the essential nucleophilic cysteinyl residue, and an identical catalytic mechanism (Tonks, 2006; Tabernero et al, 2008). All PTPs hydrolyze p-nitrophenylphosphate and show inhibition by vanadate, insensitivity to okadaic acid and lack of metal ion requirement for catalysis. LMWPTP contains two conserved adjacent tyrosines, Tyr131 and Tyr132, which are preferential sites for phosphorylation by protein tyrosine kinases and important for the regulation of its activity (Tailor et al, 1997; Buccciantini et al, 1999). This enzyme class is very important in cell signaling processes such as proliferation, adhesion and migration. It can associate with and dephosphorylate many growth factors and receptors, such as platelet-derived growth factor (PDGFR), fibroblast growth factor (FGFR), insulin receptor (IR) and ephrin receptor (Eph), causing downregulation of tyrosine kinase receptor functions and leading to cell division (Souza et al, 2009).

3.1.2 Role in prostate cancer

LMWPTP has been recognized as a positive regulator of tumor growth (Chiarugi et al., 2004). Our research group has a long-standing interest in the possible beneficial prostate cancer biological effects of LMWPTP. In this scenario, we demonstrated that a compound isolated from the Chilean tree *Persea nubigena* and from the stem bark of *Podocarpus andina* (Podocarpaceae), modulates both expression and activity of LMWPTP in prostate cancer cells (PC3) which was important for diminishing the proliferation ratio of these cells (Bispo de Jesus et al. 2008). More recently, we observed that prostate cancer cells that had LMWPTP silenced showed considerable reduction in invasiveness (unpublished data).

Thus, this enzyme is attracting great interest as a drug target. Zabell et al. (2004) described that specific inhibitors could be rationally designed according to each of the two isoform structures of this class of enzymes. Taddei et al. (2006) observed that, at least in part, the antitumoral activity of Aplidin could be due to the direct oxidation and inactivation of LMWPTP. Marzocchini et al. (2008) reported that the treatment of rats with 1,2-dimethylhydrazine provoked a significant increase in LMWPTP expression in adenocarcinomas, suggesting that this phenomenon is associated with the onset of malignancy.

3.2 SHP-1
3.2.1 Signaling features
Among all members of PTPs, SHP-1 has been suggested as a key signaling protein to control cell growth. Specifically, SHP-1 (an SH2 domain-containing cytosolic PTP) is an important modulator of intracellular phosphotyrosine level in eukaryotic cells, controlling different cell fates, such as proliferation, migration and differentiation through regulating signaling of cytokines such as IL-3R, PDGF- and EGF receptors, and other tyrosine kinase receptors (Tomic et al., 1995; Keilhack et al., 1998). Disruption on SHP-1 regulation can cause abnormal cell growth and induce different kinds of cancers such as leukemia, lymphoma, breast and prostate cancers as well. In order to validate this hypothesis, some authors have inserted the SHP-1 gene into different cancer cell lines and they reported a diminishment on growth of those cells (Zapata et al., 2002). Altogether, these data reinforce that SHP-1 acts as a tumor suppressor protein, regulating cell signaling responsible to growth of eukaryotic cells.

3.2.2 Role in prostate cancer
In men, it is known that androgen deprivation leads to development of a negative growth-regulating loop involving antiproliferative molecules like somatostatin (SST) in prostate adenocarcinoma. Physiologically, SST presents an antiproliferative effect, impairing mitogenic signals upon growth factors signaling (Patel, 1999). The SST signaling starts upon activation of a family of transmembrane receptors (SSTRs), sharing common signaling pathways such as the inhibition of adenylate cyclase, activation of PTP, and modulation of mitogen-activated protein kinase (MAPK). A number of publications support an involvement of SHP- 1 on negative regulation of cellular proliferation by SST (Lahlou et al., 2003). The expression of SHP-1 in rat prostate (Valencia et al., 1997) and in human prostate was shown as well (Tassidis et al., 2010). Despite the limitation of cell culture, some authors have defined SHP-1 as a decisive protein on determining cancer cell phenotype *in vitro* by using two classical prostate cancer cell lines: PC3 and LNCap. They determined an inverse relationship between cell proliferation and secreted somatostain amount. Briefly, SST was able to inhibit both PC-3 and LNCap cell proliferation by an autocrine/paracrine manner, suggesting its participation on blocking cell cycle signaling. Moreover, when SST secretion was blocked, the expression and activity levels of SHP-1 protein were reduced, and PC-3 cell proliferation was increased (Zapata et al., 2002). These authors suggest that SHP-1 could

play a key role in controlling prostatic cell proliferation, which also indicates that SHP-1 expression might be a therapeutic target for treatment of prostate cancer (Zapata et al., 2002). On the other hand, by using human prostate biopsies, Cariaga-Martinez et al. (2009) observed a decrease of SHP-1 and somatostatin in prostate cancer cells, and they demonstrated that this is consistent with aggressiveness of the tumor. In addition, Wu et al. (2003) proposed the diminished or abolished SHP-1 expression could be due to mutation of the SHP-1 gene, methylation of the promoter region or post-transcriptional regulation of SHP-1 protein synthesis. It might also be explained by the action of specific families of miRNAs.

3.3 CDC25
3.3.1 Signaling features
Unbalance on either expression or activity of proteins related to control of cell cycle progression provokes a wide variety of malignant diseases, including prostate cancer. Biochemically, cell cycle progression is a well orchestrated event regulated by well-defined sequential activities of cyclin-dependent kinases (CDKs), cyclins, and other proteins (Karlsson-Rosenthal and Millar, 2006). During mitosis, Cdc2/Cyclin B complexes can be dephosphorylated by the CDC25 phosphatase (a dual-specificity protein tyrosine phosphatase). CDC25 phosphatases play a critical role in regulating cell cycle progression by dephosphorylating CDKs at inhibitory residues and, therefore, have been shown to possess oncogenic potential (Karlsson-Rosenthal and Millar, 2006). In human, CDC25 proteins are encoded by a multigene family: CDC25A, CDC25B, and CDC25C (Turowski et al., 2003). It has been suggested that phosphorylation of CDC25C at Ser216 (activated Chk kinases) negatively regulate the activity of this phosphatase by an immediate cytoplasmic sequestration (Peng et al., 1997). Despite its potential role in prostate cancer, its exact involvement remains unclear.

3.3.2 Role in prostate cancer
Due to its hormone-dependent nature, prostate cancer at the metastatic stage is usually treated with hormone ablation therapy. Androgen receptor (AR) is a ligand-dependent transcription factor and its activity is regulated by numerous AR coregulators. Inadequate incidence of these AR coregulators contributes for the development of prostate cancer. Current studies have shown that AR activity is modulated by phosphorylation at specific sites performed by mitogen-activated protein kinases, Akt/PKB, and cAMP-activated protein kinase A, which control AR transcriptional activity. Guo et al. (2006) reported that AR was tyrosine-phosphorylated in prostate cancer cell lines and that an elevated level of phosphorylation was detected in hormone refractory prostate tumor xenografts, demonstrating that such AR modification may contribute to androgen-independent activation of AR. Chiu et al. (2009) demonstrated for the first time that CDC25A could interact with AR and inhibit its transcriptional activity. Since CDC25A overexpression is implicated in cancer development, their findings may provide an insight into the pathological role of CDC25A and AR in the development of prostate cancer.
In addition, CDC25A phosphatase has been implicated in the regulation of Raf-1 and the MAPK pathway. Raf-1 controls the mitogen activated protein kinase (MAPK) pathway, which has been associated with the progression of prostate cancer to the more advanced and androgen-independent disease. Nemoto et al. (2004) showed that Raf-1 interacts with

CDC25A in PC-3 and LNCap cells and CDC25A inhibitors induced both extracellular signal-regulated kinase (Erk) activation and augmented Raf-1 tyrosine phosphorylation. These results indicate that CDC25A phosphatase regulates Raf-1/MEK/Erk kinase activation in human prostate cancer cells. Indeed, CDC25A controls proliferation and survival signaling, culminating on modulation of prostate cancer progression and aggressiveness.

Moreover, to determine whether CDC25C activity is altered in prostate cancer, Ozen and Ittman (2005) have examined the expression of CDC25C and an alternatively spliced variant in human prostate cancer samples and cell lines. Interestingly, they showed that an active dephosphorylated form of CDC25C was up-regulated in prostate cancer in comparison with normal prostate tissue. In addition, they showed that at the transcriptional level, CDC25C and alternatively spliced variants were both overexpressed in prostate cancer. Finally, their findings suggest that expression of the spliced variants is correlated with biochemical recurrence.

Regarding CDC25B, Ngan et al. (2003) described that its overexpression is associated with the stage of prostate cancer, transiting from a hormone-dependent to a hormone-independent state and contributing to prostate cancer development and progression.

3.4 Acid phosphatase
3.4.1 Signaling features

Acid phosphatases (EC 3.1.3.2), enzymes that catalyze the hydrolysis of a wide range of orthophosphate monoesters, are largely distributed in nature and have been studied in numerous organisms and tissues (Granjeiro et al, 1997; Ferreira et al, 1998a, 1998b; Granjeiro et al, 1999; Fernandes et al, 2003; Jonsson et al, 2007). The enzyme found in mammalian tissues occurs in multiple forms that differ in regard to molecular mass, substrate specificity and sensitivity to inhibitors (Granjeiro et al, 1997). Low relative molecular mass (Mr) enzymes (Mr < 20.0 kDa) are insensitive to tartrate and fluoride and strongly inhibited by SH-reacting compounds. High Mr acid phosphatases (Mr > 100.0 kDa) are inhibited by tartrate and intermediary Mr enzymes (30.0 kDa < Mr<60.0 kDa) by fluoride. In contrast to high Mr acid phosphatases, low Mr enzymes present more restricted substrate specificity, preferentially hydrolyzing p-nitrophenylphosphate, flavin mononucleotide and tyrosine-phosphorylated proteins.

In 1985, Chernoff and Li reported several similarities between the low molecular weight acid phosphatase and one class of protein tyrosine phosphatase (PTP), the low molecular weight protein tyrosine phosphatase (LMWPTP).

The phosphatidic acid phosphatase (PAP) is a key enzyme in both glycerolipid biosynthesis and cellular signal transduction. It was observed that the plasma membrane-bound type 2 PAP, now known as lipid phosphate phosphatase, participates in germ cell migration, epithelial differentiation and other signaling processes (Kanoh et al, 1997; Brindley and Pilquil, 2009).

3.4.2 Role in prostate cancer

Altered acid phosphatase activities can be related to several pathological processes, such as those involving infectious, inflammatory or tumoral processes. For instance, high and intermediary molecular weight acid phosphatases levels are increased in the serum of patients with prostate carcinoma (Hudson et al. 1955), of patients suffering from spleen disorders (Kumar and Gupta, 1971), of patients with endothelial reticulum leukemia (Ketcham et al, 1985), etc.

Human prostatic acid phosphatase has been used as a valuable marker for prostate cancer, before the evaluation by the prostate-specific antigen (PSA). Increased prostatic acid phosphatase serum levels are well correlated with metastatic prostate cancer (Ahmann and Schifman, 1987). In normal human prostate epithelial cells, human prostatic acid phosphatase expression is very high and guarantees the slow proliferation rate of those cells (Goldfarb et al., 1986; Veeramani et al, 2005). On the other hand, decreased activity of this phosphatase correlates with the poor differentiation of high-grade prostate cancer. One possible mechanism by which this phosphatase regulates the proliferation of prostate cancer is due to the dephosphorylation of the receptor HER-2. Uncontrolled phosphorylation of HER-2 leads to increased hormone-refractory growth of prostate cancer cells (Chuang et al, 2010).

3.5 PTEN
3.5.1 Signaling features
PTEN is a tumor suppressor protein, acting as a dual-specificity protein phosphatase. It is one of several enzymes with the ability to dephosphorylate tyrosine-, serine- and threonine-phosphorylated residues (Pulido & van Huijsduijnen, 2008). It also presents lipid phosphatase activity, mainly towards phosphatidylinositol-3,4,5-triphosphate (Maehama & Dixon, 1998). This is crucial to its tumor suppressor function, since it opposes the survival and proliferative actions of many growth factors (Uzoh et al., 2008).

PTEN was first described in 1997. Mutations in its encoding gene were detected, at the time, in several human cancer tissues and cell lines, including prostate cancer (Li et al., 1997). Its loss has been associated mainly with activation of the PI3K/Akt/mTOR pathway, leading to proliferation and survival of cancer cells (Hollander et al., 2011).

3.5.2 Role in prostate cancer
The lack of PTEN has been implicated in the resistance of prostate cancer cells to conventional chemo- and radiotherapy, as well as androgen-independence (Uzoh et al., 2008; Huang et al., 2001; Priulla et al., 2007; Anai et al., 2006; Shen & Abate-Shen, 2007). In a mouse model of prostate cancer, PTEN inactivation was shown to induce growth arrest through the p53-dependent cellular senescence pathway both *in vitro* and *in vivo* (Chen et al., 2005).

Chemo- and radiotherapy resistance is linked to overexpression of Bcl-2, an anti-apoptotic protein that blocks PTEN-mediated apoptosis. Huang et al. showed this overexpression to be related to PTEN-loss, as well as establishing an association between PTEN-induced chemosensitivity and inhibition of Bcl-2 expression (Huang et al., 2001).

mTOR inhibition has also been shown to sensitize Pten-null prostate cancer cells to chemo- and radiotherapy (Grunwald et al., 2002; Cao et al., 2006), pointing to PTEN's role in resistance. Interestingly, Cao and colleagues used an mTOR inhibitor other than rapamycin (RAD001 - everolimus) to enhance the cytotoxic effects of radiotherapy on two prostate cancer cell lines (PC-3 and DU145). They found that the increased susceptibility to radiation presented by both cell lines was due to autophagy, instead of apoptosis. They also showed that blocking apoptosis with caspase inhibition and Bax/Bak small interfering RNA leads to the same effects (Cao et al., 2006). TORC1/TORC2 inhibition in association with docetaxel and cisplatin also led to promising results in mice with chemoresistant prostate cancer (Gravina et al., 2011).

PTEN loss effects also extend to the androgen receptor (AR) activity, associated to androgen-independence. AR is shown to be inhibited by PTEN through blockage of the Akt pathway (Shen & Abate-Shen, 2007; Nan et al., 2003). However, a recent study points to the opposite activities of AR and PI3K signaling pathways and their cross-regulation, with inhibition of one activating the other, maintaining cancer cell survival by distinct means. Through combined pharmacological inhibition of both pathways, the authors could achieve near-complete prostate cancer regressions in a PTEN-deficient murine model and in human xenografts (Carver et al., 2011).

Recent studies have also implicated PTEN loss in chemokine receptor 4 (CXCR4)- mediated prostate cancer progression and metastasis, as well as showing that reactive oxygen species (ROS) can increase this outcome through direct inactivation of PTEN by active site oxidation (Chetram et al., 2011).

3.6 DUSP
3.6.1 Signaling features
Dual-specificity phosphatases (DUSPs) are enzymes able to dephosphorylate both tyrosine and serine/threonine residues within their substrate (Patterson et al., 2009). There are 49 gene products characterized as human DUSPs in the Gene Ontology database (The Gene Ontology Consortium, 2000). These are divided into subgroups, according to their substrate specificity. MKPs, one of the best-characterized subgroups, are able to dephosphorylate mitogen-associated protein kinases (MAPKs), which are in turn increasingly implicated in the development and progression of several cancers, including prostate cancer. Another subgroup is named atypical DUSPs. Some of them also show a preference for MAPKs as substrates, but, unlike MKPs, they are mostly of low-molecular mass and lack the N-terminal CH2 (Cdc25 homology 2) domain (Patterson et al., 2009).

In spite of some clear links between some DUSPs, their substrates and specific cancer types, there is still variability in respect to their role in distinct tissue environments. The existing reports regarding prostate cancer are diverse, sometimes even antagonistic. Thus, the precise role of DUSPs in carcinogenesis remains to be clarified (Arnoldussen & Saatcioglu, 2009).

DUSP1 is a member of the MKP group. It is able to dephosphorylate all members of the MAPK family, although displaying preference for p38 and JNK substrates (Magi-Galluzzi et al., 1997; Sun et al., 1993; Franklin & Kraft, 1997).

DUSP3 is an atypical dual-specificity phosphatase that has controversial substrate specificity. ERK 1/2 and JNK were identified as direct substrates for DUSP3 (Todd et al., 1999; Todd et al., 2002), although a later report points to ERK2 as an unlikely substrate for DUSP3 (Zhou et al., 2002). STAT5 was also identified as a substrate for DUSP3 (Hoyt et al., 2007).

DUSP10 is a MKP with preference for p38 and JNK rather than ERK as substrates. It has been implicated in the regulation of innate and adaptive immune responses (Zhang et al., 2004) and also has been shown to have a potent anti-inflammatory activity in prostate cells (Nonn et al., 2007).

DUSP18 is a member of the atypical subgroup of dual-specificity phosphatases whose mRNA expression was identified in several cancer tissues and cell lines, including prostate, among others (Patterson et al., 2009; Wu et al., 2006). It presents phosphatase activity against ERK, JNK and p38 synthetic substrates, with a preference for ERK and JNK (Hood et al., 2002).

3.6.2 Role in prostate cancer

DUSP1 mRNA was found to be overexpressed in the early phases of prostate cancer, but this did not prevent high ERK-1 expression (Loda et al., 1996). Overall, ERK appears to increase DUSP1 expression, decreasing JNK activity and inhibiting apoptosis. In a 2008 study it was shown that coordinate inhibition of AKT/mTOR and ERK-1/MAPK pathways leads to reduced cell growth and proliferation, as well as upregulation of the apoptotic regulator Bcl-2-interacting mediator of cell death (Bim) in a preclinical mouse model of hormone-refractory prostate cancer (Kinkade et al., 2008). Accordingly, a later study showed DUSP1 mRNA expression to be lower in hormone-refractory prostate carcinomas than in benign prostate hyperplasia (BPH) or untreated prostate carcinomas. Higher DUSP1 protein levels were found in BPH, normal prostate and high-grade prostate intraepithelial neoplasia (Rauhala et al., 2005). Consistent with the low levels of DUSP1 in response to androgen ablation, DUSP1 mRNA was found to be upregulated upon androgen treatment of LNCaP cells (Arnoldussen et al., 2008) The androgen receptor (AR) has been identified as responsible for increased expression of DUSP1 (and several other DUSPs) upon interaction with testosterone. However, DUSP1 implication in prostate cancer is not yet fully resolved, since there have been reports showing that both high and low levels of DUSP1 may have an antiapoptotic effect, depending on which MAP kinase DUSP1 is targeting (Rauhala et al., 2005).

Similarly, androgens protect LNCaP cells from 12-O-tetradecanoylphorbol-13-acetate- and thapsigargin-induced apoptosis via down-regulation of JNK activity through an increase in DUSP3 expression. This effect was not observed in androgen-independent DU145 cells (Arnoldussen et al., 2008). Expression analysis in human prostate cancer specimens also show that DUSP3 is increased in prostate cancer compared with normal prostate, evidencing a direct DUSP3 role in prostate cancer progression through JNK-mediated apoptosis inhibition (Arnoldussen et al, 2008).

Another DUSP that has been related to prostate cancer is DUSP10. DUSP10 presents anti-inflammatory activity and its expression is increased after treatment with calcitriol, the hormonally active form of vitamin D. This results in the subsequent inhibition of p38 stress kinase signaling and the attenuation of the production of pro-inflammatory cytokines (Nonn, et al., 2006; Krishnan & Feldman, 2010).

4. Concluding remarks

Deciphering the molecular networks that distinguish progressive from non-progressive prostate cancer will bring light on the biology of this tumor, as well as lead to the identification of biomarkers that will aid to the selection of better-suited treatments for each patient. For this, it is crucial to characterize and integrate the molecular mediators involved in prostate cancer biology. In this chapter we pointed out some evidences of the contribution of protein tyrosine phosphatases for prostate cancer pathogenesis. PTPs, as a large enzyme family, can act as prostate cancer suppressors or promoters, depending on their target protein (Table 2). However, studies quantifying PTPs on gene and protein levels in prostate cancer have been limited. New efforts to raise this kind of combinatory data might reveal a spectacular relationship between genotype and PTP activity levels and lead to an understanding of the fundamental role of this enzyme family in controlling malignant cell transformation. This, in turn, may open new avenues to treat prostate cancer based on PTP activity modulation.

Phosphatase	Prostate cancer cell localization	Main action	Main targets in prostate cancer
LMWPTP	cytosol	cancer promoter	unknown
SHP-1	cytosol	cancer suppressor	IL-3R, PDGF- and EGF receptors
CDC25B and CDC25C	nucleus	cancer promoter	unknown
CDC25A	nucleus	cancer suppressor	Androgen receptor (AR)
Acid phosphatase	cytosol	cancer suppressor	Her-2
PTEN	cytosol and nucleus	cancer suppressor	phosphatidylinositol-3,4,5-triphosphate
DUSP	nucleus	cancer promoter	JNK, p38 and ERK

Table 2. Prostate cancer protein tyrosine phosphatases

5. Acknowledgment

Our research on this field is supported by Fundação de Amparo à Pesquisa do Estado de São Paulo (FAPESP), Coordenação de Aperfeiçoamento de Pessoal de Nível Superior (CAPES) and Conselho Nacional de Desenvolvimento Científico e Tecnológico (CNPq).

6. References

Ahmann, F.R. and Schifman, R.B. (1987) Prospective comparison between serum monoclonal prostate specific antigen and acid phosphatase measurements in metastatic prostatic cancer. *J. Urol.* 137, 431-434.

Alonso, A., Sasin, J., Bottini, N., Friedberg, I., Friedberg, I., Osterman, A., Godzik, A., Hunter, T., Dixon, J. and Mustelin, T. (2004) Protein tyrosine phosphatases in the human genome. *Cell* 117, 699-711

Anai, S et al. (2006) Combination of PTEN gene therapy and radiation inhibits the growth of human prostate cancer xenografts. *Hum Gene Ther* 17, 975-984.

Andersen, J.N., Jansen, P.G., Echwald, S.M., Mortensen, O.H., Fukada, T., Del Vecchio, R., Tonks, N.K., Moller, N.P. (2004) A genomic perspective on protein tyrosine phosphatases: gene structure, pseudogenes, and genetic disease linkage, *FASEB J.* 18, 8-30.

Arnoldussen, Y.J., Lorenzo, P.I., Pretorius, M.E., Waehre, H., Risberg, B., Maelandsmo, G.M., Danielsen, H.E., Saatcioglu, F. (2008) The mitogen-activated protein kinase phosphatase vaccinia H1-related protein inhibits apoptosis in prostate cancer cells and is overexpressed in prostate cancer. *Cancer Res* 68, 9255-9264.

Arnoldussen, YJ & Saatcioglu, F (2009) Dual specificity phosphatases in prostate cancer. *Mol Cell Endocrinol* 309, 1-7.

Bialy, L., Waldmann, H. Inhibitors of protein tyrosine phosphatases: next-generation drugs? (2005) *Angew. Chem. Int. Ed. Engl.* 44, 3814-3839.

Bispo de Jesus, M., Zambuzzi, W.F., Ruela de Sousa, R.R., Areche, c., Souza, A.C.S., Aoyama, H., Schmeda-Hirschmann, G., Rodrigues, J.A., Brito, A.R.M.S., Peppelenbosch, M.P., den Hertog, J., de Paula, E. and Ferreira, C.V. (2008) Ferruginol suppresses survival signaling pathways in androgen-independent prostate cancer cells. *Biochimie* 90, 843-854.

Brindley, D.N. and Pilquil, C. (2009) Lipid phosphate phosphatases and signaling. *J. Lipid Res.*, S225-S230.

Bucciantini, M., Chiarugi, P., Cirri, P. Taddei, L., Stefani, M., Raugei, G., Nordlund, P. and Ramponi, G. (1999) The low Mr phosphotyrosine protein phosphatase behaves differently when phosphorylated at Tyr131 and Tyr132 by Src kinase. *FEBS Lett.* 456, 73-78.

Cao, C., Subhawong, T., Albert, J.M., Kim, K.W., Geng, L., Sekhar, K.R., Gi, Y.J., Lu, B. (2006) Inhibition of mammalian target of rapamycin or apoptotic pathway induces autophagy and radiosensitizes PTEN null prostate cancer cells. *Cancer Res* 66, 10040-10047.

Cariaga-Martinez AE, Lorenzati MA, Riera MA, Cubilla MA, de La Rossa A, Giorgio EM, Tiscornia MM, Gimenez EM, Rojas ME, Chaneton BJ, Rodríguez DI, Zapata PD. (2009) Tumoral prostate shows different expression pattern of somatostatin receptor 2 (SSTR2) and phosphotyrosine phosphatase SHP-1 (PTPN6) according to tumor progression. *Adv Urol.* 723831.

Carver, B.S., Chapinski, C., Wongvipat, J., Hieronymus, H., Chen, Y., Chandarlapaty, S., Arora, V.K., Le, C., Koutcher, J., Scher, H., Scardino, P.T., Rosen, N., Sawyers, C.L. (2011) Reciprocal feedback regulation of PI3K and androgen receptor signaling in PTEN-deficient prostate cancer. *Cancer Cell* 19, 575-586.

Chen, Z., Trotman, L.C., Shaffer, D., Lin, H.K., Dotan, Z.A., Niki, M., Koutcher, J.A., Scher, H.I., Ludwig, T., Gerald, W., Cordon-Cardo, C., Pandolfi, P.P. (2005) Crucial role of p53-dependent cellular senescence in suppression of Pten-deficient tumorigenesis. *Nature* 436, 725-730.

Chernoff, J. and Li, H.-C. (1985). A major phosphotyrosyl-protein phosphatase from bovine heart is associated with a low-molecular-weigth acid phosphatase. *Arch. Biochem. Biophys.*, 240:135-45.

Chetram, M.A., Don-Salu-Hewage, A.S., Hinton, C.V. (2011) ROS enhances CXCR4-mediated functions through inactivation of PTEN in prostate cancer cells. *Biochem Biophys Res Commun* doi:10.1016/j.bbrc.2011.05.074 Epub ahead of print.

Chiarugi, P., Taddei, M.L., Schiavone, N., Papucci, L., Giannoni, L., Fiaschi, T., Capaccioli, S., Raugei, G., Ramponi, G. (2004) LMW-PTP is a positive regulator of tumor onset and growth, *Oncogene* 23, 3905e3914.

Chiu YT, Han HY, Leung SC, Yuen HF, Chau CW, Guo Z, Qiu Y, Chan KW, Wang X, Wong YC, Ling MT. (2009) CDC25A functions as a novel Ar corepressor in prostate cancer cells. *J Mol Biol.* 385, 446-456.

Chuang, T.D., Chen, S.J., Lin, F.F., Veeramani, S., Kumar, S., Batra, S.K., Tu, Y. and Lin, M.F. (2010) Human prostatic acid phosphatase, an authentic tyrosine phosphatase, dephosphorylates ErbB-2 and regulates prostate cancer cell growth. *J. Biol. Chem.* 285, 23598-23606.

Denu, J.M., Stuckey, J.A., Saper, M.A., Dixon, J.E. (1996) Form and function in protein dephosphorylation, *Cell* 87, 361-364.

Fauman, E.B., Saper, M.A. (1996) Structure and function of the protein tyrosine phosphatases, *Trends Biochem. Sci.* 21, 413-417.

Fernandes, E.C., Granjeiro, J.M., Taga, E.M., Meyer-Fernandes, J.R. and Aoyama, H. (2003) Phosphatase activity characterization on the surface of intact bloodstream forms of Trypanosoma brucei. *FEMS Microbiol. Lett.* 220, 197-206.

Ferreira, C. V., Justo, G. Z., Souza, A. C. S., Queiroz, K. C., Zambuzzi, W. F., Aoyama, H. and Peppelenbosch M. P. (2006) Natural compounds as a source of protein tyrosine phosphatase inhibitors: application to the rational design of small-molecule derivatives. *Biochimie* 88, 1859-1873

Ferreira, C.V., Granjeiro, J.M., Taga, E.M. and Aoyama, H. (1998a). Multiple forms of soybean seed acid phosphatases. Purification and characterization. *Plant Physiol. Biochem.*, 36, 487-494.

Ferreira, C.V., Granjeiro, J.M., Taga, E.M. and Aoyama, H. (1998b).Soybean seeds acid phosphatases. Unusual optimum temperature and thermal stability studies. *Biochem. Biophys. Res. Commun.* 242, 282-286.

Ferreira, C.V., Justo, G.Z., Souza, A.C., Queiroz, K.C.S., Zambuzzi, W.F., Aoyama, H. and Peppelenbosch, M.P. (2006) Natural compounds as a source of protein tyrosine phosphatase inhibitors: application to the rational design of small-molecule derivatives. *Biochimie* 88, 1859-1873.

Franklin, C.C. & Kraft, A.S. (1997) Conditional expression of the mitogen-activated protein kinase (MAPK) phosphatase MKP-1 preferentially inhibits p38 MAPK and stress-activated protein kinase in U937 cells. *J Biol Chem* 272, 16917-16923.

Gee, G.E., Mansuy, I.M. (2005) Protein phosphatases and their potential implications in neuroprotective processes, *Cell. Mol. Life Sci.* 62, 1120-1130.

Goldfarb, D.A., Stein, B.S., Shamszadeh, M. & Petersen, R.O. (1986) Age-related changes in tissue levels of prostatic acid phosphatase and prostate specific antigen. *Journal of Urology* 136, 1266–1269.

Granjeiro, J.M., Ferreira, C.V., Granjeiro, P.A., Silva, C.C., Taga, E.M., Volpe, P.L.O. and Aoyama, H. (2002) Inhibition of bovine kidney low molecular mass phosphotyrosine protein phosphatase by uric acid. *J. Enzyme Inhib. Med. Chem.* 5, 345-350.

Granjeiro, J.M., Ferreira. C.V., Jucá, M.B., Taga, E.M. and Aoyama, H. (1997). "Bovine kidney low molecular weight acid phosphatase: FMN-dependent kinetics". *Biochem. Mol. Biol. Int.* 41, 1201-1208.

Granjeiro, P.A., Ferreira, C.V., Granjeiro, J.M., Taga, E.M. and Aoyama, H. (1999). Purification and kinetic properties of a castor bean seed acid phosphatase containing sulfhydryl groups. *Physiol. Plant.* 107, 151-158.

Gravina, G.L., Marampon, F., Petini, F., Biordi, L.A., Sherris, D., Jannini, E.A., Tombolini, V., Festuccia, C. (2011) The TORC1/TORC2 inhibitor, Palomid 529, reduces tumor growth and sensitizes to docetaxel and cisplatin in aggressive and hormone refractory prostate cancer cells. *Endocr Relat Cancer* ERC-11-0045 Epub ahead of print.

Grunwald, V., DeGraffenried, L., Russel, D., Friedrichs, W.E., Ray, R.B., Hidalgo, M. (2002) Inhibitors of mTOR reverse doxorubicin resistance confered by PTEN status in prostate cancer cells. *Cancer Res* 62, 6141-6145.

Guo Z, Dai B, Jiang T, Xu K, Xie Y, Kim O, Nesheiwat I, Kong X, Melamed J, Handratta VD, Njar VC, Brodie AM, Yu LR, Veenstra TD, Chen H, Qiu Y. (2006) Regulation of androgen receptor activity by tyrosine phosphorylation. *Cancer Cell.* 10, 309-319.

Hoffman, B.T., Nelson, M.R., Burdick, K., Baxter, S.M. (2004) Protein tyrosine phosphatases: strategies for distinguishing proteins in a family containing multiple drug targets and anti-targets. *Curr. Pharm. Des.* 10, 1161-1181.

Hollander, M.C., Blumenthal, G.M., Dennis, P.A. (2011) PTEN loss in the continuum of common cancers, rare syndromes and mouse models. *Nature Rev Cancer* 11, 289-301.

Hood, K.L., Tobin, J.F., Yoon, C. (2002) Identification and characterization of two novel low-molecular-weight dual specificity phosphatases. *Biochem Biophys Res Commun* 298, 545-551.

Hooft van Huijsduijnen, R., Bombrun, A., Swinnen, D. (2002) Selecting protein tyrosine phosphatases as drug targets. *Drug Discov. Today* 7, 1013-1019.

Hoyt, R., Zhu, W., Cerignoli, F., Alonso, A., Mustelin, T., David, M. (2007) Cutting edge: selective tyrosine phosphorylation of interferon-activated nuclear STAT5 by the VHR phosphatase. *J Immunol* 179, 3402-3406.

Huang, H., Cheville, J.C., Pan, Y., Roche, P.C., Schmidt, L.J., Tindall, D.J. (2001) PTEN induces chemosensitivity in PTEN-mutated prostate cancer cells by suppression of Bcl-2 expression. *J Biol Chem* 276, 38830-38836.

Hudson, P.B., Tsuboi, K.K. and Mittelman, A. (1955) Prostatic cancer: extremely elevated serum acid phosphatase associated with altered liver function. *Am. J. Med.*, 19, 895-901.

Hunter, T., (1987) A thousand and one protein kinases. *Cell* 50, 823-829

Jonnson, C.M. and Aoyama, H. (2007) In vitro effect of agriculture pollutants and their joint action on Pseudokirchneriella subcapitata acid phosphatase. *Chemosphere*, 69, 849-855.

Kanoh, H., Kai, M, and Wada, I, (1997) Phosphatidic acid phosphatase from mammalian tissues: discovery of channel-like proteins with unexpected functions. *Biochim. Biophys. Acta* 1348, 56-62.

Karlsson-Rosenthal C, Millar JB. (2006) Cdc25: mechanisms of checkpoint inhibition and recovery. *Trends Cell Biol.* 16, 285-292.

Keilhack, H., Tenev, T., Nyakatura, E., Godovac-Zimmermann, J., Nielsen, L., Seedorf, K., Bohmer, F.D. (1998) Phosphotyrosine 1173 mediates binding of the protein-tyrosine phosphatase SHP-1 to the epidermal growth factor receptor and attenuation of receptor signaling J Biol Chem 273, 24839–24846.

Ketcham, C.M., Baumbach, G.A., Bazer, F.W., and Roberts, R.M. (1985) The type 5, acid phosphatase from spleen of humans with hairy cell leukemia. *J. Biol. Chem.*, 260, 5768-5776.

Kinkade, C.W., Castillo-Martin, M., Puzio-Kuter, A., Yan, J., Foster, T.H., Gao, H., Sun, Y., Ouyang, X., Gerald, W.L., Cordon-Cardo, C., Abate-Shen, C. (2008) Targeting AKT/mTOR and ERK MAPK signaling inhibits hormone-refractory prostate cancer in a preclinical mouse model. *J Clin Invest* 118, 3051-3064.

Krebs, E.G. and Beavo, J.A. (1979) Phosphorylation-dephosphorylation of enzymes. *Annu Rev Biochem.* 48, 923-959

Krishnan, AV & Feldman, D (2010) Molecular pathways mediating the anti-inflammatory effects of calcitriol: implications for prostate cancer chemoprevention and treatment. *Endocr Relat Cancer* 17, R19-38.

Kristjansdottir, K., Rudolph, J. (2004) Cdc25 phosphatases and cancer, *Chem. Biol.* 11, 1043-51.

Kumar, M. and Gupta, R.K. (1971) Evaluation of serum acid phosphatase activity in kidney diseases. *J. Indian Med. Assoc.*, 56: 89-94.

Lahlou H, Saint-Laurent N, Estève JP, Eychène A, Pradayrol L, Pyronnet S, Susini C. (2003) sst2 Somatostatin receptor inhibits cell proliferation through Ras-, Rap1-, and B-Raf-dependent ERK2 activation. *J Biol Chem.* 278, 39356-3971.

Li, J., Yen, C., Liaw, D., Podsypanina, K., Bose, S., Wang, S.I., Puc, J., Miliaresis, C., Rodgers, L., McCombie, R., Bigner, S.H., Giovanella, B.C., Ittmann, M., Tycko, B., Hibshoosh, H., Wigler, M.H., Parsons, R. (1997) PTEN, a putative protein tyrosine phosphatase gene mutated in human brain, breast and prostate cancer. *Science* 275, 1943-1947.

Maehama, T & Dixon, JE (1998) The tumor suppressor, PTEN/MMAC1, dephosphorylates the lipid second messenger, phosphatidylinositol-3,4,5-triphosphates. *J Biol Chem* 273, 13375-13378.

Magi-Galluzzi, C., Mishra, R., Fiorentino, M., Montironi, R., Yao, H., Capodieci, P., Wishnow, K., Kaplan, I., Stork, P.J., Loda, M. (1997) Mitogen-activated protein phosphatase 1 is overexpressed in prostate cancers and is inversely related to apoptosis. *Lab Invest* 76, 37-51.

Malentacchi, F., Marzocchini, R., Gelmini, S., Orlando, C., Serio, M., Ramponi, G., Raugei, G. (2005) Up-regulated expression of low molecular weight protein tyrosine phosphatases in different human cancers. *Biochem. Biophys. Res. Commun.* 334, 875-883.

Marzocchini, R., Malentacchi, F., Biagini, M., Cirelli, D., Luceri, C., Carderni, G. And Raugei, G. (2008) The expression of low molecular weight protein tyrosine phosphatase is up-regulated in 1,2-dimethylhydrazine-induced colon tumours in rats. *Int. J. Cancer* 122, 1675-1678.

Miranda, M.A., Okamoto, A.K., Ferreira, C.V., Silva, T.L., Granjeiro, J.M. and Aoyama, H. (2006) Differential effects of flavonoids on bovine kidney low molecular mass protein tyrosine phosphatase. *J. Enzyme Inhib. Med. Chem.* 21, 419-425.

Nan, B., Snabboon, T., Unni, E., X-J, Yuan, Whang, Y.E., Marcelli, M. (2003) The PTEN tumor suppressor is a negative modulator of androgen receptor transcriptional activity. *J Mol Endocrinol* 31, 169-183.

Nemoto, K., Vogt, A., Oguri, T., Lazo, J.S. (2004) Activation of the Raf-1/MEK/Erk kinase pathway by a novel Cdc25 inhibitor in human prostate cancer cells. *Prostate.* 58, 95-102.

Ngan, E.S., Hashimoto, Y., Ma, Z.Q., Tsai, M.J., Tsai, S.Y. (2003) Overexpression of Cdc25B, an androgen receptor coactivator, in prostate cancer. *Oncogene* 22, 734-739.

Nonn, L., Peng, L., Feldman, D., Peehl, D.M. (2006) Inhibition of p38 by vitamin D reduces interleukin-6 production in normal prostate cells via mitogen-activated protein kinase phosphatase 5: implications for prostate cancer prevention by vitamin D. *Cancer Res* 66, 4516-4524.

Nonn, L., Duong, D., Peehl, D.M. (2007) Chemopreventive anti-inflammatory activities of curcumin and other phytochemicals mediated by MAP kinase phosphatase-5 in prostate cells. *Carcinogenesis* 28, 1188-1196.

Östman, A., Helberg, C. and Böhmer, F.D. (2006) Protein-tyrosine phosphatases and cancer. *Nature Reviews Cancer.* 6, 307-320.

Ozen, M., Ittmann, M. (2005) Increased expression and activity of CDC25C phosphatase and an alternatively spliced variant in prostate cancer. *Clin Cancer Res.* 11, 4701-4706.

Patel, Y.C. (1999) Somatostatin and its receptor family. *Front Neuroendocrinol.* 20, 157-198.

Patterson, K.I., Brummer, T., O'Brien, P.M., Daly, R.J. (2009) Dual-specificity phosphatases: critical regulators with diverse cellular targets. *Biochem J* 418, 475-489.

Peng, C.Y., Graves, P.R.,Thoma, R.S.,Wu, Z.Q., Shaw, A.S., Piwnica-Worms, H. (1997) Mitotic and G(2) checkpoint control: regulation of14-3-3 protein binding by phosphorylation of Cdc25C on serine-216. *Science* 277, 1501-1505.

Priulla, M., Calastretti, A., Bruno, P., Azzariti, A., Paradiso, A., Canti, G., Nicolin, A. (2007) Preferential chemosensitization of PTEN-mutated prostate cells by silencing the Akt kinase. *Prostate* 67, 782-789.

Pulido, R & van Huijsduijnen, RH (2008) Protein tyrosine phosphatases: dual-specificity phosphatases in health and disease. *FEBS Journal* 275, 848-866.

Pytel, D., Sliwinski, T., Poplawski, T., Ferriola, D. and Majsterek, I. (2009) Tyrosine kinase blockers: new hope for successful cancer therapy. *Anti-Cancer Ag. Med. Chem.* 9, 66-76.

Quintero, I.B., Araujo, C.L., Pulkka, A.E., Wirkkala, R.S., Herrala, A.M., Eskelinen, E.L., Jokitalo, E., Hellstrom, P.A., Tuominen, H.J., Hirvikoski, P.P. and Vihko, P.T. (2007) Prostatic acid phosphatase is not a prostate specific target. *Cancer Res.* 67, 6549–6554.

Rauhala, H.E., Porkka, K.P., Tolonen, T.T., Martikainen, P.M., Tammela, T.L., Visakorpi, T. (2005) Dual-specificity phosphatase 1 and serum/glucocorticoid-regulated kinase are downregulated in prostate cancer. *Int J Cancer* 117, 738-745.

Rayapureddi, J.P., Kattamuri, C., Steinmetz, B.D., Frankfort, B.J. , Ostrin, E.J., Mardon, G., Hegde, R.S. (2003) Eyes absent represents a class of protein tyrosine phosphatases, *Nature* 426, 295-298.

Shen, K., Kui, Q. and Stiff, L. (2010) Peptidomimetic competitive inhibitors of protein tyrosine phosphatases. *Cur. Pharmac, Design* 16, 3101-3117.

Shen, MM & Abate-Shen, C (2007) PTEN inactivation and the emergence of androgen-independent prostate cancer. *Cancer Res* 67, 6535-6538.

Souza, A.C.S., Azoubel, S., Queiroz, K.C.s., Peppelenbosch, M.P. and Ferreira, C.V. (2009) From immune response to cancer: a spot on the low molecular weight protein tyrosine phosphatase. *Cell. Mol. Life Sci.* 66, 1140-1153.

Sun, H., Charles, C.H., Lau, L.F., Tonks, N.K. (1993) MKP-1 (3CH134), an immediate early gene product, is a dual specificity phosphatase that dephosphorylates MAP kinases in vivo. *Cell* 75, 487-493.

Tabernero, L., Aricescu, A.R., Jones, E.Y. and Szedlacsek, S.E. (2008) *FEBS J.* 275, 867-882.

Taddei, M.L., Chiarugi, P., Cuevas, C., Ramponi, G. And Raugei, G. (2006) Oxidation and inactivation of low molecular weight protein tyrosine phosphatase by the anticancer drug Aplidin. *Int. J. Cancer* 118, 2082-2088.

Tailor, P. Gilman, J., Williams, S., Couture, C. and Mustelin, T. (1997) Regulation of low molecular weight phosphotyrosine phosphatase by phosphorylation at tyrosines 131 and 132. *J. Biol. Chem.* 272, 5371-5374.

Tassidis H, Brokken LJ, Jirström K, Ehrnström R, Pontén F, Ulmert D, Bjartell A, Härkönen P, Wingren AG. (2010) Immunohistochemical detection of tyrosine phosphatase SHP-1 predicts outcome after radical prostatectomy for localized prostate cancer. *Int J Cancer.* 126, 2296-2307.

Tautz, L. and Mustelin, T. (2007) Strategies for developing protein tyrosine phosphatase inhibitors. Methods 42, 250-260.

The Gene Ontology Consortium. (2000) Gene Ontology: tool for the unification of biology. *Nat Genet* 25, 25-29.

Todd, J.L., Tanner, K.G., Denu, J.M. (1999) Extracellular regulated kinases (ERK) 1 and ERK2 are authentic substrates for the dual-specificity protein-tyrosine phosphatase VHR: a novel role in down-regulating the ERK pathway. *J Biol Chem* 274, 13271-13280.

Todd, J.L., Rigas, J.D., Rafty, L.A., Denu, J.M. (2002) Dual-specificity protein tyrosine phosphatase VHR down-regulates c-Jun N-terminal kinase (JNK). *Oncogene* 21, 2573-2583.

Tomic, S., Greiser, U., Lammers, R., Kharitonenkov, A., Imyanitov , E., Ullrich, A., Bohmer, F.D. (1995) Association of SH2 domain protein tyrosine phosphatases with the epidermal growth factor receptor in human tumor cells. Phosphatidic acid activates receptor dephosphorylation by PTP1C. *J BiolChem* 270, 21277–21284.

Tonks, N.K. (2006) Protein tyrosine phosphatases: from genes, to function, to disease. *Nature Rev. Mol. Cell Biol.* 7, 833-846.

Turowski, P., Franckhauser, C., Morris, M.C., Vaglio, P., Fernandez, A., Lamb, N.J.C. (2003) Functional cdc25C dual specificity phosphatase is required for S-phase entry in human cells. *Mol Biol Cell* 14, 2984-2998.

Umezawa, K., Kawakami, M. and Watanabe, T. (2003) Molecular design and biological activities of protein tyrosine phosphatase inhibitors. *Pharmacol. & Therap.* 99, 15-24.

Uzoh, C.C., Perks, C.M., Bahl, A., Holly, J.M., Sugiono, M., Persad, R.A. (2009) PTEN-mediated pathways and their association with treatment-resistant prostate cancer. *British J Urol Intl* 104, 556-561.

Valencia, A.M., Oliva, J.L., Bodega, G. (1997) Identification of a protein-tyrosine phosphatase (SHP1) different from that associated with acid phosphatase in rat prostate. *FEBS Letters*, 406, 42–48.

Veeramani, S., Yuan, T.C., Chen, S.J., Lin, F.F., Petersen, J.E., Shaheduzzaman, S., Srisvatava, S., MacDonald, R.G. and Lin,M.F. (2005) Cellular prostatic acid phosphatase: a protein tyrosine phosphatase involved in androgen-independent proliferation of prostate cancer. *Endocrine-Rel. Cancer* 12, 805-822.

Wishart, M.J., Dixon, J.E. (2002) PTEN and myotubularin phosphatases: from 3-phosphoinositide dephosphorylation to disease, Trends Cell Biol. 12, 579-585.

Wu, C., Sun, M., Liu, L., Zhou, G.W. (2003) The function of the protein tyrosine phosphatase SHP-1 in cancer. *Gene.* 306, 1-12.

Wu, Q., Huang, S., Sun, Y., Gu, S., Lu, F., Dai, J., Yin, G., Sun, L., Zheng, D., Dou, C., Feng, C., Ji, C., Xie, Y., Mao, Y.. (2006) Dual specificity phosphotase 18, interacting with SAPK, dephosphorylates SAPK and inhibits SAPK/JNK signal pathway *in vivo*. *Front Biosci* 11, 2714-2724.

Zabell, A.P.R., Forden, S., Helquist, P., Stauffacher, C.V. and Wiest, O. (2004) Inhibition studies with rationally designed inhibitors of the human low molecular weiht protein tyrosine phosphatase. *Biorg. & Med. Chem.* 12, 1867-1880.

Zambuzzi, W.F., Coelho, P.G., Alves, G.G., Granjeiro, J.M. (2011) Intracellular signal transduction as a factor in the development of "smart" biomaterials for bone tissue engineering. *Biotechnol Bioeng.* 108, 1246-1250

Zambuzzi, W.F., Milani, R., Teti, A. (2011) Expanding the role of Src and protein-tyrosine phosphatases balance in modulating osteoblast metabolism: lessons from mice. *Biochimie.* 92, 327-332.

Zapata, P.D., Ropero, R.M., Valencia, A.M., Buscail, L., López, J.I., Martín-Orozco, R.M., Prieto, J.C., Angulo, J., Susini, C., López-Ruiz, P., Colás, B. (2002) Autocrine regulation of human prostate carcinoma cell proliferation by somatostatin through the modulation of the SH2 domain containing protein tyrosine phosphatase (SHP)-1. *J Clin Endocrinol Metab.* 87, 915-926.

Zhang, Y *et al.* (2004) Regulation of innate and adaptive immune responses by MAP kinase phosphatase 5. *Nature* 430:793-797.

Zhang, Z.-Y. (2003) Chemical and mechanistic approaches to the study of protein tyrosine phosphatases. *Acc. Chem. Res.* 36, 385-392.

Zhang, Z.-Y. (1997) Structure, mechanism, and specificity of protein-tyrosine phosphatases. *Curr. Top. Cell. Regul.* 35, 21-68.

Zhou, B., Wang, Z.X., Zhao, Y., Brautigan, D.L., Zhang, Z.Y. (2002) The specificity of extracellular signal-regulated kinase 2 dephosphorylation by protein phosphatases. *J Biol Chem* 277, 31818-31825.

TRP-Channels and Human Prostate Carcinogenesis

V'yacheslav Lehen'kyi and Natalia Prevarskaya
INSERM, Laboratoire de Physiologie Cellulaire, Equipe labellisée par la Ligue contre le cancer, Villeneuve d'Ascq and Université de Lille 1, Villeneuve d'Ascq
France

1. Introduction

Malignant transformation of cells resulting from enhanced proliferation, aberrant differentiation, and impaired ability to die is the prime reason for abnormal tissue growth, which can eventually turn into uncontrolled expansion and invasion, characteristic of cancer (Hanahan and Weinberg, 2011). Such transformation is often accompanied by changes in ion channel expression and, consequently, by abnormal progression of the cellular responses with which they are involved. The first important role ascribed to plasma membrane ion channels, over 60 years ago, was their participation in cellular electrogenesis and electrical excitability. However, numerous subsequent studies have firmly established the contribution of ion channels to virtually all basic cellular behaviors, including such crucial ones for maintaining tissue homeostasis as proliferation, differentiation, and apoptosis (Lang et al., 2005; Razik and Cidlowski, 2002; Schonherr, 2005). The major mechanisms via which ion channels contribute to these crucial processes include: providing the influx of essential signaling ions, regulating cell volume, and maintaining membrane potential. Malignant transformation of cells resulting from enhanced proliferation, aberrant differentiation, and impaired ability to due is the prime reason for abnormal tissue growth, which can eventually turn into uncontrolled expansion and invasion, characteristic of cancer (Chaffer and Weinberg, 2011). This review focuses on the aspects prostate tumour carcinogenesis influenced by various ion channels belonging to a large superfamily of Transient Receptor Potential (TRP) channels and how dysfunctions and/or misregulations of these channels may influence the development and progression of prostate cancer.

2. TRP-channels and epithelial cell homeostasis

Transient Receptor Potential (TRP) channels are a recently discovered superfamily of non-selective cationic channels defined firstly as mechanoreceptors. They are predominantly expressed in epithelial tissues and carry a plethora of functions including but not limited to sensation of chemical, mechanical, and thermo stimuli (for review see (Clapham et al., 2001)). According to a growing number of articles, non-voltage dependent cationic channels of the Transient Receptor Potential (TRP) channel family are key players in ion homeostasis. All TRPs contain six putative transmembrane domains, which are thought to assemble as homo- or hetero-tetramers to form cation selective channels. All TRPs are cation channels, although the permeability for different mono- and divalent cations varies greatly between isoforms. Based on amino acid homologies, the mammalian TRP channel superfamily can be divided into seven families. About thirty members of the TRP superfamily identified in mammals are classified in six different families: TRPC for «Canonical», TRPV for «Vanilloid», TRPM for «Melastatin», TRPML for «Mucolipins», TRPP for «Polycystins» and TRPA for «Ankirin transmembrane», and the TRPN (no mechanoreceptor potential C, or NOMPC). The characteristic feature of TRP channels is their ability to be activated by a wide range of chemical and mechanical stimuli. TRP channels are activated by a wide range of stimuli including intra- and extracellular messengers, chemical, mechanical and osmotic stress, and some probably by the filling state of intracellular Ca2+ stores (Clapham, 2003). As such, they can be envisioned as the polymodal molecular sensors of the cell.

For instance, all channels of the TRPC family are activated by stimulation of receptors that activate different isoforms of PLC, i.e. PLCβ after activation of G-protein coupled receptors (GPCRs), and PLCγ after activation of receptor tyrosine kinases (RTKs) (Clapham, 2003). TRPCs have also been widely proposed to be regulated by the filling status of intracellular Ca2+ stores, and consequently to be the elusive molecular candidates for store-operated Ca2+ entry channels (SOCs) (Clapham et al., 2001). However, both store-depletion dependent and independent mechanisms have been suggested for all members of the TRPC family, and at variance with a physiological role as SOCs, there is evidence that TRPC1, TRP4/5 and TRPC3/6/7 can function as receptor-operated channels that are mostly insensitive to store depletion (Lintschinger et al., 2000; Nilius, 2004; Plant and Schaefer, 2003).

At the same time TRPV1–4 are non-selective cation channels which are thermosensitive, although TRPV1 and 4, can also be activated by numerous other stimuli (Nilius et al., 2003). TRPV3, and to a lesser extend also TRPV2 and TRPV1, but not TRPV4, can be activated by 2-aminoethoxydiphenyl borate (2-APB), which, in contrast, blocks some TRPC and TRPM channels (Hu et al., 2004). Other members as TRPV5 and TRPV6 are highly expressed in the kidney and intestine, respectively, where they form highly selective Ca2+ channels essential for Ca2+ reabsorption (Nijenhuis et al., 2003).

TRPM channels exhibit highly varying permeability to Ca2+ and Mg2+, from Ca2+-impermeable (TRPM4 and 5) to highly Ca2+ and Mg2+ permeable (TRPM6 and 7). In contrast to that of TRPCs and TRPVs, the TRPM sequence does not contain ankyrin repeats. TRPM channel has a vide pattern of expression in human body and many of them are also temperature sensitive (Clapham, 2003).

The TRPML proteins are relative small (less than 600 residues), and have relatively low sequence homology to other TRP families. TRPML1 is widely expressed, and appears to reside in late endosomes/lysosomes (LaPlante et al., 2004). TRPML1-mediated control of lysosomal Ca2+ levels plays an important role in proper lysosome formation and recycling (Piper and Luzio, 2004).

A significant body of evidence indicates that TRPP1 and TRPP2 are physically coupled and act as a signaling complex which is necessary for localization of TRPP2 to the plasma membrane (Hanaoka et al., 2000), and in which the association of TRPP1 and TRPP2 suppresses the G-protein stimulating activity of TRPP1 as well as the constitutive channel activity of TRPP2 (Delmas et al., 2004). It should be noted that TRPP2 likely has roles independent of TRPP1, as TRPP2 expression and TRPP2-like activity has been detected in left ventricular myocytes in the absence of TRPP1 (Volk et al., 2003).

The TRPA family currently comprises just one mammalian member, TRPA1, which has been shown to be expressed in in hair cells (Corey et al., 2004), and in DRG and TG neurons (Story et al., 2003). TRPA1 exhibits intruiging gating promiscuity, and might be involved in pain perception, temperature sensing, and mechanosensation, e.g. hearing (Voets et al., 2005). This subfamily TRPN comprises a single member, found in C. elegans, Drosophila and zebra fish whereas the mammalian genome appears to lack the TRPN gene (Corey et al., 2004).

A large number of TRP channel binding partners have recently been described, many of which have been assigned important roles in the regulation and function of TRP channels. All TRPs also contain consensus sites for direct phosphorylation by serine/threonine and tyrosine kinases, although the role of phosphorylation in channel function remains to be fully elucidated. Also, in addition to regulatory modes activating TRP channels resident in the plasma membrane, several TRPs appear to be constitutively open, and may be regulated by vesicular insertion (Bezzerides et al., 2004; Iwata et al., 2003). Most, but not all, of the TRP channels function as Ca2+ pathways, cause cell depolarization, and also form intracellular pathways for Ca2+ release from various intracellular stores, such as the endo- and sarcoplasmic reticulum, lysosomes, and endosomes (Clapham et al., 2001). Beyond their sensory functions, they are broadly involved in diverse homeostatic functions. It is not surprising, therefore, that dysfunctions of these TRP channels are involved in the pathogenesis of several diseases (Tsavaler et al., 2001; Wissenbach et al., 2001). Many TRP channels have so far been described in the genitourinary tract (Peng et al., 2001b; Tsavaler et al., 2001) and more specifically in the prostate, where they are suggested to play a role in normal prostate physiology and prostate diseases, most importantly in prostate carcinogenesis.

3. TRPM channels and their possible implication in prostate cancer initiation

In 2009 a new TRPM channel, TRPM2, has been identified in prostate cancer cell lines (Zeng et al., 2010). TRPM2 encodes a non-selective cation-permeable ion channel and it has benn found that selectively knocking down TRPM2 with the small interfering RNA technique inhibited the growth of prostate cancer cells but not of non-cancerous cells. The subcellular localization of this protein is also remarkably different between cancerous and non-cancerous cells. In BPH-1 (benign), TRPM2 protein is homogenously located near the plasma membrane and in the cytoplasm, whereas in the cancerous cells (PC-3 and DU-145), a significant amount of the TRPM2 protein is located in the nuclei in a clustered pattern (Zeng et al., 2010).

TRPM4 levels were shown to be elevated in prostate cancer (Armisen et al., 2011). However, whether such changes in TRPM4 expression may be relevant to genesis or progression of prostate cancer remains unknown.

The last member of this family TRPM8 channel has been firstly cloned in 2001 as a novel prostate-specific gene by screening a prostate cDNA library (Tsavaler et al., 2001). Later on, it was shown that TRPM8 encodes for a cold- and menthol-sensitive ion channel in trigeminal ganglion and dorsal root ganglion neurons (TGN and DRG) (Voets et al., 2007). Moreover, the mRNA levels in BPH and PCa appeared to be higher than in the normal prostate (Tsavaler et al., 2001). Several groups have studied the expression of TRPM8 in different PCa cell lines. In primary cultures of prostate epithelial cells, the density of the TRPM8 membrane current was increased in cancerous compared to normal cells (Bidaux et al., 2007). Moreover, RT-PCR analysis of these cells revealed an up-regulation of TRPM8 in PCa-derived cells (Bidaux et al., 2007). Also in tumoral cell lines, such as LNCaP ("lymph node carcinoma of the prostate", a widely used cell line derived from a supraclavicular lymph node metastasis expressing the androgen receptor [AR] (Horoszewicz et al., 1983)), TRPM8 was detected by RT-PCR (Tsavaler et al., 2001). Zhang and Barritt also suggested a functional role for TRPM8 in LNCaP cells, since temperatures below 28°C or application of 100 µM menthol, which is sufficient for TRPM8 activation, led to an increase in [Ca2+]cyt (Zhang and Barritt, 2004). Regarding the localization of TRPM8 in LNCaP, Thebault et al. reported that TRPM8 was almost exclusively expressed in the endoplasmic reticulum (Thebault et al., 2005), whereas Mahieu et al. reported a mainly plasmamembrane localization of TRPM8 (Mahieu et al., 2007).

Bidaux et al. reported that TRPM8 expression requires a functional AR. Transfection of the AR into PNT1A cells, which lack the expression of the AR in normal physiological conditions, induced the appearance of TRPM8 that could be reversed by incubation of siRNA-AR (Bidaux et al., 2005). Primary cultures of prostate epithelial cells expressed the AR, TRPM8, CK8, and CK18 after 12 days, but after 20 days, the cultured cells displayed a more basal epithelial phenotype, expressing CK5 and CK14, but not the AR and TRPM8 (Bidaux et al., 2007). Moreover, it seems that the AR regulates the membranic translocation of TRPM8, since TRPM8 resides in the ER in the absence of the AR, and only appears in the plasmamembrane when the AR is expressed. The authors postulated the hypothesis of a shift of plasma membrane TRPM8 in normal apical fully differentiated epithelial cells to endoplasmic reticulum TRPM8 in a metastatic PCa cell during prostate carcinogenesis (Bidaux et al., 2007).

Several studies using quantitative RT-PCR revealed a significantly increased expression of TRPM8 mRNA in malignant prostate samples in comparison to nonmalignant tissue, suggesting that the level of TRPM8 in biopsy specimens could be used in the diagnosis of PCa (Fuessel et al., 2003). This elevation seemed to be statistically significant, unlike the relative transcript-level elevation of PSA mRNA (Fuessel et al., 2003). However, no clear correlation of TRPM8 expression with the pathological grade of PCa could be found (Kiessling et al., 2003). Moreover, Henshall et al. showed a strong correlation between the level of TRPM8 mRNA expression and disease relapse after radical prostatectomy, as loss of TRPM8 was associated with a significantly shorter time to PSA relapse-free survival (Henshall et al., 2003).

4. TRPC channels in prostate cancer cell survival

The first TRPC channel which has been described in the prostate was TRPC3. Using Northern blot analysis, the expression of this gene was described in the normal prostate (Zhu et al., 1996). On the other hand, a more extensive quantitative TRP expression study in human prostate samples revealed the abundant expression of TRPC1, TRPC4, and TRPC6, whereas TRPC3, TRPC5, and TRPC7 were hardly detected (Riccio et al., 2002). In addition to normal prostate, immunohistochemistry revealed expression of TRPC6 in BPH and, more importantly, a significant overexpression in PCa specimens. Higher pathological stages of PCa tended to have increased TRPC6 expression, but these differences were not statistically significant among pT2, pT3, and pT4 PCa (Yue et al., 2009). Human primary prostate epithelial cell cultures expressed TRPC1A, a TRPC1 splice variant, TRPC3, TRPC4 (and the splice variant TRPC4β), and TRPC6 (and the splice variant TRPC6γ) at the mRNA level (Thebault et al., 2006). In LNCaP, the presence of TRPC1, TRPC3, TRPC5, and TRPC7 was detected; TRPC6, however, seemed not to be present (Pigozzi et al., 2006).

The functional role of TRPC channels in the prostate has been investigated in human primary prostate epithelial cell cultures, using antisense assays of TRPC1, TRPC3, TRPC4, and TRPC6 (Thebault et al., 2006). It was postulated that TRPC1 and TRPC4 were exclusively involved in ATP-stimulated, store-dependent Ca2+ entry (SOCE), whereas TRPC6 was the diacylglycerol-gated, channel mediating α1-AR (α1-adrenergic receptor) agonist–stimulated Ca2+ influx (store independent). Moreover, treatment of the cultures with α1-AR agonists enhanced cell proliferation, in contrast to ATP, which had an inhibitory effect. Therefore, authors concluded that TRPC6 is a crucial mediator of the proliferative effects of α1-AR agonists. TRPC1 and TRPC4, on the other hand, are the major contributors of SOC activation in response to ATP (Thebault et al., 2006). In LNCaP, TRPC1 and TRPC3 were overexpressed after prolonged intracellular Ca2+ store depletion due to the decreased levels of [Ca2+]cyt. LNCaP cells overexpressing TRPC1 and TRPC3 showed an increased [Ca2+]cyt response to α-adrenergic stimulation, but SOCE entry remained unaffected. Thus, expression of TRPC1 and TRPC3 is not sufficient for SOC formation (Pigozzi et al., 2006), though the other authors have considered TRPC1 as the most likely molecular candidate for the formation of prostate-specific endogenous SOCs which could participate to enhanced proliferation and apoptosis resistance (Vanden Abeele et al., 2003).

5. TRPV channels as a hallmark of advanced prostate cancer

Vanilloid receptor subtype-1 (TRPV1), the founding member of the vanilloid receptor-like transient receptor potential channel family, is a non-selective cation channel that responds to noxious stimuli such as low pH, painful heat and irritants. It has been shown that the vanilloid TRPV1 receptor is expressed in the prostate epithelial cell lines PC-3 and LNCaP as well as in human prostate tissue (Sanchez et al., 2005). The contribution of the endogenously expressed TRPV1 channel to intracellular calcium concentration increase in the prostate cells showed that the addition of capsaicin, (R)-methanandamide and resiniferatoxin to prostate cells induced a dose-dependent increase in the intracellular calcium concentration that was reversed by the vanilloid TRPV1 receptor antagonist capsazepine. These results indicate that the vanilloid TRPV1 receptor is expressed and functionally active in human prostate cells (Sanchez et al., 2005).

Capsaicin-treated PC-3 cells increased the synthesis and secretion of IL-6 which was abrogated by the transient receptor potential vanilloid receptor subtype 1 (TRPV1) antagonist capsazepine, as well as by inhibitors of PKC-α, phosphoinositol-3 phosphate kinase (PI-3K), Akt and extracellular signal-regulated protein kinase (ERK) (Malagarie-Cazenave et al., 2011). Furthermore, incubation of PC-3 cells with an anti-TNF-α antibody blocked the capsaicin-induced IL-6 secretion. These results raise the possibility that capsaicin-mediated IL-6 increase in prostate cancer PC-3 cells is regulated at least in part by TNF-α secretion and signaling pathway involving Akt, ERK and PKC-α activation (Malagarie-Cazenave et al., 2011).

The nonselective cationic channel transient receptor potential vanilloid 2 (TRPV2) is a distinctive feature of castration-resistant PCa (Monet et al., 2010). TRPV2 transcript levels were higher in patients with metastatic cancer (stage M1) compared with primary solid tumors (stages T2a and T2b). Introducing TRPV2 into androgen-dependent LNCaP cells enhanced cell migration along with expression of invasion markers matrix metalloproteinase (MMP) 9 and cathepsin B. Consistent with the likelihood that TRPV2 may affect cancer cell aggressiveness by influencing basal intracellular calcium levels, small interfering RNA-mediated silencing of TRPV2 reduced the growth and invasive properties of PC3 prostate tumors established in nude mice xenografts, and diminished expression of invasive enzymes MMP2, MMP9, and cathepsin B. These findings establish a role for TRPV2 in PCa progression to the aggressive castration-resistant stage, prompting evaluation of TRPV2 as a potential prognostic marker and therapeutic target in the setting of advanced PCa (Monet et al., 2010). Though the physiological role, the mechanisms of activation, as well as the endogenous regulators for the non-selective cationic channel TRPV2 are not clear far. It was shown that endogenous lysophospholipids such as lysophosphatidylcholine

(LPC) and lysophosphatidylinositol (LPI) induce a calcium influx via TRPV2 channel (Monet et al., 2009). TRPV2-mediated calcium uptake stimulated by LPC and LPI occurred via Gq/Go-protein and phosphatidylinositol-3,4 kinase (PI3,4K) signalling. The activation of TRPV2 channel by LPC and LPI leads to an increase in the cell migration of the prostate cancer cell line PC3 (Monet et al., 2009).

TRPV6, an epithelium TRP channel highly selective for Ca2+ in organs that reabsorb Ca2+, was originally cloned from rat duodenum as a Ca2+ transport protein (Wissenbach and Niemeyer, 2007). In 2001, using Northern blot and in situ hybridization, Wissenbach et al. described that TRPV6 was present in PCa tissue specimens and in lymph node metastasis, but not in BPH or in normal prostate. The most elevated levels of TRPV6 mRNA were found in high-grade, locally advanced (pT3a/b) prostate tumors, whereas no TRPV6 mRNA was detectable in low-grade PCa, suggesting that TRPV6 could be a promising prostate tumor marker (Wissenbach et al., 2001). The onset of PCa seemed to be independent of the TRPV6 genotype (Kessler et al., 2009). In 2001, Peng et al. (Peng et al., 2001a) confirmed these results via in situ hybridization experiments, but claimed that TRPV6 was also expressed in normal epithelial cells, BPH tissue, and LNCaP cells. Interestingly, TRPV6 mRNA expression correlated significantly with the Gleason score and the pathological stage (TRPV6 was absent in normal prostate, BPH, and pT1a/b lesions, but appeared in higher pathological stages)(Fixemer et al., 2003). Androgen Regulation of TRPV6 Peng et al. suggested in 2001 that TRPV6 expression was androgen controlled, showing that the administration of AR antagonists to LNCaP cells resulted in a twofold increase of TRPV6 mRNA levels, whereas adding dihydrotestosterone (DHT) decreased TRPV6 levels (Peng et al., 2001b). In contrast, TRPV6 mRNA expression studies revealed decreased TRPV6 expression levels in androgen-deprived human prostates (Fixemer et al., 2003). Other authors found that the application of AR antagonists or DHT had no significant effects on TRPV6 expression in LNCaP cells at all (Lehen'kyi et al., 2007). siRNA knockdown of the AR, however, induced a significant decrease of TRPV6 expression. Moreover, it was suggested that TRPV6 was regulated by the AR in a ligand-independent manner and that the AR constituted an essential cofactor of TRPV6 gene transcription in LNCaP cells (Lehen'kyi et al., 2007).

From the other side, it's known that cell hyperpolarization will always increase the driving force for Ca2+ entry via Ca2+-permeable ion channels, such as TRPV6. Ca2+ entry via these channels depends on coactivation of the intermediate-conductance, calcium-activated, potassium channels (IKCa or according to the IUPHAR nomenclature KCa3.1 or SK41) (Alexander et al., 2007), which are expressed in LNCaP cells as well as in primary prostate epithelial cultures. Moreover, KCa3.1 seemed to be preferentially expressed in PCa tissue, leading to hyperpolarization of the plasma membrane, after which TRPV6 is opened and Ca2+ influx occurs. siRNA knockdown of KCa3.1 and blocking of KCa3.1 led to a decreased cell proliferation in LNCaP (Lallet-Daher et al., 2009). Role of TRPV6 in Prostate Authors suggested a role for TRPV6 in cell proliferation. TRPV6 increased the proliferation rate of HEK cells in a Ca2+-dependent manner. As TRPV6 slightly enhanced global resting [Ca2+]cyt, these small changes could indeed increase proliferation rate. This suggests a causal relationship between PCa progression and TRPV6 expression (Schwarz et al., 2006). Lehen'kyi et al. showed that silencing assays of TRPV6 in LNCaP led to a decreased number of viable cells. They suggested a role for TRPV6 in LNCaP proliferation by mediating Ca2+ entry, which is followed by the activation of Ca2+-dependent NFAT ("nuclear factor of activated T cells", a nuclear transcription factor) signaling pathways. As such, TRPV6 increased cell survival and induced apoptosis resistance (Lehen'kyi et al., 2007).

6. Conclusions

TRP channels are multifunctional sensors of environmental factors in the form of physical and chemical stimuli. They are widely expressed in the central nerve system and peripheral cell types, and are involved in numerous fundamental cell functions. In accordance with this, an increasing number of important pathological conditions are now being linked to TRP dysfunction. Though several TRP channels have been identified in the human prostate using non- or semi-quantitative methods, no TRP channels have definite, clear roles in prostate physiology or carcinogenesis. The majority of the TRP expression studies in the human prostate have used random prostate tissue, whereas the prostate itself is an extremely heterogeneous organ. There is a definite need for more appropriate prostate epithelial cell models, such as primary cultures of prostate epithelial cells, but the latter should be more thoroughly characterized. Many aspects of the physiology and regulation of TRPs are, however, still elusive, especially for some of the novel TRP family members. It is to be expected that the further evaluation of the cellular functions, regulation, and binding partners of TRPs, and their genetic and molecular properties may have an enormous impact in human prostate pathopysiology and disease and will become an urgent priority in biomedical sciences.

Finally, the use of some of TRP channels as cancer biomarkers has been proposed and for some of them (as TRPV2 and TRPV6) the role as potential pharmaceutical targets has been predicted. Nevertheless, further studies using *in vivo* models are needed to establish this TRP channels as potential pharmaceutical targets for the future interventions in the treatment of the early and the late prostate cancer stages.

7. References

Alexander, S. P., Mathie, A., and Peters, J. A. (2007). Guide to Receptors and Channels (GRAC), 2nd edition (2007 Revision). Br J Pharmacol *150 Suppl 1*, S1-168.

Armisen, R., Marcelain, K., Simon, F., Tapia, J. C., Toro, J., Quest, A. F., and Stutzin, A. (2011). TRPM4 enhances cell proliferation through up-regulation of the beta-catenin signaling pathway. Journal of cellular physiology *226*, 103-109.

Bezzerides, V. J., Ramsey, I. S., Kotecha, S., Greka, A., and Clapham, D. E. (2004). Rapid vesicular translocation and insertion of TRP channels. Nat Cell Biol *6*, 709-720.

Bidaux, G., Flourakis, M., Thebault, S., Zholos, A., Beck, B., Gkika, D., Roudbaraki, M., Bonnal, J. L., Mauroy, B., Shuba, Y., *et al.* (2007). Prostate cell differentiation status determines transient receptor potential melastatin member 8 channel subcellular localization and function. J Clin Invest *117*, 1647-1657.

Bidaux, G., Roudbaraki, M., Merle, C., Crepin, A., Delcourt, P., Slomianny, C., Thebault, S., Bonnal, J. L., Benahmed, M., Cabon, F., *et al.* (2005). Evidence for specific TRPM8 expression in human prostate secretory epithelial cells: functional androgen receptor requirement. Endocrine-related cancer *12*, 367-382.

Chaffer, C. L., and Weinberg, R. A. A perspective on cancer cell metastasis. (2011). Science (New York, NY 331, 1559-1564.

Clapham, D. E. (2003). TRP channels as cellular sensors. Nature *426*, 517-524.

Clapham, D. E., Runnels, L. W., and Strubing, C. (2001). The TRP ion channel family. Nat Rev Neurosci *2*, 387-396.

Corey, D. P., Garcia-Anoveros, J., Holt, J. R., Kwan, K. Y., Lin, S. Y., Vollrath, M. A., Amalfitano, A., Cheung, E. L., Derfler, B. H., Duggan, A., *et al.* (2004). TRPA1 is a candidate for the mechanosensitive transduction channel of vertebrate hair cells. Nature 432, 723-730.

Delmas, P., Nauli, S. M., Li, X., Coste, B., Osorio, N., Crest, M., Brown, D. A., and Zhou, J. (2004). Gating of the polycystin ion channel signaling complex in neurons and kidney cells. FASEB J 18, 740-742.

Fixemer, T., Wissenbach, U., Flockerzi, V., and Bonkhoff, H. (2003). Expression of the Ca2+-selective cation channel TRPV6 in human prostate cancer: a novel prognostic marker for tumor progression. Oncogene 22, 7858-7861.

Fuessel, S., Sickert, D., Meye, A., Klenk, U., Schmidt, U., Schmitz, M., Rost, A. K., Weigle, B., Kiessling, A., and Wirth, M. P. (2003). Multiple tumor marker analyses (PSA, hK2, PSCA, trp-p8) in primary prostate cancers using quantitative RT-PCR. Int J Oncol 23, 221-228.

Hanahan, D., and Weinberg, R. A. (2011). Hallmarks of cancer: the next generation. Cell 144, 646-674.

Hanaoka, K., Qian, F., Boletta, A., Bhunia, A. K., Piontek, K., Tsiokas, L., Sukhatme, V. P., Guggino, W. B., and Germino, G. G. (2000). Co-assembly of polycystin-1 and -2 produces unique cation-permeable currents. Nature 408, 990-994.

Henshall, S. M., Afar, D. E., Hiller, J., Horvath, L. G., Quinn, D. I., Rasiah, K. K., Gish, K., Willhite, D., Kench, J. G., Gardiner-Garden, M., et al. (2003). Survival analysis of genome-wide gene expression profiles of prostate cancers identifies new prognostic targets of disease relapse. Cancer research 63, 4196-4203.

Horoszewicz, J. S., Leong, S. S., Kawinski, E., Karr, J. P., Rosenthal, H., Chu, T. M., Mirand, E. A., and Murphy, G. P. (1983). LNCaP model of human prostatic carcinoma. Cancer research 43, 1809-1818.

Hu, H. Z., Gu, Q., Wang, C., Colton, C. K., Tang, J., Kinoshita-Kawada, M., Lee, L. Y., Wood, J. D., and Zhu, M. X. (2004). 2-aminoethoxydiphenyl borate is a common activator of TRPV1, TRPV2, and TRPV3. The Journal of biological chemistry 279, 35741-35748.

Iwata, Y., Katanosaka, Y., Arai, Y., Komamura, K., Miyatake, K., and Shigekawa, M. (2003). A novel mechanism of myocyte degeneration involving the Ca2+-permeable growth factor-regulated channel. J Cell Biol 161, 957-967.

Kessler, T., Wissenbach, U., Grobholz, R., and Flockerzi, V. (2009). TRPV6 alleles do not influence prostate cancer progression. BMC Cancer 9, 380.

Kiessling, A., Fussel, S., Schmitz, M., Stevanovic, S., Meye, A., Weigle, B., Klenk, U., Wirth, M. P., and Rieber, E. P. (2003). Identification of an HLA-A*0201-restricted T-cell epitope derived from the prostate cancer-associated protein trp-p8. The Prostate 56, 270-279.

Lallet-Daher, H., Roudbaraki, M., Bavencoffe, A., Mariot, P., Gackiere, F., Bidaux, G., Urbain, R., Gosset, P., Delcourt, P., Fleurisse, L., et al. (2009). Intermediate-conductance Ca2+-activated K+ channels (IKCa1) regulate human prostate cancer cell proliferation through a close control of calcium entry. Oncogene 28, 1792-1806.

Lang, F., Foller, M., Lang, K. S., Lang, P. A., Ritter, M., Gulbins, E., Vereninov, A., and Huber, S. M. (2005). Ion channels in cell proliferation and apoptotic cell death. The Journal of membrane biology 205, 147-157.

LaPlante, J. M., Ye, C. P., Quinn, S. J., Goldin, E., Brown, E. M., Slaugenhaupt, S. A., and Vassilev, P. M. (2004). Functional links between mucolipin-1 and Ca2+-dependent membrane trafficking in mucolipidosis IV. Biochemical and biophysical research communications 322, 1384-1391.

Lehen'kyi, V., Flourakis, M., Skryma, R., and Prevarskaya, N. (2007). TRPV6 channel controls prostate cancer cell proliferation via Ca(2+)/NFAT-dependent pathways. Oncogene 26, 7380-7385.

Lintschinger, B., Balzer-Geldsetzer, M., Baskaran, T., Graier, W. F., Romanin, C., Zhu, M. X., and Groschner, K. (2000). Coassembly of Trp1 and Trp3 proteins generates diacylglycerol- and Ca2+-sensitive cation channels. The Journal of biological chemistry 275, 27799-27805.

Mahieu, F., Owsianik, G., Verbert, L., Janssens, A., De Smedt, H., Nilius, B., and Voets, T. (2007). TRPM8-independent menthol-induced Ca2+ release from endoplasmic reticulum and Golgi. The Journal of biological chemistry 282, 3325-3336.

Malagarie-Cazenave, S., Olea-Herrero, N., Vara, D., Morell, C., and Diaz-Laviada, I. (2011). The vanilloid capsaicin induces IL-6 secretion in prostate PC-3 cancer cells. Cytokine 54, 330-337.

Monet, M., Gkika, D., Lehen'kyi, V., Pourtier, A., Vanden Abeele, F., Bidaux, G., Juvin, V., Rassendren, F., Humez, S., and Prevarsakaya, N. (2009). Lysophospholipids stimulate prostate cancer cell migration via TRPV2 channel activation. Biochimica et biophysica acta 1793, 528-539.

Monet, M., Lehen'kyi, V., Gackiere, F., Firlej, V., Vandenberghe, M., Roudbaraki, M., Gkika, D., Pourtier, A., Bidaux, G., Slomianny, C., et al. (2010). Role of cationic channel TRPV2 in promoting prostate cancer migration and progression to androgen resistance. Cancer research 70, 1225-1235.

Nijenhuis, T., Hoenderop, J. G., van der Kemp, A. W., and Bindels, R. J. (2003). Localization and regulation of the epithelial Ca2+ channel TRPV6 in the kidney. J Am Soc Nephrol 14, 2731-2740.

Nilius, B. (2004). Store-operated Ca2+ entry channels: still elusive! Sci STKE 2004, pe36.

Nilius, B., Watanabe, H., and Vriens, J. (2003). The TRPV4 channel: structure-function relationship and promiscuous gating behaviour. Pflugers Arch 446, 298-303.

Peng, J. B., Brown, E. M., and Hediger, M. A. (2001a). Structural conservation of the genes encoding CaT1, CaT2, and related cation channels. Genomics 76, 99-109.

Peng, J. B., Zhuang, L., Berger, U. V., Adam, R. M., Williams, B. J., Brown, E. M., Hediger, M. A., and Freeman, M. R. (2001b). CaT1 expression correlates with tumor grade in prostate cancer. Biochem Biophys Res Commun 282, 729-734.

Pigozzi, D., Ducret, T., Tajeddine, N., Gala, J. L., Tombal, B., and Gailly, P. (2006). Calcium store contents control the expression of TRPC1, TRPC3 and TRPV6 proteins in LNCaP prostate cancer cell line. Cell calcium 39, 401-415.

Piper, R. C., and Luzio, J. P. (2004). CUPpling calcium to lysosomal biogenesis. Trends Cell Biol 14, 471-473.

Plant, T. D., and Schaefer, M. (2003). TRPC4 and TRPC5: receptor-operated Ca2+-permeable nonselective cation channels. Cell calcium 33, 441-450.

Razik, M. A., and Cidlowski, J. A. (2002). Molecular interplay between ion channels and the regulation of apoptosis. Biological research 35, 203-207.

Riccio, A., Medhurst, A. D., Mattei, C., Kelsell, R. E., Calver, A. R., Randall, A. D., Benham, C. D., and Pangalos, M. N. (2002). mRNA distribution analysis of human TRPC family in CNS and peripheral tissues. Brain Res Mol Brain Res 109, 95-104.

Sanchez, M. G., Sanchez, A. M., Collado, B., Malagarie-Cazenave, S., Olea, N., Carmena, M. J., Prieto, J. C., and Diaz-Laviada, I. I. (2005). Expression of the transient receptor potential vanilloid 1 (TRPV1) in LNCaP and PC-3 prostate cancer cells and in human prostate tissue. European journal of pharmacology 515, 20-27.

Schonherr, R. (2005). Clinical relevance of ion channels for diagnosis and therapy of cancer. The Journal of membrane biology 205, 175-184.

Schwarz, E. C., Wissenbach, U., Niemeyer, B. A., Strauss, B., Philipp, S. E., Flockerzi, V., and Hoth, M. (2006). TRPV6 potentiates calcium-dependent cell proliferation. Cell calcium 39, 163-173.

Story, G. M., Peier, A. M., Reeve, A. J., Eid, S. R., Mosbacher, J., Hricik, T. R., Earley, T. J., Hergarden, A. C., Andersson, D. A., Hwang, S. W., et al. (2003). ANKTM1, a TRP-like channel expressed in nociceptive neurons, is activated by cold temperatures. Cell 112, 819-829.

Thebault, S., Flourakis, M., Vanoverberghe, K., Vandermoere, F., Roudbaraki, M., Lehen'kyi, V., Slomianny, C., Beck, B., Mariot, P., Bonnal, J. L., et al. (2006). Differential role of transient receptor potential channels in Ca2+ entry and proliferation of prostate cancer epithelial cells. Cancer research 66, 2038-2047.

Thebault, S., Lemonnier, L., Bidaux, G., Flourakis, M., Bavencoffe, A., Gordienko, D., Roudbaraki, M., Delcourt, P., Panchin, Y., Shuba, Y., et al. (2005). Novel role of cold/menthol-sensitive transient receptor potential melastatine family member 8 (TRPM8) in the activation of store-operated channels in LNCaP human prostate cancer epithelial cells. The Journal of biological chemistry 280, 39423-39435.

Tsavaler, L., Shapero, M. H., Morkowski, S., and Laus, R. (2001). Trp-p8, a novel prostate-specific gene, is up-regulated in prostate cancer and other malignancies and shares high homology with transient receptor potential calcium channel proteins. Cancer Res 61, 3760-3769.

Vanden Abeele, F., Shuba, Y., Roudbaraki, M., Lemonnier, L., Vanoverberghe, K., Mariot, P., Skryma, R., and Prevarskaya, N. (2003). Store-operated Ca2+ channels in prostate cancer epithelial cells: function, regulation, and role in carcinogenesis. Cell calcium 33, 357-373.

Voets, T., Owsianik, G., and Nilius, B. (2007). Trpm8. Handb Exp Pharmacol, 329-344.

Voets, T., Talavera, K., Owsianik, G., and Nilius, B. (2005). Sensing with TRP channels. Nat Chem Biol 1, 85-92.

Volk, T., Schwoerer, A. P., Thiessen, S., Schultz, J. H., and Ehmke, H. (2003). A polycystin-2-like large conductance cation channel in rat left ventricular myocytes. Cardiovasc Res 58, 76-88.

Wissenbach, U., and Niemeyer, B. A. (2007). Trpv6. Handb Exp Pharmacol, 221-234.

Wissenbach, U., Niemeyer, B. A., Fixemer, T., Schneidewind, A., Trost, C., Cavalie, A., Reus, K., Meese, E., Bonkhoff, H., and Flockerzi, V. (2001). Expression of CaT-like, a novel calcium-selective channel, correlates with the malignancy of prostate cancer. J Biol Chem 276, 19461-19468.

Yue, D., Wang, Y., Xiao, J. Y., Wang, P., and Ren, C. S. (2009). Expression of TRPC6 in benign and malignant human prostate tissues. Asian J Androl 11, 541-547.

Zeng, X., Sikka, S. C., Huang, L., Sun, C., Xu, C., Jia, D., Abdel-Mageed, A. B., Pottle, J. E., Taylor, J. T., and Li, M. (2010). Novel role for the transient receptor potential channel TRPM2 in prostate cancer cell proliferation. Prostate Cancer Prostatic Dis 13, 195-201.

Zhang, L., and Barritt, G. J. (2004). Evidence that TRPM8 is an androgen-dependent Ca2+ channel required for the survival of prostate cancer cells. Cancer research 64, 8365-8373.

Zhu, X., Jiang, M., Peyton, M., Boulay, G., Hurst, R., Stefani, E., and Birnbaumer, L. (1996). trp, a novel mammalian gene family essential for agonist-activated capacitative Ca2+ entry. Cell 85, 661-671.

8

Clinical Relevance of Circulating Nucleic Acids in Blood of Prostate Cancer Patients

Heidi Schwarzenbach

Department of Tumour Biology, Center of Experimental Medicine, University Medical Center Hamburg-Eppendorf, Hamburg
Germany

1. Introduction

The prostate carcinoma is the most frequent cancer of men. In contrast to the second most lung cancer, there are no self-caused risk factors. Hence, the cause of prostate cancer is still unknown. Nevertheless, there are men having a higher risk to get prostate cancer than other men. In the early stage the disease is symptom-free, whereas in the advanced stage complaints, such as difficulty in urination, miction pains and bone pains may occur. If symptoms emerge, metastases, primarily in the local lymph nodes or the bone marrow, may frequently be diagnosed (Knudsen & Vasioukhin, 2010). A successive treatment is only possible if the tumour tissue did not metastasize. So far, the early diagnosis of prostate cancer is difficult and challenging. Usually, the diagnosis is associated with several prostate biopsies. The current standard screening method is carried out by measuring the level of the prostate specific antigen (PSA) in blood, combined with a digital rectal examination (Jones & Koeneman, 2008). However, in men starting from 50 years an increased PSA value can indicate benign prostatic hyperplasia or prostate cancer. Moreover, the increase in the blood level of PSA (biochemical recurrence) cannot differentiate between local and metastatic tumours (Jansen et al., 2008). Therefore, an increased PSA value has to be absolutely clarified. Moreover, most prostate tumours are initially sensitive to androgen ablation therapy. If the treatment is not curative, patients can become hormonal refractory. Although docetaxel-based chemotherapy remains the standard treatment for hormone-refractory prostate cancer (Tannock et al., 2004), few predictive factors for the efficacy of chemotherapy has been reported. Thus, new strategies of early prostate cancer diagnosis and prognosis should be developed.

During the last years, nucleic acids, such as DNA, RNA and microRNAs (miRs), which circulate in high concentrations in blood of cancer patients, have gained increasing attention and their potential value as possible biomarkers has been highlighted. To avoid tumour biopsies by invasive methods, cell-free nucleic acids in plasma or serum could serve as a "liquid biopsy" useful for diagnostic application of prostate cancer. This minimally invasive procedure delivers the possibility of taking repeated blood samples, consequently allowing the changes in cell-free nucleic acids to be traced during the natural course of the disease or during anti-cancer treatment. The current chapter focuses on the clinical utility of cell-free nucleic acids as blood-based biomarkers for prostate cancer, considering the genetic and epigenetic alterations that can be detected in circulating DNA as well as the modulated levels of miRs. The relationship between cell-free nucleic acids and micrometastatic cells is also discussed.

As a result of increased apoptotic and necrotic cell deaths during carcinogenesis, nucleic acids are released into the blood circulation (Jahr et al., 2001). The concentrations of these tumour-associated, cell-free nucleic acids may associate with tumour load and malignant progression towards metastatic relapse, and discriminate between men with localized prostate cancer and benign prostatic hyperplasia (Muller et al., 2006). Analyses of cell-free DNA allow the detection of tumour-specific genetic and epigenetic alterations of genes relevant to prostate cancer development and progression. In particular, DNA hypermethylation of pi-class glutathione S-transferase genes may be an additional blood-based biomarker relevant for prostate cancer. Combining the scrutiny of tumour-specific blood DNA with the screening of disseminated tumour cells - the putative precursor cells of metastases - in blood and bone marrow, may provide additional information for monitoring tumour progression and metastases, and support the molecular staging of prostate tumours (Schwarzenbach & Pantel, 2008; Ellinger et al., 2011). The approach could also favour an early intervention to therapy, and contribute to identify those patients with a higher risk for a recurrence. In addition, miRs involved in the regulatory networks of protein expression by binding to and repressing the translation of specific target mRNAs are frequently deregulated in cancer (Ozen et al., 2008). Recent measurements have shown that these small RNA molecules may become potential blood-based biomarkers for prostate cancer patients (Wang et al., 2009).

2. History and biology of circulating nucleic acids

In 1948, Mandel and Métais described the presence of cell-free nucleic acids in human blood for the first time (Mandel & Métais, 1948). This attracted little attention in the scientific community, and it was not until 1994 that the importance of circulating nucleic acids was recognized as a result of the detection of mutated RAS gene fragments in blood of cancer patients (Sorenson et al., 1994; Vasioukhin et al., 1994). Two years later, also microsatellite alterations on cell-free DNA could be detected in the blood (Nawroz et al., 1996). These findings were the beginning of increasing attention that has during the past decade been paid to cell-free nucleic acids, such as DNA and RNA, which are present at high concentrations in blood of cancer patients. The first study on cell-free DNA in blood of prostate cancer was published in 2004, and showed higher plasma DNA levels in patients with metastatic disease than in patients with clinically localized prostate cancer (Jung et al., 2004).

Investigations of DNA fragmentation patterns in blood of cancer patients revealed that this DNA shows an apoptotic as well as a necrotic pattern (Jahr et al., 2001), as a result of cell death of tumour and wild type cells or of active secretion. It is unknown, whether besides the increased cell turnover in cancer patients, the clearance time also contributes to the higher levels of cell-free DNA. The degradation of cell-free DNA from the bloodstream occurs usually rapidly, e.g., the half-life time of fetal DNA in blood of mothers after delivery was approximately 16 minutes (Lo et al., 1999). Conversely, miRs appear highly stable, as they are small nucleotide fragments resistant to enzymes and incorporated in microvesicles (Kosaka et al., 2010). The nuclease activity in blood may be one of the important factors for the turnover of cell-free nucleic acids. However, this area of physiology remains unclear and needs further examination. The elimination of cell-free nucleic acids occurs by renal and hepatic mechanisms (Botezatu et al., 2000; Minchin et al., 2001).

3. Quantification of cell-free genomic and mitochondrial DNA

In blood of patients with prostate cancer, increased levels of cell-free DNA consisting of genomic and mitochondrial DNA have been assessed by different fluorescence-based methods using PicoGreen or SybrGreen and quantitative real-time PCR amplifying different genes. It is difficult to compare the DNA concentrations reported by various groups of investigators, since different techniques and plasma or serum were used. Plasma DNA seems to reflect the in vivo concentrations of cell-free DNA better than serum DNA. In respect to the quantification of DNA released from haematopoietic cells during the clotting process, the DNA concentrations in serum were essentially higher than those in plasma (Lee et al., 2001). Table 1 summarizes the diagnostic and prognostic relevance of cell-free DNA in plasma and serum of prostate

n>50	Cell-free nucleic acids	Diagnostic	Prognostic	Refs.
64	DNA quantification	x		Altimari et al., 2008
78	DNA quantification	x		Boddy et al., 2005
91	DNA quantification		x	Jung et al., 2004
161	DNA quantification	x		Chun et al., 2006
192	DNA quantification		x	Bastian et al., 2007
252	DNA quantification	x		Gordian et al., 2010
168	PTGS2 DNA	x	x	Ellinger et al., 2008a
75	mitochondrial DNA		x	Mehra et al., 2007
100	mitochondrial DNA		x	Ellinger et al., 2008c
57	microsatellite assay	x		Schwarzenbach et al., 2007
65	microsatellite assay	x		Muller et al., 2006
71	microsatellite assay	x		Muller et al., 2008
81	microsatellite assay	x		Schwarzenbach et al., 2009
83	microsatellite assay	x		Sunami et al., 2009
230	microsatellite assay	x		Schwarzenbach et al., 2008
76	DNA methylation		x	Okegawa et al., 2010
83	DNA methylation	x		Sunami et al., 2009
85	DNA methylation	x		Bastian et al., 2005
210	DNA methylation	x		Bastian et al., 2008
91	DNA methylation	x		Schwarzenbach et al., 2010
142	DNA methylation	x		Payne et al., 2009
168	DNA methylation	x		Ellinger et al., 2008b
171	DNA methylation	x		Ellinger et al., 2008a
61	Histone modification	x		Deligezer et al., 2010
50	miR 21	x		Zhang et al., 2010
51	miR 21, 141, 221	x		Yaman Agaoglu et al., 2011
71	miR 375, 141	x		Brase et al., 2010

Table 1. Detection of cell-free DNA with its genetic and epigenetic alterations and quantification of miRs in patients with prostate cancer

cancer patients, and represents different forms of cell-free nucleic acids analyzed in studies including more than 50 prostate cancer patients (n>50). This table is based on my review of publications deemed as significant clinical translational events.

3.1 Cell-free genomic DNA

The first systematic investigation on the quantitative changes of circulating DNA in prostate cancer patients was the study by Jung et al. (Jung et al., 2004). In this publication increased DNA concentrations were only observed in patients with lymph node and distant metastases. Whereas the DNA concentrations measured in patients with organ-confined cancer did not differ from those in healthy controls, the concentrations in patients with benign prostate hyperplasia (BPH) were elevated. These enquiries suggested that high DNA levels in patients with prostatic diseases can be considered neither as cancer-specific nor as sensitive marker for prostate cancer. In contrast to the lacking diagnostic relevance, the prognostic value of DNA concentrations as survival indicator could be shown and was comparable with the established marker PSA or with a reliable bone marker like osteoprotegerin (Jung et al., 2004). Besides, Boddy et al. found higher DNA levels in prostate cancer patients than in either healthy controls or men at low risk of having prostate cancer (low PSA or normal digital rectal examination). However, the elevated levels were not of diagnostic value during the management of prostate cancer, because those men with benign prostatic pathology had significantly higher DNA yields than the prostate cancer group (Boddy et al., 2005). Although the diagnostic relevance of cell-free DNA levels has been reported by other studies, most of those studies have not examined benign prostatitis. My laboratory compared the plasma DNA levels in prostate cancer and BPH patients and showed that the preoperative DNA level is a highly accurate and informative predictor in uni- and multivariate models for the presence of prostate cancer on needle biopsy. The median plasma concentration of cell-free DNA was 267 ng/mL in men with BPH versus 709 ng/mL in men with prostate cancer, and could consequently discriminated between men with localized prostate cancer and BPH (Chun et al., 2006). In another study, the median serum DNA concentration of prostate cancer patients was 5.3 ng/mL. Concentrations of ≥5.75 ng/mL were associated with an increased risk of PSA recurrence within 2 years of radical prostatectomy (Bastian et al., 2007). A cut off value of 8 ng/mL of plasma DNA was reported to discriminate between patients and healthy control subjects with a sensitivity of 80% and specificity of 82%, but in comparison to the other studies, these DNA measurements were very low. In addition, high levels of cell-free DNA correlated with pathologic tumour stage (Altimari et al., 2008). It was also reported, that patients with PSA of ≤10 ng/mL and cell-free DNA of > 180 ng/mL were at increased risk for prostate cancer compared with those with DNA of ≤180 ng/mL. Summing up, these findings show that cell-free DNA improved the specificity of prostate cancer screening and might, therefore, reduce the number of unnecessary prostate biopsies (Gordian et al., 2010).

Ellinger et al. designed a study to evaluate the apoptosis index which expresses the ratio of prostaglandin-endoperoxide synthase 2 (PTGS2) to Reprimo DNA fragments. Concentrations of apoptotic PTGS2 fragments discriminated between BPH and prostate cancer patients with a sensitivity of 88% and specificity of 64%, whereas the apoptosis index was more specific with 82% but less sensitive with 70%. Following radical prostatectomy apoptotic PTGS2 fragments and the apoptosis index correlated with PSA recurrence (Ellinger et al., 2008a).

3.2 Cell-free mitochondrial DNA

Apart from genomic DNA, mitochondrial DNA can also be quantified in blood of prostate cancer patients. Indicating the different nature of these circulating DNA types, the levels of cell-free genomic and mitochondrial DNA did not correlate (Mehra et al., 2007). In contrast to two copies of genomic DNA, a single cell contains up to several hundred copies of mitochondrial DNA. Whereas genomic DNA circulates mostly in a cell-free form and has also been isolated from microvesicles (which include exosomes and apoptotic bodies (Orozco & Lewis, 2010), mitochondrial DNA circulates mainly in microvesicles (Chiu et al., 2003). As diagnostic and prognostic marker in prostate cancer patients the amplification of mitochondrial nucleic acids has been reported to display increased sensitivity and specificity over genomic DNA. Advanced prostate cancer patients with high plasma mitochondrial nucleic acids (DNA and RNA) had a poorer survival than patients with low levels. Thus, mitochondrial RNA seems to be a strong predictor of overall survival and an independent prognostic factor for cancer-related death (Mehra et al., 2007). A further study showed that circulating mitochondrial DNA levels did not distinguish between prostate cancer and BPH patients. However, there was a significant increase in short mitochondrial DNA fragments including apoptotic DNA in patients with early PSA recurrence after radical prostatectomy (Ellinger et al., 2008c).

4. Genetic analyses of cell-free DNA

The development of prostate cancer is associated with genetic and epigenetic alterations accumulating during tumour growth and disease progression. The loss of particular sequences encoding for tumour suppressors can lead to the loss of a tumour-protective function of the appropriate gene product. Such gene defects may have an influence on cell cycle, cell adhesion or apoptosis. Cytogenetic and molecular genetic methods have identified numerous tumour-associated chromosomal regions playing a role in the tumourigenesis of prostate cancer.

Genetic alterations on cell-free DNA, including loss of heterozygosity (LOH), can be detected by PCR-based fluorescence microsatellite assays using microsatellite DNA (Fig. 1). Microsatellite DNA consists of short highly repetitive DNA sequences and is widely spread in the genome. In maternal and paternal chromosomes microsatellite DNA frequently differs in its length, corresponding to the number of repetitive sequences. This allows the separation of both alleles by gel or capillary electrophoresis and their analyses. Although similar plasma- and serum-based detection methods have been used, a great variability in detection of LOH on cell-free DNA has been reported. Besides the concordance of tumour-related LOH on cell-free DNA in blood with LOH on DNA from matched primary tumour tissues, discrepancies have also been found (Fleischhacker & Schmidt, 2007). These contradictory LOH data derived from blood and tumour tissue and the low incidence of LOH on cell-free DNA have been explained in part by technical problems and the dilution of tumour-associated cell-free DNA in blood by DNA released from normal cells (Muller et al., 2008; Schwarzenbach et al., 2008; Schmidt et al., 2006). Moreover, abnormal proliferation of benign cells, due to inflammation or tissue repair processes, also leads to an increase in apoptotic cell death, the accumulation of small, fragmented DNA in blood and the masking of LOH (Schulte-Hermann et al., 1995). In spite of these evident restrictions, plasma DNA may be a more appropriate source for genetic analyses than tumour tissue because blood may be a pool of tumour-specific DNA derived from focal areas of the heterogeneous primary prostate tumour harbouring different genetic alterations

(Bonkhoff & Remberger, 1998). Furthermore, the possibility of taking repeated blood samples allows tracing genetic alterations during treatment.

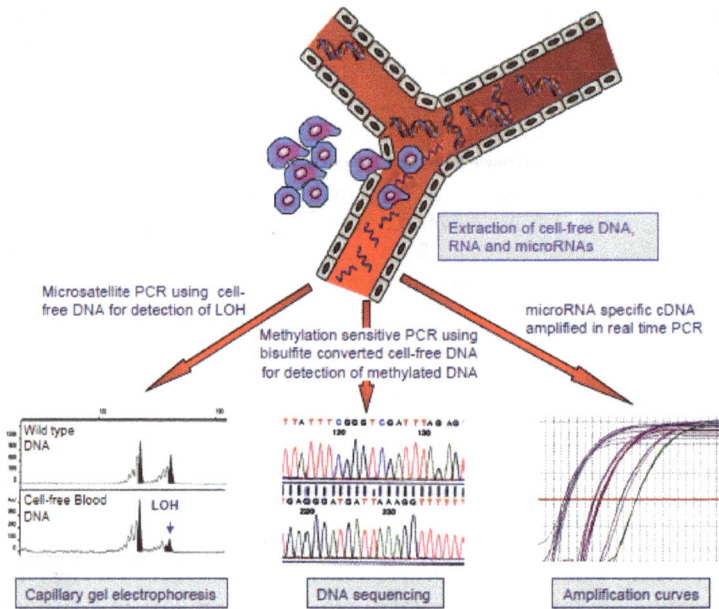

Fig. 1. Detection of genetically and epigenetically altered DNA and quantification of microRNAs in blood

To detect LOH on cell-free DNA, extracted DNA is amplified in a PCR-based fluorescence microsatellite analysis using a gene-specific primer set binding to tumour suppressor genes. The fluorescence-labeled PCR products can be separated by capillary gel electrophoresis and detected by a fluorescence laser. In the diagram (left) the abscissa indicates the length of the PCR product, whereas the ordinate gives information on the fluorescence intensity represented as peaks. The upper and lower part of the diagram show the PCR products derived from wild type DNA (from leukocytes) and plasma DNA, respectively. As depicted by the two peaks of the amplified wild type DNA, both alleles are intact, whereas the lower peak of the PCR product derived from the plasma DNA shows LOH (indicated by an arrow). To detect cell-free methylated DNA, extracted DNA is denatured and treated by sodium bisulfite. In a methylation-sensitive PCR the modified DNA is amplified with gene-specific primers. Since sodium bisulfite converts unmethylated cytosine residues into uracil, in contrast to methylated cytosine, the methylation pattern can be determined by DNA sequencing (middle). To quantify miRs, extracted total RNA is subscribed into cDNA which is then amplified with miR-specific primers in a quantitative real-time PCR reaction (right).

To investigate the potential significance of LOH on cell-free DNA, my laboratory compared the LOH incidence at 5 polymorphic microsatellite markers in plasma of prostate cancer and BPH patients. We found that LOH was frequently detected in prostate cancer patients and rarely observed in BPH patients indicating for the first time that microsatellite analysis using plasma DNA may be an interesting tool for molecular screening of prostate cancer patients (Muller et al., 2006). When the LOH frequency in blood plasma was compared with the incidence in tumour tissues and bone marrow aspirates of prostate cancer patients without clinical signs of overt metastases, we found that the concordance of LOH aberrations was 65% in blood plasma and 55% in bone marrow plasma samples with the analogous primary tumours. Our findings show that at least part of the cell-free DNA in blood and bone marrow may originate from the primary tumour. The subsets of LOH in blood and bone marrow plasma, which were not concordant with the detected tumour alterations, might be due to the known heterogeneity of the prostate tumours and the presence of wild type DNA in the plasma (Schwarzenbach et al., 2007). Moreover, we analyzed LOH at a panel of 13 polymorphic microsatellite markers in a large cohort of 230 prostate cancer and 43 BPH patients. The overall incidence was significantly higher in primary tumours (34%) than in blood plasma samples from prostate cancer patients (11%). Although LOH was also found in BPH plasma samples, its frequency of 2% was low. The highest concordance of LOH between tumour and plasma samples was 83% at the chromosomal locus 8p21 (Schwarzenbach et al., 2008). These findings provoked us to optimize the DNA extraction method to increase the detection rate of LOH on cell-free DNA in blood.

Comparing two DNA extraction techniques, Wang et al. demonstrated that the guanidine/Promega resin method significantly enhanced the sensitivity of detection of k-ras mutations on circulating serum DNA from colorectal cancer patients in comparison to the commonly used QIAamp DNA blood kit from the manufacturer Qiagen (Wang et al., 2004). The most abundant DNA detected in the Qiagen preparation was high-molecular-weight DNA, in contrast to mono-, di-, and trinucleosomal DNA isolated by the guanidine/Promega resin method (Wang et al., 2004). These findings lead to the suggestion that tumour-specific DNA might be enriched in the DNA portion containing shorter fragments, and to optimize the PCR-based fluorescence microsatellite method, we established a method to fractionate plasma DNA in short and long fragments (Muller et al., 2008). For preparation of the first fraction containing high-molecular-weight DNA, we isolated plasma DNA by Qiagen DNA Mini columns, and for the second fraction containing low-molecular-weight DNA, we used the flow-through of the first fraction and purified it on Promega columns. Because low-molecular-weight DNA may interfere with assay sensitivity, it was necessary to improve the assay conditions. By adding tetramethylammonium chloride (TMAC) (Hung et al., 1990; Chevet et al., 1995) as a general and essential enhancer to the PCR reactions, our results could be stabilized and ambiguous allelic losses could be largely avoided. Our data showing an enhancement of the detection rate of LOH in the low-molecular-weight plasma DNA from prostate cancer patients, point out that tumour-specific plasma DNA seems to mainly consist of short fragments. However, for practical plasma-based diagnostic tests the presence of LOH in both fractions should be considered (Muller et al., 2008).

Table 1 summarizes the diagnostic relevance of genetically altered DNA in plasma and serum of prostate cancer patients.

5. Epigenetic analyses of cell-free DNA

The epigenetic process includes DNA methylation and chromatin histone modifications. In chromosomal regions of tumour-associated genes epigenetic alterations may affect important regulatory mechanisms for the pathogenesis of malignant transformation (Klose

& Bird, 2006). Inactivation of tumour suppressor genes by promoter hypermethylation is thought to play a crucial role in this process (Esteller & Herman, 2002). DNA methylation of the cytosine base in CpG dinucleotides, which are found as isolated or clustered CpG islands, induces gene repression by inhibiting the access of transcription factors to their binding sites, and by recruiting methyl-CpG binding proteins (MBDs) to methylated DNA together with histone modifying enzymes (Hendrich & Tweedie, 2003). This leads to configurational changes in chromatin histone proteins and a compact packing of nucleosomes that are implicated in transcriptional regulation, as well (Zheng et al., 2008; Cedar & Bergman, 2009). DNA methylation on cell-free DNA can be detected by methylation-sensitive PCR using bisulfite-converted DNA (Fig. 1, Table 1).

CpG hypermethylation within the regulatory region of the π-class glutathione S-transferase gene (GSTP1) has been observed to be the most prevalent somatic genome abnormality in human prostate cancer, whereas this methylated GSTP1 is rarely detected in other organs. GSTP1 encodes an enzyme that acts as a carcinogen detoxifier by catalyzing conjugation reactions with reduced glutathione (Lee et al., 1994). Using a restriction endonuclease quantitative PCR technique, Bastian et al. (Bastian et al., 2005) addressed the question whether circulating cell-free DNA hypermethylation of GSTP1 can be evaluated as a prognostic biomarker for prostate cancer. They did not detect circulating hypermethylated GSTP1 in serum of men with a negative prostate biopsy, but they detected hypermethylation in 12% of men with clinically localized disease and 28% of men with metastatic cancer. Thus, they saw a continuing increase in DNA methylation during tumour progression. Moreover, they showed that men with clinically localized prostate cancer displaying CpG hypermethylation of GSTP1 in their preoperative serum were at significant risk to experience PSA recurrence within the following years after radical prostatectomy. These data suggest that hypermethylation of GSTP1 in blood may be an important DNA-based prognostic serum biomarker for prostate cancer (Bastian et al., 2005). The same laboratory also assessed the hypermethylation profile of several other genes including multidrug resistance 1 (MDR1), endothelin receptor B (EDNRB), CD44, NEP (neutral endopeptidase), PTGS2, Ras association domain family 1 isoform A (RASSF1A), retinoic acid receptor-ß (RAR-ß) and ESR1 (estrogen receptor 1) in serum of men with clinically localized prostate cancer, hormone refractory metastatic disease or a negative prostate biopsy (Bastian et al., 2008). Hypermethylation of MDR1 was positive in 38% of the cases without PSA recurrence and in 16% of those with biochemical recurrence after radical prostatectomy. DNA hypermethylation of the other genes was not detected in the serum. No single gene was observed to be consistently hypermethylated in patients with hormone refractory disease. In serum from men with metastatic prostate cancer, hypermethylation was detected at MDR1 in 83%, EDNRB in 50%, RAR-ß in 39%, and NEP as well as RASSF1A in 17% of the cases. The hypermethylation of CD44, PTGS2 or ESR1 was not detected in any samples (Bastian et al., 2008). These finding show that along with the hypermethylation of GSTP1, the hypermethylation status of a defined panel of genes may represent convenient targets for men with prostate cancer.

Using real-time PCR and sodium bisulfite-modified DNA, Payne et al. compared DNA methylation of the biomarkers GSTP1, RASSF2, histone 1H4K (HIST1H4K) and transcription factor AP2E (TFAP2E) in matched plasma and urine samples collected prospectively. The DNA methylation of the biomarkers in urine and plasma correlated significantly with each other. Surprisingly, the measurements of the biomarkers in urine were more sensitive for prostate cancer detection than those in plasma (Payne et al., 2009). Ellinger et al. compared the CpG hypermethylation of GSTP1, TIG1, PTGS2 and Reprimo in prostate cancer and BPH patients using a restriction endonuclease real-time PCR. They detected a higher methylation frequency in serum of prostate cancer patients than in BPH patients. The hypermethylation in serum distinguished between both patient cohorts in a highly specific but less sensitive manner (Ellinger et al., 2008b).

It is also possible to detect tumour-related altered histone modifications in blood of prostate cancer patients (Table 1). The utility of plasma levels of circulating bone-morphogenetic protein-6-specific (BMP6) mRNA and histone H3 lysine 27 trimethylation (H3K27me3) in discriminating metastatic prostate cancer from organ confined, local disease was evaluated at the end of therapy of the patients. Higher levels of BMP6 mRNA were found in the patients with metastases than in those with localized or local advanced disease. H3K27me3 displayed an inverse distribution compared to BMP6 mRNA and was significantly lower in patients with metastatic disease than in those with localized or local advanced disease. This study provides evidence that post-treatment analysis of cBMP6 mRNA and H3K27me3 in plasma may be used to distinguish metastatic prostate cancer from organ confined, local disease (Deligezer et al., 2010).

6. Combined genetic and epigenetic analyses of cell-free DNA

Sunami et al. hypothesized that circulating multimarker DNA assays detecting both genetic and epigenetic markers in serum would be more useful in assessing prostate cancer patients. They examined DNA methylation of RASSF1, RAR-ß2 and GSTP1 using a methylation-specific PCR assay and a panel of six microsatellite markers (D6S286 at 6q14, D8S261 at 8p22, D8S262 at 8p23, D9S171 at 9p21, D10S591 at 10p15 and D18S70 at 18q23). The combination of these two DNA assays increased the number of prostate cancer patients positive for at least one marker and detected the presence of prostate cancer regardless of AJCC (American Joint Cancer Committee) stage or PSA concentration. When these DNA assays were combined with PSA measurements, they reached a sensitivity of 89%. This pilot study demonstrated that the combined circulating DNA multimarker assay may yield information independent of AJCC stage or PSA concentration (Sunami et al., 2009).

7. Cell-free tumour DNA as a marker for circulating tumour cells

Currently, PSA blood serum levels are measured repeatedly after the primary treatment of prostate cancer. However, approximately 25% of patients with clinically localized prostate cancer will eventually experience biochemical evidence of tumour recurrence after surgical resection of the primary tumour. A possible explanation for this clinical observation may be an early occult onset of tumour cell dissemination to the blood circulation in these men. Even if overt metastases are subsequently confirmed by current imaging technologies, such as bone scans, these patients have become already incurable (Pantel et al., 2009). Therefore, a biomarker indicating early spread of tumour cells as the potential seed for future metastases is highly desirable.

The precise sources of tumour-related cell-free DNA in the peripheral blood are still unknown, but it has been postulated that this DNA may originate from primary and metastatic tumours. The most common view is that apoptotic and necrotic tumour cells shed their DNA into the blood circulation. Dying circulating tumour cells (CTCs) may also contribute to the high levels of circulating DNA in the blood. This assumption provoked scientists to investigate the relation between cell-free tumour-related DNA and CTCs.

Since different patterns of LOH may affect cancer progression toward metastases, we assessed the relationship of the occurrence of LOH on cell-free DNA with the presence of CTCs in peripheral blood of prostate cancer patients (Schwarzenbach et al., 2009). The presence of CTCs, which was detected by an epithelial immunospot assay, significantly correlated with the increase in LOH at the microsatellite markers D8S137, D9S171, and D17S855, which are located in the chromosomal regions of the cytoskeletal protein dematin (Lutchman et al., 1999), the inhibitor of the cyclin dependent kinase CDKN2/p16 (Perinchery et al., 1999) and BRCA1 (Gao et al., 1995), respectively. Identification of LOH in these regions may contribute to a better understanding of early steps in the metastatic cascade in prostate cancer. Dematin is localized in the junctional complex bundling actin filaments in a phosphorylation-dependent manner. Its biological function is to regulate the cell shape, and changes in cell plasticity are thought to be important for the dissemination of tumour cells (Thiery & Sleeman, 2006). CDKN2/p16 is a protein of the cell cycle regulating the G_1-S phase transition. It can be inactivated by mutations, deletions, or transcriptional silencing during pathogenesis of a variety of human malignancies and seems to be involved in the tumourigenesis of prostate cancer (Fernandez et al., 2002). BRCA1 has been implicated in a number of cellular processes including DNA repair and recombination, cell cycle checkpoint control, chromatin remodelling, ubiquitination, and apoptosis (Murray et al., 2007). Deletions in the BRCA1 gene have recently been implicated in metastatic spread and tumour progression in prostate cancer (Bednarz et al., 2010).

A comparative genetic profiling of isolated PSA-positive CTCs and multifocal prostate tumour tissues was performed by Schmidt et al. They showed that the detection of LOH at the BRCA1 locus in CTCs and primary tumours was associated with an early biochemical recurrence (Schmidt et al., 2006). In a recent study, Okegawa et al. determined for the first time the relation between CTCs detected on the CellSearch System and circulating tumour-related methylated DNA using a sensitive SYBR green methylation-specific PCR (Okegawa et al., 2010). In blood of patients with hormone-refractory prostate cancer hypermethylation of adenomatosis polyposis coli (APC), GSTP1, PTGS2, MRD1 and RASSF1A was analyzed. With the exception of PTGS2, the presence of CTCs significantly correlated with the presence of methylated APC, GSTP1, MDR1 and RASSF1A. Patients with CTCs and methylated DNA in their blood had a shorter median overall survival time, which was significantly different from that of patients without either molecular markers or with one of both markers. In addition, patients with CTCs or tumour-related methylated DNA had a poorer outcome than patients without these blood markers, and patients with both markers had the worst outcome. These findings indicate the high relapse risk and aggressiveness of tumours in patients with high levels of CTCs and DNA methylation in the blood (Okegawa et al., 2010).

Although the findings discussed above are still preliminary, they emphasize that cell-free tumour-related DNA may also stem from CTCs that have undergone cell death in the circulatory system.

8. Circulating microRNAs

MiRs are a class of naturally occurring small non-coding RNA molecules. They modulate post-transcriptionally the expression of numerous genes, such as tumor suppressor genes, by binding sequence-specifically to their target mRNA and inhibiting their translation into proteins or degrading the mRNA. Mature miRs consist of 19 to 25 nucleotides and are derived from hairpin precursor molecules of 70-100 nucleotides. As half of human miRs are localized in fragile chromosomal regions, which may exhibit DNA amplifications, deletions or translocations during tumour development, their expression is frequently deregulated in cancer (Croce, 2009). MiRs have, therefore, important roles in repression of protein expression in cancer (Bartel, 2009). To date, studies on solid cancers (ovarian, lung, breast and colorectal cancer) reported that miRs are involved in the regulation of different cellular processes, such as apoptosis, cell proliferation, epithelial to mesenchymal transition and metastases (Heneghan et al., 2009). In blood, miRs appear highly stable, because most of them are included in apoptotic bodies, microvesicles, or exosomes and can withstand known mRNA degradation factors (Asaga et al., 2011; Kosaka et al., 2010). Quanitative real-time PCR can be used to measure circulating miRs with miR-specific TaqMan MicroRNA assays (Fig. 1, Table 1).

Circulating miRs have recently been indicated as practicable and promising biomarkers for minimally invasive diagnosis in prostate cancer. Quantification of miR 21 targeting the tumour suppressor gene phosphatase and tensin homolog deleted (PTEN) and programmed cell death 4 (PDCD4) has been reported to be a useful biomarker for prostate cancer patients during disease progression (Zhang et al., 2010). Patients with hormone-refractory prostate cancer expressed higher serum miR 21 levels than those with androgen-dependent and localized prostate cancer. Androgen-dependent prostate cancer patients with low serum PSA levels had similar serum miR 21 levels to patients with localized prostate cancer or BPH. The highest serum miR 21 levels were found in hormone-refractory prostate cancer patients who were resistant to docetaxel-based chemotherapy when compared to those sensitive to chemotherapy. These findings suggest that miR 21 is an indicator of the transformation to hormone refractory disease and a potential predictor for the efficacy of docetaxel-based chemotherapy (Zhang et al., 2010). Quantification of miR-21 together with miR 141 and 221 revealed varying patterns in blood of the clinical subgroups. The differences in plasma between the control group and the patients were highly significant for miR 21 and 221 but not for miR 141. In patients diagnosed with metastatic prostate cancer, levels of all three miRs were significantly higher than in patients with localized and local advanced disease (Yaman Agaoglu et al., 2011). After screening of 667 miRs in serum samples from patients with metastatic and localized prostate cancer by microaarray analyses, five upregulated miRs were selected for further validation. Circulating miR 375 and 141 turned out to be the most pronounced markers for high-risk tumours. Their levels also correlated with high Gleason score and lymph-node positive status. These observations suggest that the release of miR 375 and 141 into the blood circulation is associated with advanced cancer disease (Brase et al., 2010).

Although there is only a few literatures on circulating miRs in blood of prostate cancer patients, the findings discussed above highlight their potential clinical utility (Table 1).

9. Conclusion

It took decades to attract attention to circulating cell-free nucleic as a surrogate for molecular analysis in the management of cancer patients, but their clinical relevance gains more and more in importance. Cell-free nucleic acids may be a reflection of the pathological processes during prostate cancer development, progression and metastasis. Besides these attributes, nucleic acids play also important biological roles. An intriguing hypothesis, the so-called genometastasis hypothesis describes that extracellular DNA and RNA from cancer cells may transform normal cells. Thus, metastases could develop in distant organs as a result of horizontal transfer of dominant oncogenes released from the primary tumour by susceptible cells (Garcia-Olmo et al., 2004). Whether this biological function has relevance in human blood in prostate cancer patients is an aspect to be considered in the future.

Since tumour-associated nucleic acids are easily accessible from plasma/serum and may be derived from several different sources, e.g. primary tumour, lymph nodes or CTCs, their detection could provide more information on prostate tumour biology. Although there is a number of biomarkers, e.g. PSA, commonly used for prostate cancer, these markers are also elevated in BPH patients, and their levels are dependent on prostate volume and age of the men. To date, the screening of cancer patients relies on early diagnosis, precise tumour staging, and monitoring of therapies. Histological evaluation of tumour tissues obtained from biopsies is the gold standard of diagnosis at present. Minimally invasive blood analyses of cell-free nucleic acids could have the potential to complement the existing biomarkers, such as PSA, and current clinical methods. These minimally invasive assays could serve as a "liquid biopsy" that can be repeated many times in an individual patient to assure a real-time monitoring of the disease course and assess the efficacy of anti-cancer therapies. In combination with the detection of CTCs, this assay might allow following metastatic progression and to predict the outcome of prostate cancer patients. The emerging biological role of miRs in the regulation of different cellular processes, e.g. apoptosis, cell proliferation, tumour progression, epithelial-mesenchymal transition and metastasis suggests that they may have a great potential as novel blood-based biomarkers and may also be considered as future therapeutic targets.

However, there are also some drawbacks. As the prevalence of wild type nucleic acids in blood hampers the genetic analyses of cell-free tumour DNA, better extraction procedures are required. This also implicates that the pre-analytical parameters, such as blood collection, processing of plasma or serum, storage and accurate clinical conditions need to be improved. The quantification of cell-free nucleic acids using different methods ia a further problem. To date, no approach has been developed that is consistent, robust, reproducible, and validated on a large-scale prostate cancer patient population. If these problems could be solved, these issues would provide better universal standardization for comparison of results and address clinical utility of the assays. Another issue is that after extraction of nucleic acids, different assays varying in assay sensitivity and specificity are used for analysis. A standardized PCR-based assay is needed in validating clinical biomarkers. This implicates that the slowed down progress of new cancer blood-based biomarkers in the last decade could be pushed.

10. References

Altimari, A., Grigioni, A.D., Benedettini, E., Gabusi, E., Schiavina, R., Martinelli, A., Morselli-Labate, A.M., Martorana, G., Grigioni, W.F. & Fiorentino, M. (2008). Diagnostic role of circulating free plasma DNA detection in patients with localized prostate cancer. *Am J Clin Pathol*, Vol.129, No.5, (May), pp. 756-762

Asaga, S., Kuo, C., Nguyen, T., Terpenning, M., Giuliano, A.E. & Hoon, D.S. (2011). Direct serum assay for microRNA-21 concentrations in early and advanced breast cancer. *Clin Chem*, Vol.57, No.1, (Jan), pp. 84-91, ISBN 1530-8561

Bartel, D.P. (2009). MicroRNAs: Target recognition and regulatory functions. *Cell*, Vol.136, No.2, (Jan 23), pp. 215-233

Bastian, P.J., Palapattu, G.S., Lin, X., Yegnasubramanian, S., Mangold, L.A., Trock, B., Eisenberger, M.A., Partin, A.W. & Nelson, W.G. (2005). Preoperative serum DNA gstp1 cpg island hypermethylation and the risk of early prostate-specific antigen recurrence following radical prostatectomy. *Clin Cancer Res*, Vol.11, No.11, (Jun 1), pp. 4037-4043

Bastian, P.J., Palapattu, G.S., Yegnasubramanian, S., Lin, X., Rogers, C.G., Mangold, L.A., Trock, B., Eisenberger, M., Partin, A.W. & Nelson, W.G. (2007). Prognostic value of preoperative serum cell-free circulating DNA in men with prostate cancer undergoing radical prostatectomy. *Clin Cancer Res*, Vol.13, No.18 Pt 1, (Sep 15), pp. 5361-5367

Bastian, P.J., Palapattu, G.S., Yegnasubramanian, S., Rogers, C.G., Lin, X., Mangold, L.A., Trock, B., Eisenberger, M.A., Partin, A.W. & Nelson, W.G. (2008). Cpg island hypermethylation profile in the serum of men with clinically localized and hormone refractory metastatic prostate cancer. *J Urol*, Vol.179, No.2, (Feb), pp. 529-534; discussion 534-52

Bednarz, N., Eltze, E., Semjonow, A., Rink, M., Andreas, A., Mulder, L., Hannemann, J., Fisch, M., Pantel, K., Weier, H.U., Bielawski, K.P. & Brandt, B. (2010). Brca1 loss preexisting in small subpopulations of prostate cancer is associated with advanced disease and metastatic spread to lymph nodes and peripheral blood. *Clin Cancer Res*, Vol.16, No.13, (Jul 1), pp. 3340-3348, ISBN 1078-0432

Boddy, J.L., Gal, S., Malone, P.R., Harris, A.L. & Wainscoat, J.S. (2005). Prospective study of quantitation of plasma DNA levels in the diagnosis of malignant versus benign prostate disease. *Clin Cancer Res*, Vol.11, No.4, (Feb 15), pp. 1394-1399

Bonkhoff, H. & Remberger, K. (1998). Morphogenetic concepts of normal and abnormal growth in the human prostate. *Virchows Arch*, Vol.433, No.3, (Sep), pp. 195-202, ISBN 0945-6317

Botezatu, I., Serdyuk, O., Potapova, G., Shelepov, V., Alechina, R., Molyaka, Y., Ananev, V., Bazin, I., Garin, A., Narimanov, M., Knysh, V., Melkonyan, H., Umansky, S. & Lichtenstein, A. (2000). Genetic analysis of DNA excreted in urine: A new approach for detecting specific genomic DNA sequences from cells dying in an organism. *Clin Chem*, Vol.46, No.8 Pt 1, (Aug), pp. 1078-1084, ISBN 0009-9147

Brase, J.C., Johannes, M., Schlomm, T., Falth, M., Haese, A., Steuber, T., Beissbarth, T., Kuner, R. & Sultmann, H. (2011). Circulating miRNAs are correlated with tumor progression in prostate cancer. *Int J Cancer*, Vol.128, No.3, (Feb 1), pp. 608-616, ISBN 1097-0215

Cedar, H. & Bergman, Y. (2009). Linking DNA methylation and histone modification: Patterns and paradigms. *Nat Rev Genet*, Vol.10, No.5, (May), pp. 295-304, ISBN 1471-0064

Chevet, E., Lemaitre, G. & Katinka, M.D. (1995). Low concentrations of tetramethylammonium chloride increase yield and specificity of pcr. *Nucleic Acids Res*, Vol.23, No.16, (Aug 25), pp. 3343-3344, ISBN 0305-1048

Chiu, R.W., Chan, L.Y., Lam, N.Y., Tsui, N.B., Ng, E.K., Rainer, T.H. & Lo, Y.M. (2003). Quantitative analysis of circulating mitochondrial DNA in plasma. *Clin Chem*, Vol.49, No.5, (May), pp. 719-726, ISBN 0009-9147

Chun, F.K., Muller, I., Lange, I., Friedrich, M.G., Erbersdobler, A., Karakiewicz, P.I., Graefen, M., Pantel, K., Huland, H. & Schwarzenbach, H. (2006). Circulating tumour-associated plasma DNA represents an independent and informative predictor of prostate cancer. *BJU Int*, Vol.98, No.3, (Sep), pp. 544-548

Croce, C.M. (2009). Causes and consequences of microRNA dysregulation in cancer. *Nat Rev Genet*, Vol.10, No.10, (Oct), pp. 704-714, ISBN 1471-0064

Deligezer, U., Yaman, F., Darendeliler, E., Dizdar, Y., Holdenrieder, S., Kovancilar, M. & Dalay, N. (2010). Post-treatment circulating plasma bmp6 mrna and h3k27 methylation levels discriminate metastatic prostate cancer from localized disease. *Clin Chim Acta*, Vol.411, No.19-20, (Oct 9), pp. 1452-1456, ISBN1873-3492

Ellinger, J., Bastian, P.J., Haan, K.I., Heukamp, L.C., Buettner, R., Fimmers, R., Mueller, S.C. & von Ruecker, A. (2008a). Noncancerous ptgs2 DNA fragments of apoptotic origin in sera of prostate cancer patients qualify as diagnostic and prognostic indicators. *Int J Cancer*, Vol.122, No.1, (Jan 1), pp. 138-143

Ellinger, J., Haan, K., Heukamp, L.C., Kahl, P., Buttner, R., Muller, S.C., von Ruecker, A. & Bastian, P.J. (2008b). Cpg island hypermethylation in cell-free serum DNA identifies patients with localized prostate cancer. *Prostate*, Vol.68, No.1, (Jan 1), pp. 42-49

Ellinger, J., Muller, S.C., Stadler, T.C., Jung, A., von Ruecker, A. & Bastian, P.J. (2011). The role of cell-free circulating DNA in the diagnosis and prognosis of prostate cancer. *Urol Oncol*, Vol.29, No.2, (Mar-Apr), pp. 124-129, ISBN 1873-2496

Ellinger, J., Muller, S.C., Wernert, N., von Ruecker, A. & Bastian, P.J. (2008c). Mitochondrial DNA in serum of patients with prostate cancer: A predictor of biochemical recurrence after prostatectomy. *BJU Int*, Vol.102, No.5, (Aug 5), pp. 628-632

Esteller, M. & Herman, J.G. (2002). Cancer as an epigenetic disease: DNA methylation and chromatin alterations in human tumours. *J Pathol*, Vol.196, No.1, (Jan), pp. 1-7

Fernandez, P.L., Hernandez, L., Farre, X., Campo, E. & Cardesa, A. (2002). Alterations of cell cycle-regulatory genes in prostate cancer. *Pathobiology*, Vol.70, No.1, pp. 1-10

Fleischhacker, M. & Schmidt, B. (2007). Circulating nucleic acids (cnas) and cancer--a survey. *Biochim Biophys Acta*, Vol.1775, No.1, (Jan), pp. 181-232

Gao, X., Zacharek, A., Salkowski, A., Grignon, D.J., Sakr, W., Porter, A.T. & Honn, K.V. (1995). Loss of heterozygosity of the brca1 and other loci on chromosome 17q in human prostate cancer. *Cancer Res*, Vol.55, No.5, (Mar 1), pp. 1002-1005

Garcia-Olmo, D.C., Ruiz-Piqueras, R. & Garcia-Olmo, D. (2004). Circulating nucleic acids in plasma and serum (CNAPS) and its relation to stem cells and cancer metastasis: state of the issue. *Histol Histopathol*, Vol. 19, No.2, (Apr), pp. 575–583

Gordian, E., Ramachandran, K., Reis, I.M., Manoharan, M., Soloway, M.S. & Singal, R. (2010). Serum free circulating DNA is a useful biomarker to distinguish benign versus malignant prostate disease. *Cancer Epidemiol Biomarkers Prev*, Vol.19, No.8, (May), pp. 1984-1991, ISBN 1538-7755

Hendrich, B. & Tweedie, S. (2003). The methyl-cpg binding domain and the evolving role of DNA methylation in animals. *Trends Genet*, Vol.19, No.5, (May), pp. 269-277

Heneghan, H.M., Miller, N., Lowery, A.J., Sweeney, K.J. & Kerin, M.J. (2009). MicroRNAs as novel biomarkers for breast cancer. *J Oncol*, Vol.2009, pp. 950201, ISBN 1687-8450

Hung, T., Mak, K. & Fong, K. (1990). A specificity enhancer for polymerase chain reaction. *Nucleic Acids Res*, Vol.18, No.16, (Aug 25), pp. 4953, ISBN 0305-1048

Jahr, S., Hentze, H., Englisch, S., Hardt, D., Fackelmayer, F.O., Hesch, R.D. & Knippers, R. (2001). DNA fragments in the blood plasma of cancer patients: Quantitations and evidence for their origin from apoptotic and necrotic cells. *Cancer Res*, Vol.61, No.4, (Feb 15), pp. 1659-1665

Jansen, F.H., Roobol, M., Jenster, G., Schroder, F.H. & Bangma, C.H. (2008). Screening for prostate cancer in 2008 ii: The importance of molecular subforms of prostate-specific antigen and tissue kallikreins. *Eur Urol*, Vol.55, No.3, (Mar), pp. 563-574

Jones, M.J. & Koeneman, K.S. (2008). Local-regional prostate cancer. *Urol Oncol*, Vol.26, No.5, (Sep-Oct), pp. 516-521

Jung, K., Stephan, C., Lewandowski, M., Klotzek, S., Jung, M., Kristiansen, G., Lein, M., Loening, S.A. & Schnorr, D. (2004). Increased cell-free DNA in plasma of patients with metastatic spread in prostate cancer. *Cancer Lett*, Vol.205, No.2, (Mar 18), pp. 173-180

Klose, R.J. & Bird, A.P. (2006). Genomic DNA methylation: The mark and its mediators. *Trends Biochem Sci*, Vol.31, No.2, (Feb), pp. 89-97, ISBN Klose, R.J. & Bird, A.P.

Knudsen, B.S. & Vasioukhin, V. (2010). Mechanisms of prostate cancer initiation and progression. *Adv Cancer Res*, Vol.109, pp. 1-50, ISBN 0065-230X

Kosaka, N., Iguchi, H. & Ochiya, T. (2010). Circulating microRNA in body fluid: A new potential biomarker for cancer diagnosis and prognosis. *Cancer Sci*, Vol.101, No.10, (Oct), pp. 2087-2092, ISBN 1349-7006

Lee, T.H., Montalvo, L., Chrebtow, V. & Busch, M.P. (2001). Quantitation of genomic DNA in plasma and serum samples: Higher concentrations of genomic DNA found in serum than in plasma. *Transfusion*, Vol.41, No.2, (Feb), pp. 276-282, ISBN 0041-1132

Lee, W.H., Morton, R.A., Epstein, J.I., Brooks, J.D., Campbell, P.A., Bova, G.S., Hsieh, W.S., Isaacs, W.B. & Nelson, W.G. (1994). Cytidine methylation of regulatory sequences near the pi-class glutathione s-transferase gene accompanies human prostatic carcinogenesis. *Proc Natl Acad Sci U S A*, Vol.91, No.24, (Nov 22), pp. 11733-11737

Lo, Y.M., Zhang, J., Leung, T.N., Lau, T.K., Chang, A.M. & Hjelm, N.M. (1999). Rapid clearance of fetal DNA from maternal plasma. *Am J Hum Genet*, Vol.64, No.1, (Jan), pp. 218-224

Lutchman, M., Pack, S., Kim, A.C., Azim, A., Emmert-Buck, M., van Huffel, C., Zhuang, Z. & Chishti, A.H. (1999). Loss of heterozygosity on 8p in prostate cancer implicates a role for dematin in tumor progression. *Cancer Genet Cytogenet*, Vol.115, No.1, (Nov), pp. 65-69

Mandel, P. & Métais, P. (1948). Les acides nucléiques du plasma sanguin chez l'homme. *C R Acad Sci Paris*, Vol.142, pp. 241-243

Mehra, N., Penning, M., Maas, J., van Daal, N., Giles, R.H. & Voest, E.E. (2007). Circulating mitochondrial nucleic acids have prognostic value for survival in patients with advanced prostate cancer. *Clin Cancer Res*, Vol.13, No.2 Pt 1, (Jan 15), pp. 421-426

Minchin, R.F., Carpenter, D. & Orr, R.J. (2001). Polyinosinic acid and polycationic liposomes attenuate the hepatic clearance of circulating plasmid DNA. *J Pharmacol Exp Ther*, Vol.296, No.3, (Mar), pp. 1006-1012, ISBN 0022-3565

Muller, I., Beeger, C., Alix-Panabieres, C., Rebillard, X., Pantel, K. & Schwarzenbach, H. (2008). Identification of loss of heterozygosity on circulating free DNA in peripheral blood of prostate cancer patients: Potential and technical improvements. *Clin Chem*, Vol.54, No.4, (Apr), pp. 688-696

Muller, I., Urban, K., Pantel, K. & Schwarzenbach, H. (2006). Comparison of genetic alterations detected in circulating microsatellite DNA in blood plasma samples of patients with prostate cancer and benign prostatic hyperplasia. *Ann N Y Acad Sci*, Vol.1075, (Sep), pp. 222-229

Murray, M.M., Mullan, P.B. & Harkin, D.P. (2007). Role played by brca1 in transcriptional regulation in response to therapy. *Biochem Soc Trans*, Vol.35, No.Pt 5, (Nov), pp. 1342-1346

Nawroz, H., Koch, W., Anker, P., Stroun, M. & Sidransky, D. (1996). Microsatellite alterations in serum DNA of head and neck cancer patients. *Nat Med*, Vol.2, No.9, (Sep), pp. 1035-1037

Okegawa, T., Nutahara, K. & Higashihara, E. (2010). Association of circulating tumor cells with tumor-related methylated DNA in patients with hormone-refractory prostate cancer. *Int J Urol*, Vol.17, No.5, (May), pp. 466-475, ISBN 1442-2042

Orozco, A.F. & Lewis, D.E. (2010). Flow cytometric analysis of circulating microparticles in plasma. *Cytometry A*, Vol.77, No.6, (Jun), pp. 502-514, ISBN 1552-4930

Ozen, M., Creighton, C.J., Ozdemir, M. & Ittmann, M. (2008). Widespread deregulation of microRNA expression in human prostate cancer. *Oncogene*, Vol.27, No.12, (Mar 13), pp. 1788-1793

Pantel, K., Alix-Panabieres, C. & Riethdorf, S. (2009). Cancer micrometastases. *Nat Rev Clin Oncol*, Vol.6, No.6, (Jun), pp. 339-351, ISBN 1759-4782

Payne, S.R., Serth, J., Schostak, M., Kamradt, J., Strauss, A., Thelen, P., Model, F., Day, J.K., Liebenberg, V., Morotti, A., Yamamura, S., Lograsso, J., Sledziewski, A. & Semjonow, A. (2009). DNA methylation biomarkers of prostate cancer: Confirmation of candidates and evidence urine is the most sensitive body fluid for non-invasive detection. *Prostate*, Vol.69, No.12, (Sep 1), pp. 1257-1269, ISBN 1097-0045

Perinchery, G., Bukurov, N., Nakajima, K., Chang, J., Li, L.C. & Dahiya, R. (1999). High frequency of deletion on chromosome 9p21 may harbor several tumor-suppressor genes in human prostate cancer. *Int J Cancer*, Vol.83, No.5, (Nov 26), pp. 610-614

Schmidt, H., DeAngelis, G., Eltze, E., Gockel, I., Semjonow, A. & Brandt, B. (2006). Asynchronous growth of prostate cancer is reflected by circulating tumor cells delivered from distinct, even small foci, harboring loss of heterozygosity of the pten gene. *Cancer Res*, Vol.66, No.18, (Sep 15), pp. 8959-8965

Schulte-Hermann, R., Bursch, W., Grasl-Kraupp, B., Torok, L., Ellinger, A. & Mullauer, L. (1995). Role of active cell death (apoptosis) in multi-stage carcinogenesis. *Toxicol Lett*, Vol.82-83, (Dec), pp. 143-148, ISBN 0378-4274

Schwarzenbach, H., Alix-Panabieres, C., Muller, I., Letang, N., Vendrell, J.P., Rebillard, X. & Pantel, K. (2009). Cell-free tumor DNA in blood plasma as a marker for circulating tumor cells in prostate cancer. *Clin Cancer Res*, Vol.15, No.3, (Feb 1), pp. 1032-1038

Schwarzenbach, H., Chun, F.K., Isbarn, H., Huland, H. & Pantel, K. (2010). Genomic profiling of cell-free DNA in blood and bone marrow of prostate cancer patients. *J Cancer Res Clin Oncol*, Vol.137, No.5, (May), pp. 811-819, ISBN 1432-1335

Schwarzenbach, H., Chun, F.K., Lange, I., Carpenter, S., Gottberg, M., Erbersdobler, A., Friedrich, M.G., Huland, H. & Pantel, K. (2007). Detection of tumor-specific DNA in blood and bone marrow plasma from patients with prostate cancer. *Int J Cancer*, Vol.120, No.7, (Apr 1), pp. 1465-1471

Schwarzenbach, H., Chun, F.K., Muller, I., Seidel, C., Urban, K., Erbersdobler, A., Huland, H., Pantel, K. & Friedrich, M.G. (2008). Microsatellite analysis of allelic imbalance in tumour and blood from patients with prostate cancer. *BJU Int*, Vol.102, No.2, (Jul), pp. 253-258

Schwarzenbach, H. & Pantel, K. (2008) Methods of cancer diagnosis, therapy and prognosis. Prostate cancer: Detection of free tumor-specific DNA in blood and bone marrow., Vol 2. Springer, USA

Sorenson, G.D., Pribish, D.M., Valone, F.H., Memoli, V.A., Bzik, D.J. & Yao, S.L. (1994). Soluble normal and mutated DNA sequences from single-copy genes in human blood. *Cancer Epidemiol Biomarkers Prev*, Vol.3, No.1, (Jan-Feb), pp. 67-71, ISBN 1055-9965

Sunami, E., Shinozaki, M., Higano, C.S., Wollman, R., Dorff, T.B., Tucker, S.J., Martinez, S.R., Singer, F.R. & Hoon, D.S. (2009). Multimarker circulating DNA assay for assessing blood of prostate cancer patients. *Clin Chem*, Vol.55, No.3, (Mar), pp. 559-567

Tannock, I.F., de Wit, R., Berry, W.R., Horti, J., Pluzanska, A., Chi, K.N., Oudard, S., Theodore, C., James, N.D., Turesson, I., Rosenthal, M.A. & Eisenberger, M.A. (2004). Docetaxel plus prednisone or mitoxantrone plus prednisone for advanced prostate cancer. *N Engl J Med*, Vol.351, No.15, (Oct 7), pp. 1502-1512, ISBN 1533-4406

Thiery, J.P. & Sleeman, J.P. (2006). Complex networks orchestrate epithelial-mesenchymal transitions. *Nat Rev Mol Cell Biol*, Vol.7, No.2, (Feb), pp. 131-142

Vasioukhin, V., Anker, P., Maurice, P., Lyautey, J., Lederrey, C. & Stroun, M. (1994). Point mutations of the n-ras gene in the blood plasma DNA of patients with myelodysplastic syndrome or acute myelogenous leukaemia. *Br J Haematol*, Vol.86, No.4, (Apr), pp. 774-779, ISBN 0007-1048

Wang, L., Tang, H., Thayanithy, V., Subramanian, S., Oberg, A.L., Cunningham, J.M., Cerhan, J.R., Steer, C.J. & Thibodeau, S.N. (2009). Gene networks and microRNAs implicated in aggressive prostate cancer. *Cancer Res*, Vol.69, No.24, (Dec 15), pp. 9490-9497, ISBN 1538-7445

Wang, M., Block, T.M., Steel, L., Brenner, D.E. & Su, Y.H. (2004). Preferential isolation of fragmented DNA enhances the detection of circulating mutated k-ras DNA. *Clin Chem*, Vol.50, No.1, (Jan), pp. 211-213

Yaman Agaoglu, F., Kovancilar, M., Dizdar, Y., Darendeliler, E., Holdenrieder, S., Dalay, N. & Gezer, U. (2011). Investigation of mir-21, mir-141, and mir-221 in blood circulation of patients with prostate cancer. *Tumour Biol*, Vol.32, No.3, (Jun), pp. 583-588, ISBN 1423-0380

Zhang, H.L., Yang, L.F., Zhu, Y., Yao, X.D., Zhang, S.L., Dai, B., Zhu, Y.P., Shen, Y.J., Shi, G.H. & Ye, D.W. (2010). Serum miRNA-21: Elevated levels in patients with metastatic hormone-refractory prostate cancer and potential predictive factor for the efficacy of docetaxel-based chemotherapy. *Prostate*, Vol.71, No.3, (Feb 15), pp. 326-331, ISBN 1097-0045

Zheng, Y.G., Wu, J., Chen, Z. & Goodman, M. (2008). Chemical regulation of epigenetic modifications: Opportunities for new cancer therapy. *Med Res Rev*, Vol.28, No.5, (Sep), pp. 645-687

9

Epidermal Growth Factor Receptor (EGFR) Phosphorylation, Signaling and Trafficking in Prostate Cancer

Yao Huang and Yongchang Chang
St. Joseph's Hospital and Medical Center, Phoenix, Arizona
USA

1. Introduction

The molecular mechanisms of prostate cancer are still poorly understood, despite the threat that prostate cancer poses to the health of men worldwide. As prostate tumors are initially dependent on androgens for growth and survival, androgen deprivation therapy is the first-line treatment for prostate cancer patients. However, a hormonal-refractory (androgen independent) state often develops afterwards, and principal treatment options are palliative because of the tumor progression, which is characterized by uncontrolled growth and metastasis associated with androgen independence. To date, no effective therapy can abrogate prostate cancer progression to advanced, invasive forms. Recent evidence suggests that acquisition of androgen-independence may be due to upregulation of growth factor receptor signaling pathways, principally the epidermal growth factor receptor (EGFR)/ErbB/human epidermal receptor (HER) family (Craft et al., 1999), making it an attractive target for therapeutic intervention. EGFR/ErbB/HER signaling in cancer has been extensively studied for decades, and there have been a number of excellent reviews on the roles of ErbB receptors in the initiation and progression of a wide variety of cancers, including prostate cancer (Laskin & Sandler, 2004; Ratan et al., 2003; Yarden & Sliwkowski, 2001). Thus, this review chapter will focus more narrowly on EGFR phosphorylation, signaling, and trafficking, and their specific roles in prostate cancer development and progression (tumor growth and metastasis) given the growing literature in this area. Better understanding of the precise roles of divergent EGFR signaling pathways and their phenotypic consequences in prostate cancer (and normal prostate) will enable the development of more effective and selective therapies for this urologic disease.

2. Overview of the EGF/EGFR signaling system

2.1 The EGFR/ErbB/HER family and ligands

EGFR/ErbB1/HER1 is the prototype of the EGFR or ErbB family, which also includes other three receptor tyrosine kinases, ErbB2/HER2/Neu, ErbB3/HER3, and ErbB4/HER4 (Figure 1). All four members have in common an extracellular ligand-binding domain, a single hydrophobic transmembrane domain, and a cytoplasmic region that contains a highly conserved tyrosine kinase domain and C-terminal tail (Wells, 1999). However, ErbB3 lacks intrinsic tyrosine kinase activity due to substitutions of critical amino acids within the kinase domain (Guy et al., 1994). The extracellular domains are less conserved among the four, suggesting their ligand binding specificity (Yarden, 2001; Yarden & Sliwkowski, 2001).

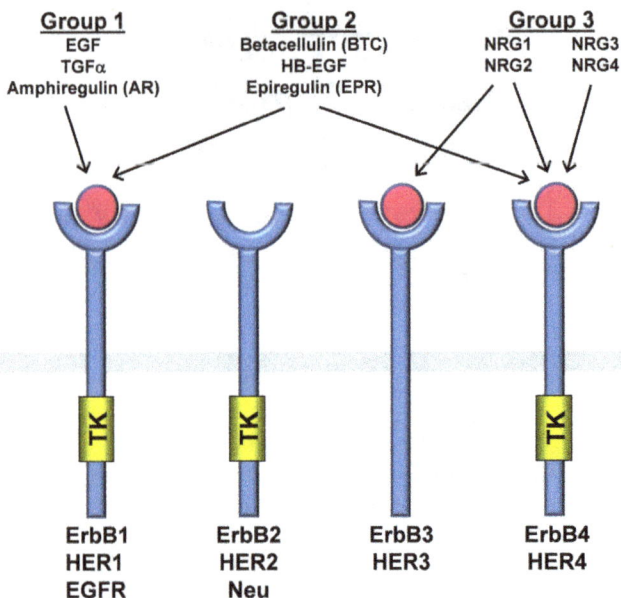

Fig. 1. The four EGFR/ErbB family members and their ligands. TK, tyrosine kinase domain. See the text for more details.

ErbB receptors are activated by a number of ligands that belong to the EGF family of peptide growth factors (Citri & Yarden, 2006; Yarden, 2001). The EGF-related growth factors are characterized by the presence of an EGF-like domain consisting of three disulfide-bonded intramolecular groups conferring binding specificity, and additional structural motifs such as immunoglobulin-like domains, heparin-binding sites and glycosylation sites. They are produced as transmembrane precursors that are biologically active and able to interact with receptors expressed on adjacent cells, and the ectodomains are processed by proteolysis, resulting in the shedding of soluble growth factors (Massagué & Pandiella, 1993). Based on their affinity for one or more ErbBs, the EGF-related growth factors are generally classified into three groups (Yarden & Sliwkowski, 2001) (Figure 1). The first group includes EGF, transforming growth factor-α (TGF-α) and amphiregulin (AR), which bind specifically to EGFR. The second group includes betacellulin (BTC), heparin-binding EGF (HB-EGF), and epiregulin (EPR), which exhibit dual specificity for both EGFR and ErbB4 (Yarden, 2001). The third group includes nuregulins (NRG, also called Neu differentiation factors (NDF) or heregulins (HRG)) that can be divided into two subgroups based on their binding specificity to both ErbB3 and ErbB4 (NRG-1 and NRG-2) or only ErbB4 (NRG-3 and NRG-4) (Harari et al., 1999; Zhang et al., 1997). Despite intensive efforts, no direct ligand for ErbB2 has yet been discovered. Increasing evidence suggests that ErbB2 primarily functions as a coreceptor for other ErbB family members (Graus-Porta et al., 1997; Tzahar et al., 1996).

2.2 Major EGF/EGFR signaling pathways

The repertoire of ErbB ligands and the combinatorial properties of ligand-induced receptor dimers give rise to the signaling diversity of the ErbB family. Ligand binding drives receptor homo- or hetero-dimerization, leading to activation of the intrinsic tyrosine kinase and subsequent auto- or trans-phosphorylation of specific tyrosine residues in the cytoplasmic tail (Citri & Yarden, 2006; Olayioye et al., 2000; Yarden & Sliwkowski, 2001), which provide the docking sites for proteins containing Src homology 2 (SH2) or phosphotyrosine binding (PTB) domains (Shoelson, 1997; Sudol, 1998). These proteins generally include the adaptor proteins such as Src homology domain-containing adaptor protein C (Shc), Crk, growth factor receptor-bound protein 2 (Grb2), Grb7, Grb2-associated binding protein 1 (Gab1), phospholipase C γ (PLCγ), Cbl, Esp15; the kinases such as Src, Chk and phosphatidylinositol-3-kinase (PI3K; via the p85 regulatory subunit); and the protein tyrosine phosphatases such as PTP1B, SHP1 and SHP2 (Olayioye et al., 2000; Sebastian et al., 2006), suggesting diversity and complexity of ErbB signaling networks. Among them, the signaling elicited by EGF-induced EGFR homodimers is perhaps the best studied and has served as the prototype for other cases.

Adaptor proteins, kinases, and phosphatases recruited by the activated EGFR transmit signals from the receptor through different downstream signaling pathways to the nucleus to regulate various biological functions such as cell proliferation, differentiation, anti-apoptosis (survival), adhesion, migration, and angiogenesis (Baselga & Hammond, 2002; Laskin & Sandler, 2004; Morandell et al., 2008; Yarden & Sliwkowski, 2001). So far with the numbers still growing, over one hundred EGFR interacting proteins have been described in the literature, of which many were discovered by proteomics approaches (Morandell et al., 2008). Approximately twenty phosphotyrosine residues located within the EGFR cytoplasmic tail have been identified as specific docking sites for above-mentioned EGFR interacting partners to engage various signaling cascades (Figure 2). The major EGF/EGFR signaling pathways include Ras/Raf/MAPK kinase (MEK)/extracellular-related kinase (ERK) and PI3K/Akt (Hirsch et al., 2003; Singh & Harris, 2005), although other pathways such as PLCγ/protein kinase C (PKC), signal transducer and activator of transcription (STAT) (Andl et al., 2004; Kloth et al., 2002), c-Jun terminal kinase (JNK) and p38 MAPKs (Johnson et al., 2005), and Ca^{2+}-calmodulin-dependent protein kinase (CaMK) (Sengupta et al., 2009) have been reported. It is also known that upon EGF binding, EGFR undergoes a process of internalization, ubiquitination (via Cbl), destruction (namely EGFR endocytosis and trafficking), resulting in temporary EGFR downregulation (Citri & Yarden, 2006; Sebastian et al., 2006; Wiley, 2003). This will be discussed in Section 3.

2.3 EGFR signaling in prostate cancer development

Both clinical and experimental data have established the importance of ErbBs, especially EGFR and ErbB2, in carcinogenesis and progression of various types of solid tumors including prostate cancer (Harari, 2004; Laskin & Sandler, 2004; Sebastian et al., 2006; Yarden & Sliwkowski, 2001). Increased expression and signaling of EGFR and/or ErbB2 are associated with a more aggressive clinical behavior of tumors, and correlate with a poor prognosis (Alroy & Yarden, 1997; Hatake et al., 2007; Lichtner, 2003; Nicholson et al., 2001). There are estimated 40-80% of prostate tumors with expressed EGFR (Kim et al., 1999; Sebastian et al., 2006). Studies mainly from breast cancer, lung cancer, and glioma have suggested many potential mechanisms related to aberrant EGFR signaling (quantitatively and/or qualitatively). These include elevated expression of ligands and/or receptors, enhanced autocrine signaling loop, constitutive activation of EGFR mutants, impaired endocytosis and trafficking of the ligand-receptor complex, hetero-dimerization with other ErbBs (Ciardiello & Tortora, 2003; Grandal & Madshus, 2008; Huang et al., 2009; Olayioye et al., 2000; Roepstorff et al., 2008; Sebastian et al., 2006; Sharma et al., 2007), as well as crosstalk with other receptor signaling systems such as type 1 insulin-like growth factor receptor (IGF-1R), G-protein-coupled receptors (GPCRs), and cytokine receptors (Adams et al., 2004; Gee et al., 2005; Prenzel et al., 2000).

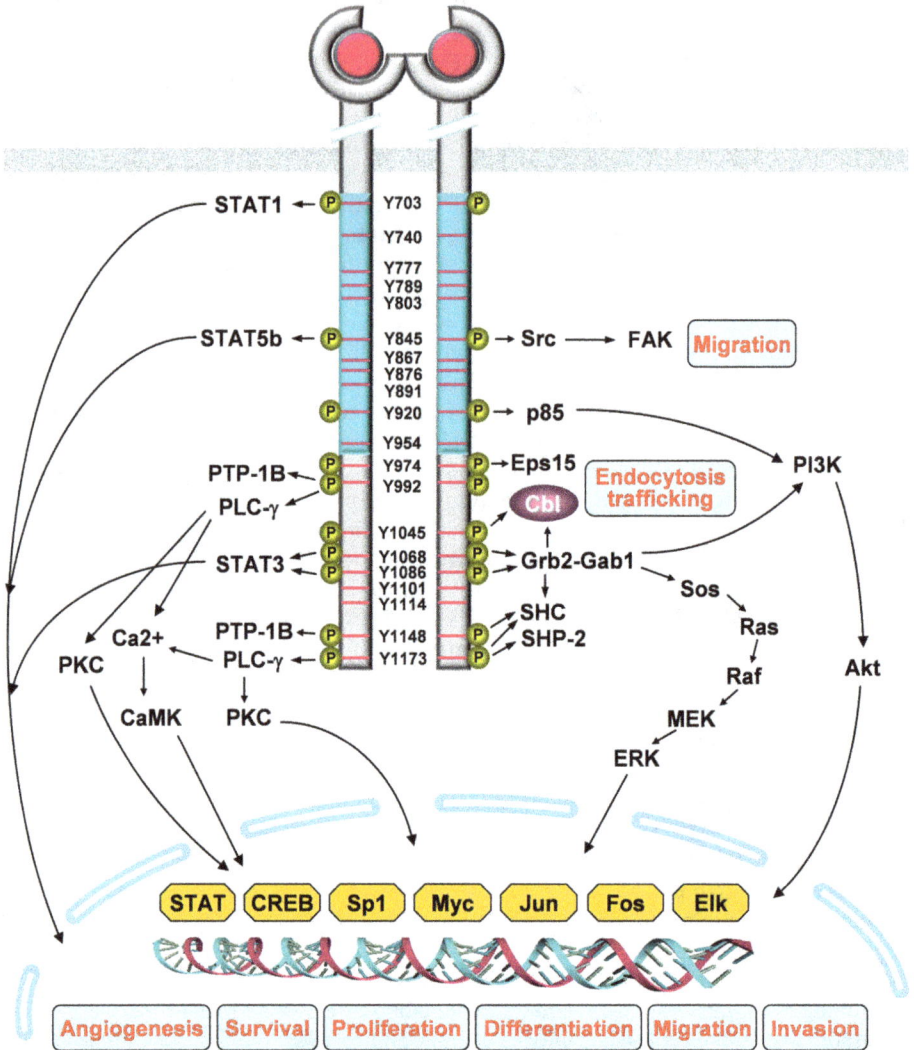

Fig. 2. EGF/EGFR-mediated signaling pathways and cellular effects. Major tyrosine phosphorylation sites in the EGFR cytoplasmic tail, possible adaptors and signaling proteins, and signaling cascades are indicated. See the text for more details.

Progression from normal prostate epithelium to an androgen-responsive tumor, and finally to hormone-refractory carcinoma is a multistep process, usually accompanied by the upregulation of growth factor receptors and/or their ligands, and downregulation of tumor suppressor gene products (Djakiew, 2000; Ware, 1999). EGFR ligands, such as EGF, HB-EGF, and TGF-α, are expressed in the prostate and prostatic carcinomas (Elson et al., 1984; Freeman et al., 1998). In particular, the expression of TGF-α (signaling merely through EGFR) has been found to be greater in some higher grade and metastatic prostate cancers than in primary low grade tumors (Scher et al., 1995). It is now more widely believed that EGF is the predominant EGFR ligand in early, localized prostate cancer, and that TGF-α becomes more abundant than EGF at advanced, metastatic stages (Liu et al., 1993; Scher et al., 1995; Seth et al., 1999). This is the so-called EGFR ligand switch (DeHaan et al., 2009). Overexpression of EGFR and/or ErbB2 would have been expected in prostate carcinomas, as seen in breast cancer (Hatake et al., 2007; Lichtner, 2003; Nicholson et al., 2001). However, current data regarding ErbB receptor overexpression in prostate cancer appear to conflict with each other, possibly due to technical reasons and lack of standardized measurement and evaluation methods (Marks et al., 2008; Neto et al., 2010; Salomon et al., 1995; Schlomm et al., 2007; Sherwood & Lee, 1995). Nevertheless, several lines of evidence strongly support the important role of EGFR signaling in prostate cancer development. For example, autocrine activation of EGFR signaling by EGF and TGF-α most likely drives the autonomous growth of human prostate cancer (Hofer et al., 1991; Scher et al., 1995). Expression of mutant EGFRs also contributes to prostate carcinogenesis and malignant progression (Cai et al., 2008; Douglas et al., 2006; He & Young, 2009; Olapade-Olaopa et al., 2000). Taken together, studies over the years have suggested that both EGFR and ErbB2 signaling play important roles in prostate cancer development and, more specifically, in the progression from an androgen-dependent to a hormone-refractory state.

3. EGF/EGFR endocytosis and trafficking

As just described, aberrant EGFR signaling is frequently associated with carcinogenesis and cancer progression. This can be the result of several unbalanced mechanisms controlling the quantitative and qualitative output of EGFR, such as elevated expression of receptors and ligands, activating receptor mutations, and impaired endocytic receptor downregulation. Proper endocytic uptake and endosomal sorting of signaling receptors have been considered as a crucial step for precisely controlling cellular processes such as growth, differentiation, and survival. Our current understanding of ligand-induced receptor endocytic downregulation is largely from the knowledge of EGFR trafficking routes following EGF binding, which has historically been and remains to be the most popular experimental system for studies in this field. In contrast, very little is known about endocytosis of ErbB2-4, as well as about EGFR endocytosis following binding of ligands other than EGF.

It is generally believed that EGFR is present at the plasma membrane as a monomer prior to activation. Ligand (EGF) binding triggers EGFR dimerization and activation of its intrinsic kinase, leading to signaling and relocation to invaginating clathrin-coated pits (CCPs) on the plasma membrane. The CCPs give rise to clathrin-coated endocytic vesicles. The vesicles are then released from the membrane and fuse with early endosomes. Thus, EGFR is delivered to this compartment by these sequential processes. From here the receptor is sorted for further transport, either back to the cell surface by recycling, or to the multivesicular bodies (MVBs), a pathway for eventual delivery of EGFR to late endosomes and lysosomes for degradation, which results in temporary EGFR downregulation (Figure 3). Under most physiological conditions, clathrin-dependent pathways are considered to be the main routes of EGFR internalization and downregulation. However, clathrin-independent pathways have also been reported and suggested as alternative mechanisms for EGFR endocytosis (Orth et al., 2006; Sigismund et al., 2005; Yamazaki et al., 2002), which will not be discussed here.

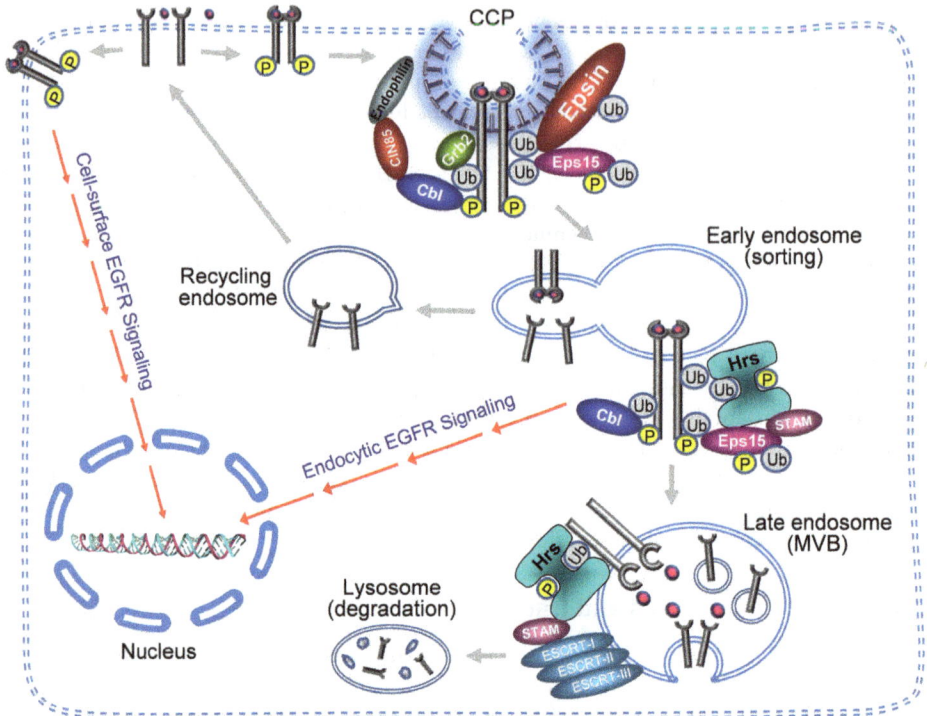

Fig. 3. EGFR endocytosis, trafficking, and turnover. EGF engagement results in EGFR activation and signaling from the cell surface. Upon EGF binding, EGFRs are internalized into clathrin-coated pits (CCP). Activated EGFR recruits the E3 ubiquitin (Ub) ligase Cbl, which ubiquitinates EGFR. EGFRs are delivered to early endosomes. From here, the receptors are sorted for either recycling back to the plasma membrane or transferring via multivesicular bodies (MVB) to late endosomes/lysosomes for degradation. The activated EGFR can continuously signal from endosomes or during its postendocytic trafficking. See the text for more details.

3.1 Ubiquitination and internalization of EGFR

Although the major steps of EGF/EGFR endocytosis and trafficking pathways are well established (Grandal & Madshus, 2008; Wiley, 2003), the molecular machinery controlling these processes remains poorly understood. It is believed that ubiquitination plays a key role in "tagging" or sorting EGFR for endocytosis and degradation (Hicke, 1999). Cbl is a ring-finger domain E3 ubiquitin ligase that is mainly responsible for EGFR ubiquitination (Levkowitz et al., 1998; Waterman et al., 1999). Upon EGF binding to EGFR, Cbl proteins are tyrosine phosphorylated by Src kinases (Feshchenko et al., 1998) and recruited rapidly to the activated EGFR to mediate the receptor ubiquitination (Sebastian et al., 2006). Cbl can bind to EGFR either directly at phosphorylated tyrosine residue 1045 (Y1045) or indirectly via adaptor protein Grb2, which binds to phosphorylated EGFR at Y1068 and Y1086 (Levkowitz et al., 1999; Waterman et al., 2002). However, these two Cbl-EGFR interaction mechanisms have different effects on EGFR endocytosis. Direct binding via Y1045 may not be necessary for EGFR endocytosis, as the Y1045F mutation of EGFR results in impaired ubiquitination but does not affect receptor internalization (Grøvdal et al., 2004; Jiang et al., 2003). In contrast, Grb2-mediated binding is essential and sufficient for EGFR internalization. This is supported by the fact that Grb2 knockdown inhibits EGFR endocytosis and a chimeric protein consisting of the Y1068/Y1086-binding domain of Grb2 fused to Cbl can rescue the EGFR internalization in Grb2-depleted cells (Huang & Sorkin, 2005).

In addition to acting as an E3 ubiquitin ligase, Cbl may have other functions in EGFR endocytic signaling. Phosphorylated Cbl can bind to the 85 kDa Cbl interacting protein (CIN85) that is constitutively associated with endophilin (Soubeyran et al., 2002), a known regulator of clathrin-mediated endocytosis (CME) (Reutens & Begley, 2002). The recruitment of CIN85 and endophilin to EGFR by Cbl plays an important role in EGF-induced EGFR internalization and downregulation (Soubeyran et al., 2002). Furthermore, Eps15 and epsin, the two adaptor proteins with ubiquitin binding capacity and known to localize to CCPs, are required for EGFR internalization and possibly form a complex with ubiquitinated EGFR (Polo et al., 2002; Roepstorff et al., 2008; Salcini et al., 1999). Interestingly, it has been reported that Esp15 localizes at the rim of CCPs (Stang et al., 2004; Tebar et al., 1996), while epsin localizes along the entire CCP curvature (Stang et al., 2004). These findings suggest that EGFR (ubiquitinated by Cbl) is captured by Eps15 and subsequently handed off to epsin deeper in the coated pits, which could be a more efficient way of EGFR progression into CCPs (Grandal & Madshus, 2008).

As shown above, many lines of evidence indicate that functional Cbl is a prerequisite for EGFR internalization and that Cbl ubiquitinates EGFR. However, the role of EGFR ubiquitination as an internalization signal remains controversial. One study reported that an ubiquitination-deficient mutant of EGFR with full kinase activity can still undergo normal internalization (Huang et al., 2007). Several studies also showed that siRNA depletion of epsin and/or Eps15 did not specifically affect the clathrin-mediated EGFR internalization (Chen & Zhuang, 2008; F. Huang et al., 2004; Sigismund et al., 2005; Vanden Broeck & De Wolf, 2006). A very recent study has demonstrated that CME of activated EGFR is regulated by four mechanisms, which function in a redundant and cooperative fashion (Goh et al., 2010). All these imply that the EGFR endocytosis is a rather complicated process whose molecular mechanisms deserve further investigation.

3.2 Ubiquitination and endosomal sorting of EGFR

Upon EGF binding, activated EGFR undergoes CME at a much enhanced rate compared to the constitutive (ligand-independent) rate (Wiley, 2003). Immediately after internalization by CME, EGFR is delivered to early endosomes for sorting to either recycled back to the plasma membrane or transferred via MVBs to late endosomes/lysosomes for degradation (Figure 3). If not recycled back to the cell surface (as in the absence of EGF stimulation), EGFRs are sorted for lysosomal degradation. The latter is initiated by forming a complex with Esp15, signal transduction adaptor molecule (STAM), and hepatocyte growth factor-regulated tyrosine kinase substrate (Hrs) (Bache et al., 2003). Hrs directs the receptors to tumor susceptibility gene-101 (TSG101). The endosomal sorting complex required for transport (ESCRT) complexes (ESCRT-I to III) are sequentially recruited. These processes eventually lead to the translocation of EGFRs into the intralumenal vesicles (ILVs) of MVBs and MVS fusion with lysosomes for receptor degradation and signal termination (Bache et al., 2006; Katzmann et al., 2002; Q. Lu et al., 2003; Williams & Urbé, 2007).

In contrast to its controversial role in EGFR internalization (see above), it is clear that Cbl-mediated EGFR ubiquitination plays a pivotal role at the early endosome to the late endosome/lysosome sorting step of EGFR downregulation (Duan et al., 2003). EGFR mutants with reduced ubiquitination display impaired downregulation or degradation (Grøvdal et al., 2004; Huang et al., 2007; F. Huang et al., 2006; Jiang & Sorkin, 2003; Levkowitz et al., 1999), and the Y1045F mutant can not translocate to ILVs (Grøvdal et al., 2004). Thus, it can be concluded from these studies that Cbl-associated ubiquitination is the signal for EGFR downregulation.

3.3 EGFR signaling from the endosome

EGF binding leads to and accelerates internalization and lysosomal degradation of EGFR. The most obvious function of receptor endocytosis is to remove activated EGF/EGFR complexes from the cell surface to achieve consumption of ligand and activated receptors and to prevent excessive signaling. Thus, the canonical view holds that endocytosis is a mechanism to attenuate receptor signaling via receptor downregulation. On the other hand, it has been known for many years that activated EGFR following EGF stimulation remains at the cell surface only briefly (5-10 min), and the majority of activated receptors are located in endosomes for a much longer time (1 h) (Lai et al., 1989; Sebastian et al., 2006; Wiley, 2003). Accumulating evidence indicates that the activated EGFR can continuously signal from endosomes or during its postendocytic trafficking (Baass et al., 1995; Carpenter, 2000; Pennock & Wang, 2003; Wang et al., 2002a).

Studies of EGFR signaling in the context of endocytosis have uncovered that endosome-associated EGFR is linked to many, if not all, of its downstream signaling cascades, suggesting the complex and multifaceted effects of EGFR endocytosis on its signaling. Early work done in rat liver parenchyma (in vivo) has demonstrated that, shortly after EGF administration (1 min), internalized activated EGFR recruits a protein complex of Shc, Grb2, and the son of sevenless (Sos) to endosomes, leading to endosomally localized activation of the Ras/Raf/MEK/ERK pathway (Di Guglielmo et al., 1994). In mice, the MEK1 binding partner (MP1), adaptor protein p14, and MEK1 form a complex in endosomes. Such endosomal p14-MP1-MEK1 signaling plays an important role in cell proliferation during tissue homeostasis (Teis et al., 2006; Teis et al., 2002). Further, appropriate trafficking of activated EGFRs through endosomes ensures spatial and temporal fidelity of MAPK signaling (Taub et al., 2007). An elegant work in which EGFR is specifically activated when it is endocytosed into endosomes, has established that internalized EGFR can exert signals from endosomes to control cell survival (Wang et al., 2002a; Wang et al., 2002b), possibly by stimulating the PI3K/Akt pathway (Haugh & Meyer, 2002; Sorkin & von Zastrow, 2009). Finally, it has been reported that EGFR endocytosis is essential for STAT3 nuclear translocation and STAT3-dependent gene regulation, suggesting that endocytosis is the transport machinery for STAT3 translocation through the cytoplasm to the nucleus (Bild et al., 2002). Collectively, ligand-activated EGFR has been demonstrated to continue to signal along the endocytic pathway, which contributes to the spatio-temporal regulation of signaling, i.e. determining the specificity of signals and controlling the strength and duration of signaling.

4. ERK-dependent EGFR phosphorylation and its impact on EGFR trafficking

4.1 Ras/Raf/MEK/ERK signaling pathway

The Ras/Raf/MEK/ERK cascade is one of the major and best studied EGFR downstream pathways, which links extracellular signals to the machinery that can regulate diverse and fundamentally important cellular processes such as cell proliferation, differentiation, migration, apoptosis, angiogenesis, and chromatin remodeling (Dunn et al., 2005; Yoon & Seger, 2006). Upon ligand binding, receptor dimerization, and EGFR intrinsic kinase activation and auto-phosphorylation, activation of the ERK pathway is triggered by Grb2 binding directly to EGFR at Y1068 and Y1086 and indirectly through Shc binding at Y1148 and Y1173 (Batzer et al., 1994; Lowenstein et al., 1992) (Figure 2). Grb2 recruits Sos guanine nucleotide exchange factor to the receptor complex and Sos mediates the route of activation of Ras proteins (H-Ras, K-Ras, and N-Ras) at the plasma membrane (Downward, 1996; Quilliam et al., 1995). Ras activation induces the activation of Raf family kinases including A-Raf, B-Raf, and C-Raf (Raf-1) (Marais et al., 1997; Marais & Marshall, 1996). The active Raf then activates MEK1 and MEK2 by phosphorylating serines 218 and 222 in the activation loop, which further phosphorylate and activate ERK1 and ERK2 (Dhillon et al., 2007; McKay & Morrison, 2007). These active ERKs phosphorylate numerous cytoplasmic and nuclear targets including kinases, phosphatases, transcription factors, and cytoskeletal proteins (Yoon & Seger, 2006). We have recently uncovered ERK activation-dependent phosphorylation of EGFR in several cell systems including human prostate cancer cells, which can have profound feedback to EGFR signaling and trafficking and EGFR-driven cell migration. These previously understudied aspects are further discussed below.

4.2 ERK activity-dependent phosphorylation of EGFR at threonine-669

As illustrated in Figure 2, EGF binding to EGFR causes activation of the receptor tyrosine kinase and phosphorylation at multiple tyrosine residues in the cytoplasmic tail. Besides the tyrosine phosphorylation events, EGFR can be phosphorylated at several serine and threonine residues (Bao et al., 2000; Countaway et al., 1990; Theroux et al., 1992a), which may influence the EGFR kinase activity (Countaway et al., 1992; Theroux et al., 1992b). We have recently uncovered a previously unappreciated type of EGFR phosphorylation induced by EGF stimulation in several cell types. By employing a state-specific monoclonal antibody (mAb), PTP101, which specifically recognizes phosphorylation of the consensus site(s) (serine or threonine residues) in the substrates for proline-directed protein kinases such as ERKs (Pearson & Kemp, 1991), we initially observed that upon EGF stimulation, both EGFR and ErbB2 undergo PTP101-reactive phosphorylation in addition to tyrosine phosphorylation in murine 3T3-F442A preadipocytes (Huang et al., 2003). Such PTP101-reactive phosphorylation seems to correlate well with EGF-induced ERK activation, as the phosphorylation can be specifically inhibited by pretreatment of the cells with two separate MEK1 inhibitors, PD98059 and UO126 (Huang et al., 2003). Furthermore, we found that peptide hormones, such as growth hormone (GH) and prolactin, can activate ERKs and cause PTP101-reactive phosphorylation of both EGFR and ErbB2 in 3T3-F442A (Huang et al., 2003) and human T47D breast cancer cells (Y. Huang et al., 2006), respectively. Previous studies suggested that serine/threonine phosphorylation of EGFR and ErbB2/Neu induced by the phorbol ester (PMA) and platelet-derived growth factor (PDGF) are attributable to the activation of PKC (Bao et al., 2000; Davis & Czech, 1985; Davis & Czech, 1987; Epstein et al., 1990; Hunter et al., 1984; Lund et al., 1990). Our data showed that neither GH-induced

ERK activation nor EGFR and ErbB2 PTP101 reactivity are affected by the PKC inhibitor (GF109203X), though the MEK1 inhibitors (PD98059 and UO126) are indeed inhibitory (Huang et al., 2003). Similar results have been obtained for prolactin-induced ERK activation and PTP101-reactivity of EGFR in T47D cells (Y. Huang et al., 2006). Collectively, our data suggests that the mAb PTP101 detects ERK-dependent, rather than PKC-dependent, serine/threonine phosphorylation of EGFR and ErbB2, and that EGF/GH/prolactin-induced and PMA-induced phosphorylation may have distinct mechanisms (Huang et al., 2003; Y. Huang et al., 2006). Interestingly, we have recently demonstrated that such an EGF-induced serine/threonine phosphorylation of EGFR also occurs in human prostate cancer cells, which requires activation of ERK pathway but not Akt pathway (Gan et al., 2010) (Figure 4).

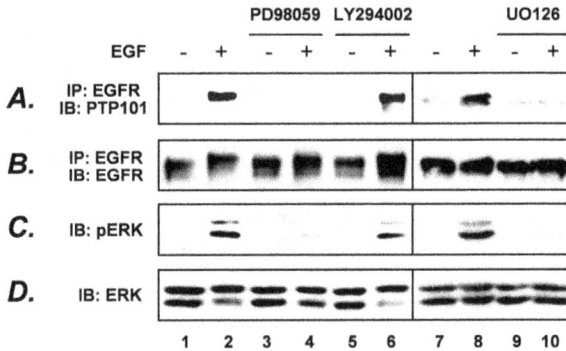

Fig. 4. EGF-induced PTP101-reactive threonine phosphorylation of EGFR is ERK pathway dependent. Serum-starved DU145 cells were pretreated with vehicle control, MEK/ERK pathway inhibitors (PD98059 or UO126) or PI3K/Akt pathway inhibitor (LY294002) for 1 h prior to stimulation with EGF for 15 min. Protein extracts were either immunoprecipitated (IP) with anti-EGFR antibody, followed by immunoblotting (IB) with PTP101 (A) or anti-EGFR (B), or directly immunoblotted with anti-phospho-ERK (C) or anti-total ERK (D). For more details see (Gan et al., 2010). Reprinted with permission from *Oncogene*.

Two major threonine phosphorylation sites are known in the EGFR juxtamembrane cytoplasmic domain, Thr-654 and Thr-669 (Davis & Czech, 1985; Heisermann & Gill, 1988; Hunter et al., 1984; Takishima et al., 1988). PKC may directly mediate Thr-654 phosphorylation (Davis & Czech, 1985; Hunter et al., 1984), whereas Thr-669 is thought to be phosphorylated by ERKs (Northwood et al., 1991; Takishima et al., 1991). The human EGFR cytoplasmic tail contains only one ERK consensus phosphorylation site [PX(S/T)P], i.e. PL^{669}TP (Li et al., 2008). In reconstituted Chinese hamster ovary (CHO) cells, we showed that only wild-type EGFR, but not EGFR mutant (EGFR-T669A in which Thr-669 is mutated to alanine), underwent PTP101-reactive phosphorylation upon EGF stimulation, although EGF can cause tyrosine phosphorylation of both forms of receptors (Li et al., 2008). In a comparison experiment, in distinction to EGFR-T669A, a different EGFR mutant (EGFR-T654A in which Thr-654 is mutated to alanine) can undergo PTP101-reactive phosphorylation after EGF treatment, which was abolished by the MEK/ERK pathway inhibitor PD98059 (Li et al., 2008). These findings indicate that Thr-669, but not Thr-654, is required for EGF-induced, ERK activity-dependent PTP101-reactive (threonine) phosphorylation of EGFR.

4.3 Impact of Thr-669 phosphorylation on EGFR tyrosine phosphorylation (activation) and trafficking

EGF binding triggers EGFR kinase activation and phosphorylation, and also initiates the process of EGFR endocytosis and degradation, leading to temporary downregulation of EGFR (Wiley, 2003; Wiley et al., 2003). Previous views held that signaling emanated only from activated cell-surface EGFRs and that internalization terminated signaling (Wells et al., 1990). However, it is now more widely believed that signaling can also emanate from the EGFR in the process of postendocytic trafficking and thus, altered postendocytic trafficking of the activated EGFR may quantitatively and/or qualitatively influence its net signaling (Burke et al., 2001; Ceresa & Schmid, 2000; Di Fiore & De Camilli, 2001; Sebastian et al., 2006; Wiley, 2003). We previously reported that GH pretreatment lessens EGF-induced EGFR downregulation in murine 3T3-F442A preadipocytes (Huang et al., 2003). Further, GH-mediated attenuation of EGF-induced EGFR downregulation is ERK pathway-dependent, correlating with GH-induced threonine phosphorylation of EGFR and signaling synergy of GH and EGF (Y. Huang et al., 2004; Huang et al., 2003). Similarly, in human T47D breast carcinoma cells, prolactin-induced, ERK activation-dependent, PTP101-reactive phosphorylation of EGFR retards subsequent EGF-induced receptor downregulation and potentiates acute EGF/EGFR signaling (Y. Huang et al., 2006). Furthermore, in T47D cells, EGF itself causes PTP101-reactive threonine phosphorylation of EGFR, and inhibition of the MEK/ERK pathway enhances EGF-induced EGFR downregulation (Y. Huang et al., 2006). Similar results were obtained in a human fibrosarcoma cell line that harbors an activating Ras mutation and subsequent basal activation of ERK and ERK-dependent PTP101-reactive EGFR phosphorylation (Li et al., 2008). Recently, we have demonstrated that in two human prostate cancer cell lines, DU145 and PC-3, pharmacological blockade of MEK/ERK pathway, but not PI3K/Akt pathway, results in accelerated EGF-induced EGFR downregulation (Figure 5), which negatively correlates with ligand-induced ERK-dependent threonine phosphorylation of EGFR (Figure 4) (Gan et al., 2010). Taken together, these results strongly suggest that ERK-mediated threonine phosphorylation of EGFR, whether accomplished by GH or prolactin (via crosstalk), or as a result of EGF-induced ERK activation, may serve as a "brake" on ligand-induced EGFR downregulation. Indeed, elimination of EGFR phosphorylation at threonine-669 by a point mutation (threonine to alanine) resulted in accelerated EGF-induced EGFR loss in CHO reconstitution cell system (Li et al., 2008).

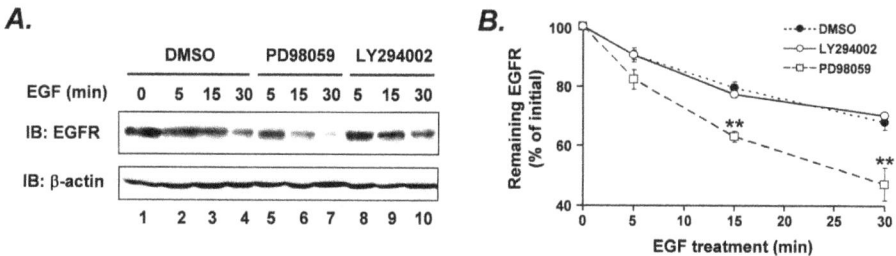

Fig. 5. Inhibition of ERK pathway but not Akt pathway accelerates EGF-induced EGFR downregulation. (*A*) Serum-starved DU145 cells were pretreated with vehicle (DMSO), PD98059 or LY294002 for 1 h prior to stimulation with EGF for 0-30 min. Protein extracts were subjected to immunoblotting (IB) with anti-EGFR or anti-β-actin. (*B*) Statistical analysis of pooled data from five independent experiments indicated that PD98059 significantly enhances EGF-induced EGFR downregulation at 15 and 30 min (**, $P < 0.01$). For more details see (Gan et al., 2010). Reprinted with permission from *Oncogene*.

Early studies of EGFR phosphorylation at serine and threonine sites, including serine-1046, serine 1047, and threonine-654, revealed that mutations at these sites can modulate EGFR signaling and downregulation (Bao et al., 2000; Countaway et al., 1990; Countaway et al., 1992; Theroux et al., 1992a). When examining the impact of ERK-mediated EGFR phosphorylation at threonine-669 on EGFR signaling, we found that in the CHO cell reconstitution system, the mutant EGFR-T669A exhibits enhanced tyrosine phosphorylation (reflecting EGFR kinase activation) compared to wild-type EGFR upon EGF stimulation (Li et al., 2008). Interestingly, coexpression of wild-type EGFR and EGFR-T669A, presumably resulting in a hybridimer of wild-type and mutant EGFR, does not dampen the propensity of EGFR-T669A to enhance EGF sensitivity (reflected in enhanced EGFR kinase activation) (Li et al., 2008). This led us to conclude that, in the hybridimer, the mutant EGFR-T669A exerts dominance regarding the EGF-induced EGFR activation (Li et al., 2008). More recently, in human prostate cancer cells (DU145 and PC-3) where the endogenous EGFR level is high, we have shown that pharmacological inhibition of the MEK/ERK pathway, but not the PI3K/Akt pathway, significantly augments the EGF-induced EGFR phosphorylation at multiple tyrosine residues including Y845, Y1045, and Y1068 (Gan et al., 2010).

The EGF-induced downregulation of EGFR is a complex, tightly regulated process, and impaired endocytic downregulation is often associated with malignancy (Grandal & Madshus, 2008; Polo et al., 2004; Roepstorff et al., 2008). The molecular machinery controlling ligand-induced EGFR endocytic trafficking remains poorly understood. It is believed that ubiquitination plays a key role in "tagging" EGFR for endocytosis. Subsequent to EGF binding to EGFR, the activated receptor is rapidly ubiquitinated by Cbl, an ubiquitin ligase that binds to phosphorylated EGFR, promoting post-internalization EGFR sorting to lysosomes for degradation (see Sections 3.1 and 3.2 for details). In human prostate cancer cells, we uncovered that blockade of the MEK/ERK pathway, but not the PI3K/Akt pathway, significantly enhanced EGF-induced ubiquitination of EGFR, correlating with increased Cbl tyrosine phosphorylation level and degree of physical association between tyrosine phosphorylated Cbl and activated EGFR (Gan et al., 2010). This phenomenon in prostate cancer cells resembles the effects of mutant EGFR-T669A in the CHO reconstitution system, in which EGFR-T669A underwent more robust ubiquitination than wild-type EGFR did upon EGF stimulation, due to the loss of phosphorylation at Thr-669 in EGFR-T669A cells (Li et al., 2008).

Emerging evidence suggests that Cbl can bind to EGFR directly at phosphorylated Y1045 or indirectly through Grb2, which binds to phosphorylated Y1068 and Y1086 in the EGFR cytoplasmic tail (Levkowitz et al., 1999; Waterman et al., 2002). As described above, our data in prostate cancer cells indicated that inhibition of ERK activity enhances the EGF-induced tyrosine phosphorylation of EGFR at multiple sites, at least including Y1045 and Y1068 (Gan et al., 2010). This raises several interesting questions, such as through which site(s) or tyrosine residue(s) within the EGFR cytoplasmic domain is the effect of the ERK activation-dependent Thr-669 phosphorylation exerted; whether Cbl is the sole factor in EGFR ubiquitination or are there any other contributors, such as CIN85, Grb2, Eps15, epsin, Hrs, and ESCRT complexes (see Sections 3.1 and 3.2 for details); and finally whether two completely different types of EGFR phosphorylation (tyrosine versus threonine phosphorylation) exist and how they are balanced under physiological and pathological conditions. More detailed studies are required to decipher these mechanisms. Taken together, our recent experimental data from multiple cell systems strongly support the notion that ERK-mediated Thr-669 phosphorylation of EGFR may serve as a "brake" on EGF-induced EGFR activation, signaling, and trafficking (ubiquitination and downregulation) (Figure 6).

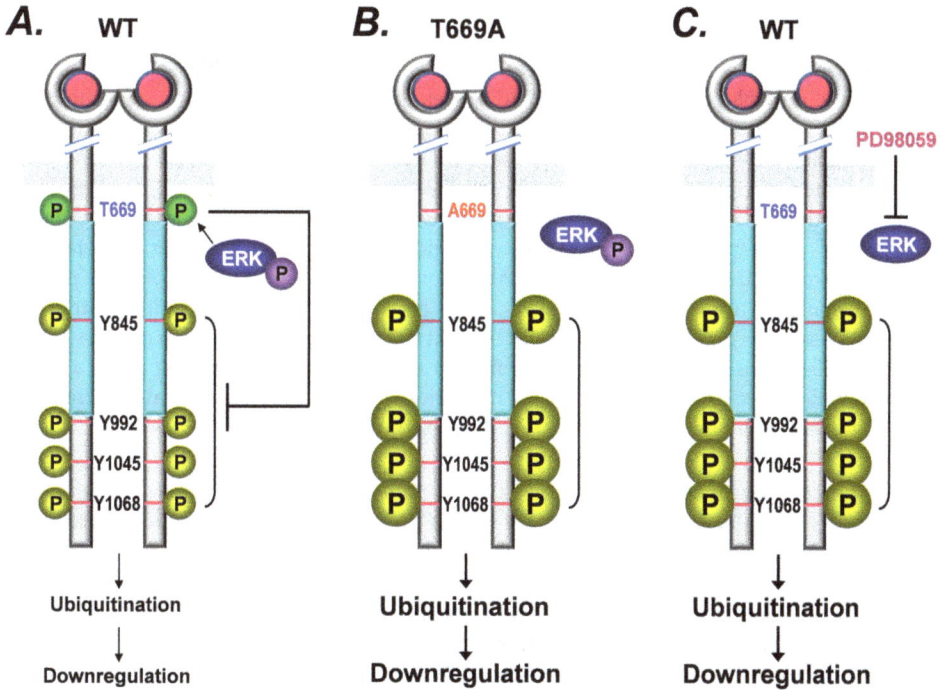

Fig. 6. Schematic model of how ERK activity-dependent threonine phosphorylation of EGFR modulates EGF-induced EGFR ubiquitination and downregulation. Based on our published data (Gan et al., 2010; Huang et al., 2003; Y. Huang et al., 2006; Li et al., 2008), ERK activation results in PTP101-reactive phosphorylation of EGFR at Thr-669. Such threonine phosphorylation serves as a "brake" on EGF-induced EGFR tyrosine phosphorylation (kinase activation), ubiquitination, and downregulation (A). Mutation of Thr-669 to alanine (B), or blockade of the ERK pathway by PD98059 (C) abolishes the threonine phosphorylation of EGFR, which releases the "brake", resulting in enhanced EGF-induced EGFR tyrosine phosphorylation/activation, ubiquitination, and downregulation.

5. Akt signaling, EGF/EGFR-driven epithelial-mesenchymal transition (EMT) and tumor metastasis

5.1 PI3K/Akt signaling pathway

The PI3K/Akt pathway plays an important role in human cancers including prostate carcinoma (Chin & Toker, 2009; de Souza et al., 2009; Morgan et al., 2009; Qiao et al., 2008). Akt was initially identified as an oncogene within the murine leukemia virus AKT8 (Staal, 1987; Staal & Hartley, 1998). It is a serine/threonine kinase and also called protein kinase B (PKB) because its catalytic domain is related to PKA and PKC family members (Jones et al., 1991). In humans, there are three highly homologous isoforms of Akt (Akt1, Akt2, and Akt3) (Nicholson & Anderson, 2002). However, it remains controversial whether all three are equally important in human malignancies (Chin & Toker, 2009; Le Page et al., 2006; Maroulakou et al., 2008). PI3K and the tumor suppressor, phosphatase and tensin homolog deleted on chromosome 10 (PTEN), are two well-known upstream components of Akt. Receptor tyrosine kinases such as EGFR and IGF-1R can activate PI3K at the cell membrane, initiating the PI3K/Akt signaling cascade. Once activated, PI3K phosphorylates phosphatidylinositol-4,5-diphosphate (PIP2), leading to accumulation of phosphatidylinositol-3,4,5-triphosphate (PIP3) (Morgan et al., 2009). PIP3 recruits Akt and phosphoinositide dependent protein kinase 1 (PDK1) to the cell membrane, where Akt is phosphorylated at Thr-308 by PDK1 and at Ser-473 via an unknown mechanism (de Souza et al., 2009). Activated Akt translocates to the nucleus, resulting in downstream effects, such as cell survival (anti-apoptosis), cell motility, angiogenesis, proliferation, and metabolism (Chin & Toker, 2009; de Souza et al., 2009; Morgan et al., 2009). PTEN is the primary negative regulator of Akt (Li et al., 1997). Loss of PTEN or PTEN mutation is the most common cause of hyperactivation of the PI3K/Akt pathway in many human cancers (Sansal & Sellers, 2004). Most recently, we have demonstrated that the Akt pathway plays a central role in EGFR-driven prostate cancer cell migration by activating epithelial-mesenchymal transition (EMT) (Gan et al., 2010), which is discussed in detail below.

5.2 EMT and tumor metastasis

EMT is a pivotal physiological process involved in embryogenesis, wound healing, and tissue remodeling (Thiery, 2003), and is regulated by complex signaling networks (Thiery & Sleeman, 2006). It is now recognized that EMT may be an important mechanism for carcinoma progression given EMT-like phenotypes of epithelial cancers (Klymkowsky & Savagner, 2009; Thiery, 2002). Acquisition of migratory properties is a prerequisite for cancer progression and for invasive migration of tumor cells into surrounding tissue. Within carcinoma (cancer of epithelial origin) cells, acquisition of invasiveness requires a dramatic morphological alteration similar to EMT, wherein carcinoma cells lose their epithelial characteristics of cell polarity and cell-cell adhesion and switch to a motile mesenchymal phenotype (Thiery, 2002; Thiery, 2003; Thiery & Sleeman, 2006). Disruption of cell-cell adherens junctions mediated by E-cadherin (one of the epithelial markers) is considered a crucial step in EMT and the downregulation of E-cadherin is common in metastatic carcinomas (Cavallaro & Christofori, 2004). Reduced E-cadherin expression has been found in high-grade prostate cancers and is associated with poor prognosis (Umbas et al., 1994; Umbas et al., 1992), reflective of its critical role in tumor progression. It is widely believed that downregulation of E-cadherin occurs via transcriptional repression mediated by the protein, Snail (Cano et al., 2000; Moreno-Bueno et al., 2008; Peinado et al., 2007). Accumulating evidence indicates that the EGFR family and PI3K/Akt signaling pathway can regulate Snail expression (Hipp et al., 2009; Lee et al., 2008; Qiao et al., 2008), suggesting that inhibition of the EGFR signaling pathways may prevent the loss of E-cadherin function and thereby acquisition of invasive motility (metastasis).

5.3 Role of Akt signaling in EGF/EGFR-driven EMT and prostate cancer cell migration

To understand which pathway(s) may have significant impact on EGFR-driven migration, we have recently probed this issue in human prostate cancer cells. The two cell lines, DU145 and PC-3, are both androgen insensitive (van Bokhoven et al., 2003), and are excellent models for studying EGFR signaling in hormonal-refractory prostate cancer. We showed that the two cell lines predominantly expressed EGFR but not ErbB-2 when compared to an androgen-responsive prostate cancer cell line, LnCap (van Bokhoven et al., 2003), in which both EGFR and ErbB-2 were expressed (Gan et al., 2010). EGF activated EGFR and its downstream ERK and Akt pathways, and markedly promoted cell migration in both DU145 and PC-3. Using pharmacological inhibitors, LY294002 and PD98059, to specifically block PI3K/Akt and MEK/ERK pathways, respectively, we further demonstrated that LY29004, but not PD98059, significantly inhibited EGF/EGFR-driven cell motility. In parallel, we observed that DU145 cells expressing constitutively activated (myristoylated) Akt (Myr-Akt) migrated much faster than control cells (Gan et al., 2010). Taken together, our data suggests that Akt activation is critical for EGFR-mediated prostate cancer cell migration.

As described above, tumors of epithelial origin, as they transform to malignancy, appear to exploit the innate plasticity of epithelial cells, with EMT conferring increased invasiveness and metastatic potential. Previous studies have implicated the involvement of ErbBs in EMT and E-cadherin downregulation in breast, lung, and cervical cancer cells (Lee et al., 2008; Lu et al., 2009; Z. Lu et al., 2003). Our recent work has clearly demonstrated that prostate cancer cells undergo EMT-like morphological changes after EGF treatment, accompanied by the loss of E-cadherin at cell-cell junctions (Gan et al., 2010). Interestingly, these EGF-induced phenomena were markedly prevented when the cells were exposed to the PI3K/Akt pathway inhibitor LY294002 (Figure 7). Consistent with downregulation of E-cadherin (an epithelial marker), we further showed an upregulation of vimentin (a mesenchymal marker) induced by EGF treatment. Similarly, LY294002 pretreatment abolished the EGF-induced quantitative (mass) changes of both E-cadherin and vimentin (Figure 8) (Gan et al., 2010). All these findings suggest that Akt activation is required for EGFR-driven EMT.

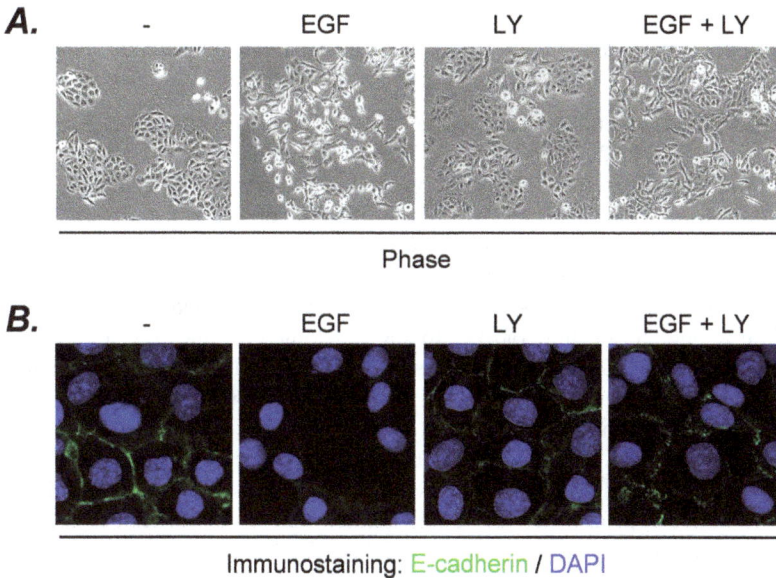

Fig. 7. Effect of inhibition of Akt pathway on EGF-induced EMT and loss of E-cadherin at cell-cell junction. Serum-starved DU145 cells were treated with vehicle (-) or EGF for 24 h in the presence or absence of LY294002. Inhibition of the Akt pathway by LY294002 prevents EGF-induced EMT (A) and loss of E-cadherin expression at cell-cell adherens junctions (B). For details see (Gan et al., 2010). Reprinted with permission from *Oncogene*.

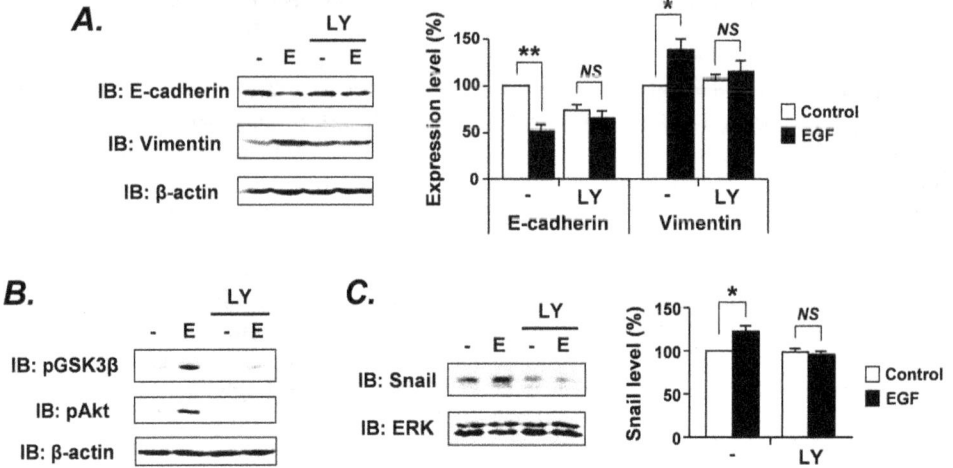

Fig. 8. Akt signaling contributes to EGF-driven EMT through the route of EGFR→Akt→GSK3β→Snail→E-cadherin. (A) LY294002 abolishes EGF-induced downregulation of E-cadherin and upregulation of vimentin. (B) LY294002 prevents EGF-induced phosphorylation (inactivation) of GSK3β via Akt inhibition. (C) LY294002 blocks EGF-induced upregulation of Snail. *, $P < 0.05$; **, $P < 0.01$; NS, not statistically significant. For details see (Gan et al., 2010). Reprinted with permission from *Oncogene*.

Snail is one of the several transcriptional factors that can suppress E-cadherin gene expression (Batlle et al., 2000; Cano et al., 2000) via binding to E-box sequences in the proximal E-cadherin promoter (Hemavathy et al., 2000). Snail is regulated by glycogen synthase kinase 3β (GSK3β, a downstream effector of Akt) by direct binding and phosphorylation, and inhibition of GSK3β results in upregulation of Snail and downregulation of E-cadherin (Zhou et al., 2004). This implies that Snail and GSK3β together, function as a molecular switch for many signaling pathways leading to EMT, and may provide a new connection of Akt to EMT. Along this line, we uncovered that in prostate cancer cells, EGF induced robust GSK3β phosphorylation (inactivation) and LY294002 markedly inhibited this phosphorylation, which correlated with the Akt activity. Consistent with Akt-mediated inactivation of GSK3β, Snail was upregulated upon EGF stimulation. Intriguingly, LY294002 pretreatment abolished such an EGF-induced upregulation of Snail, presumably by inactivating Akt and restoring GSK3β activity (Figure 8). As an alternative approach, we also demonstrated that knockdown of endogenous Snail in DU145 cells significantly prevented the EGF-induced loss of E-cadherin expression and concomitantly suppressed EGF-driven EMT, which correlated with a decrease in EGF-directed cell migration (Figure 9) (Gan et al., 2010). These results implicate Snail as a central effector of EMT and cell motility mediated by EGF/EGFR-activated Akt within prostate cancer cells. Collectively, our findings that EGF-mediated Akt signaling affects both phenotypic and molecular attributes, typical of EMT, provide new insights into the molecular mechanisms of EGFR-driven prostate cancer progression and metastasis.

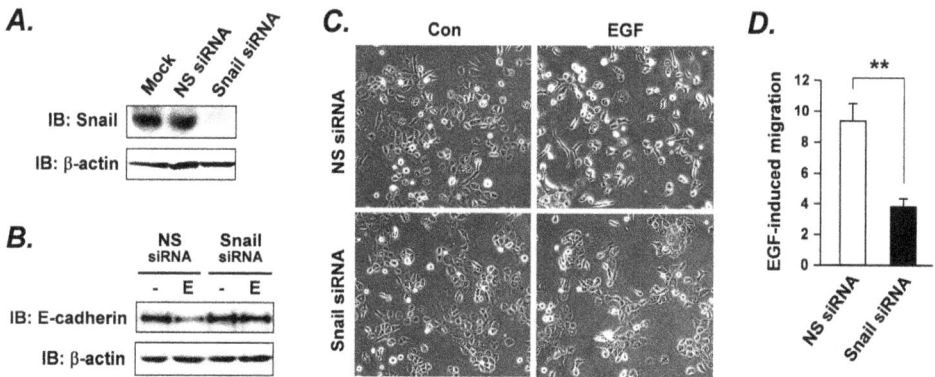

Fig. 9. Knockdown of endogenous Snail prevents EGF-induced E-cadherin loss, EMT, and cell migration. (A) Knockdown of Snail in DU145 cells. (B) Knockdown of Snail prevents EGF-induced loss of E-cadherin expression. (C) Knockdown of Snail blocks EGF-induced EMT process. (D) Knockdown of Snail reduces EGF-driven cell migration measured by transwell assay. NS siRNA, nonspecific siRNA (control); **, $P < 0.01$. For details see (Gan et al., 2010). Reprinted with permission from *Oncogene*.

6. Negative feedback loop between EGFR-directed ERK and Akt signaling

As described above, Ras/Raf/MEK/ERK and PI3K/Akt signaling pathways play central roles in many aspects related to tumorigenesis and cancer progression. Thus, inhibition of these signaling cascades could hold powerful therapeutic potentials. Given that many receptors utilize the common downstream pathways such as MEK/ERK and PI3K/Akt, targeting these kinases is expected to have greater therapeutic efficacy and broader applicability. For example, blockade of signaling through MEK offers the potential advantage of inhibiting both proliferation-promoting and anti-apoptotic signals originating from either activated receptors or mutation of RAS/Raf in breast cancer (Adeyinka et al., 2002). However, clinical studies of MEK inhibitors have only shown limited antitumor effects (Adjei et al., 2008; Rinehart et al., 2004). The underlying mechanisms remain poorly understood.

The molecular features of breast cancer cells that determine sensitivity to pharmacological inhibition of the Ras/Raf/MEK/ERK signaling pathway have been recently examined. Using a large set of human breast cancer cell lines as a model system, it was found that activation of PI3K/Akt pathway in response to MEK inhibition through a negative MEK-EGFR-PI3K feedback loop counteracts the efficacy of MEK inhibition on cell cycle and apoptosis induction (Mirzoeva et al., 2009). In concert with this finding, we uncovered that in prostate cancer cells, in contrast to inhibition of PI3K/Akt pathway, inhibition of MEK/ERK pathway rather enhanced EGF-directed cell motility, accompanied by enhanced EGF-induced Akt activation (Figure 10) (Gan et al., 2010). This phenomenon highly supports the notion that Akt is the key node in EGFR-mediated migratory pathways (see Section 5.3). It also raises a key question as to how ERK inactivation exerts its feedback effect to EGF-induced Akt activation. Based on our data, we believe that one mechanism could be through the feedback of ERK on EGFR phosphorylation (Figure 6). One can envision that inhibition of ERK activity eliminates EGFR threonine-669 phosphorylation, resulting in enhanced EGFR tyrosine phosphorylation (kinase activation), and subsequently augmented activation of the downstream PI3K/Akt pathway. The discovery of the negative feedback loop of MEK/ERK-EGFR-PI3K/Akt on several cellular aspects implies that targeting single MEK/ERK pathway in some cancers (e.g., breast and prostate carcinomas) may have undesirable outcomes, which deserves further investigation.

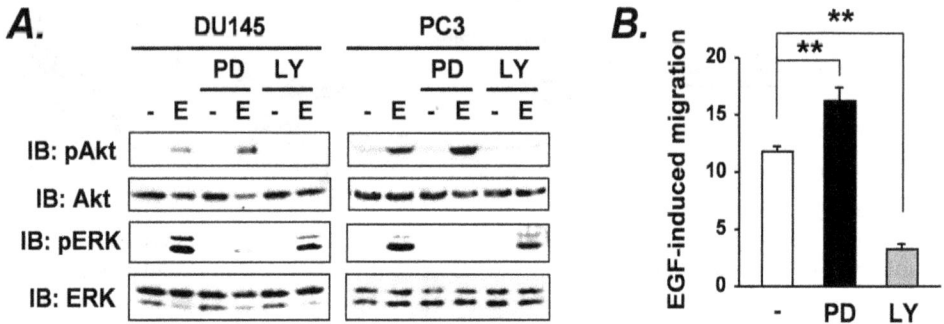

Fig. 10. Effects of ERK and Akt pathways on EGF-driven prostate cancer cell migration. (*A*) Inhibition of the ERK pathway by PD98059 augments EGF-induced Akt activation in both DU145 and PC3 cells, revealed by immunoblotting (IB) with anti-phospho-Akt antibody (*top panel*). (*B*) Transwell assay shows that blockade of the Akt pathway by LY294002 significantly inhibits EGF-driven cell migration. In contrast, blockade of the ERK pathway by PD98059 rather enhances EGF-induced migration. **, $P < 0.01$. For details see (Gan et al., 2010). Reprinted with permission from *Oncogene*.

7. Concluding remarks

Recent advances in the ErbB field have broadened our understanding of the important roles of EGFR/ErbB signaling in human cancer. However, the complexity of the ErbB signaling network, which involves numerous ligands, multiple dimerization partners, and a variety of downstream signaling components, makes it a real challenge to establish which pathways are activated or critical in the context of tumorigenesis and progression of specific cancer types. In this chapter, several aspects of EGFR/ErbB signaling and their potential roles in prostate cancer initiation and progression are discussed. In particular, we focus on the mechanisms of how Ras/Raf/MEK/ERK and PI3K/Akt pathways impact EGFR phosphorylation, trafficking, and cell motility. New insights into prostate cancer biology gained from our own work and the studies of other investigators highlight the importance of ERK activity-dependent threonine-669 phosphorylation of EGFR and its profound feedback on EGFR tyrosine phosphorylation/kinase activation, ubiquitination, and trafficking. Recent data from our group demonstrates that the Akt pathway plays a pivotal role in EGFR-driven prostate cancer cell migration by activating EMT. In particular, our results in prostate cancer (Gan et al., 2010) and data from a recent study in breast cancer (Mirzoeva et al., 2009) suggest that therapeutic targeting of ERK signaling may have undesirable outcomes. For example, inhibition of the MEK/ERK pathway conversely activates the PI3K/Akt pathway through a negative MEK/ERK-EGFR-PI3K/Akt feedback loop. We believe that ERK-mediated threonine-669 phosphorylation is critically involved in such a negative feedback and thereby contributes to invasive migration (metastasis). Thus, inhibition of the MEK/ERK-EGFR-PI3K/Akt feedback loop is likely to result in therapeutic synergism. Future detailed studies along these lines and a deeper understanding of various mechanisms of cell signaling from EGFR and other ErbBs will undoubtedly generate new avenues for drug and biomarker development to combat cancers including prostate cancer.

8. Acknowledgments

This work was supported by a St. Joseph's Foundation (SJF) Startup Fund, an American Heart Association (AHA) Beginning Grant-in-Aid Award, and a Science Foundation Arizona (SFAz) Competitive Advantage Award (to YH). The authors have nothing to disclose. Correspondence should be addressed to Dr. Yao Huang, 445 N 5th Street, Suite 110, Phoenix, Arizona, 85004, USA. E-mail: yhuang@chw.edu.

9. References

Adams, T.E.; McKern, N.M. & Ward, C.W. (2004). Signaling by the type 1 insulin-like growth factor receptor: interplay with the epidermal growth factor receptor. *Growth Factors*, 22:89-95.

Adeyinka, A.; Nui, Y.; Cherlet, T.; Snell, L.; Watson, P.H. & Murphy, L.C. (2002). Activated mitogen-activated protein kinase expression during human breast tumorigenesis and breast cancer progression. *Clin Cancer Res*, 8:1747-53.

Adjei, A.A.; Cohen, R.B.; Franklin, W.; Morris, C.; Wilson, D.; Molina, J.R.; Hanson, L.J.; Gore, L.; Chow, L.; Leong, S.; Maloney, L.; Gordon, G.; Simmons, H.; Marlow, A.; Litwiler, K.; Brown, S.; Poch, G.; Kane, K.; Haney, J. & Eckhardt, S.G. (2008). Phase I pharmacokinetic and pharmacodynamic study of the oral, small-molecule mitogen-activated protein kinase kinase 1/2 inhibitor AZD6244 (ARRY-142886) in patients with advanced cancers. *J Clin Oncol*, 26:2139-46.

Alroy, I. & Yarden, Y. (1997). The ErbB signaling network in embryogenesis and oncogenesis: signal diversification through combinatorial ligand-receptor interactions. *FEBS Lett*, 410:83-6.

Andl, C.D.; Mizushima, T.; Oyama, K.; Bowser, M.; Nakagawa, H. & Rustgi, A.K. (2004). EGFR-induced cell migration is mediated predominantly by the JAK-STAT pathway in primary esophageal keratinocytes. *Am J Physiol Gastrointest Liver Physiol*, 287:G1227-37.

Baass, P.C.; Di Guglielmo, G.M.; Authier, F.; Posner, B.I. & Bergeron, J.J. (1995). Compartmentalized signal transduction by receptor tyrosine kinases. *Trends Cell Biol*, 5:465-70.

Bache, K.G.; Raiborg, C.; Mehlum, A. & Stenmark, H. (2003). STAM and Hrs are subunits of a multivalent ubiquitin-binding complex on early endosomes. *J Biol Chem*, 278:12513-21.

Bache, K.G.; Stuffers, S.; Malerød, L.; Slagsvold, T.; Raiborg, C.; Lechardeur, D.; Wälchli, S.; Lukacs, G.L.; Brech, A. & Stenmark, H. (2006). The ESCRT-III subunit hVps24 is required for degradation but not silencing of the epidermal growth factor receptor. *Mol Biol Cell*, 17:2513-23.

Bao, J.; Alroy, I.; Waterman, H.; Schejter, E.D.; Brodie, C.; Gruenberg, J. & Yarden, Y. (2000). Threonine phosphorylation diverts internalized epidermal growth factor receptors from a degradative pathway to the recycling endosome. *J Biol Chem*, 275:26178-86.

Baselga, J. & Hammond, L.A. (2002). HER-targeted tyrosine-kinase inhibitors. *Oncology*, 63:6-16.

Batlle, E.; Sancho, E.; Francí, C.; Domínguez, D.; Monfar, M.; Baulida, J. & García De Herreros, A. (2000). The transcription factor snail is a repressor of E-cadherin gene expression in epithelial tumour cells. *Nat Cell Biol*, 2:84-9.

Batzer, A.G.; Rotin, D.; Ureña, J.M.; Skolnik, E.Y. & Schlessinger, J. (1994). Hierarchy of binding sites for Grb2 and Shc on the epidermal growth factor receptor. *Mol Cell Biol*, 14:5192-201.

Bild, A.H.; Turkson, J. & Jove, R. (2002). Cytoplasmic transport of Stat3 by receptor-mediated endocytosis. *EMBO J*, 21:3255-63.

Burke, P.; Schooler, K. & Wiley, H.S. (2001). Regulation of epidermal growth factor receptor signaling by endocytosis and intracellular trafficking. *Mol Biol Cell*, 12:1897-910.

Cai, C.Q.; Peng, Y.; Buckley, M.T.; Wei, J.; Chen, F.; Liebes, L.; Gerald, W.L.; Pincus, M.R.; Osman, I. & Lee, P. (2008). Epidermal growth factor receptor activation in prostate cancer by three novel missense mutations. *Oncogene*, 27:3201-10.

Cano, A.; Pérez-Moreno, M.A.; Rodrigo, I.; Locascio, A.; Blanco, M.J.; del Barrio, M.G.; Portillo, F. & Nieto, M.A. (2000). The transcription factor snail controls epithelial-mesenchymal transitions by repressing E-cadherin expression. *Nat Cell Biol*, 2:76-83.

Carpenter, G. (2000). The EGF receptor: a nexus for trafficking and signaling. *Bioessays*, 22:697-707.

Cavallaro, U. & Christofori, G. (2004). Cell adhesion and signalling by cadherins and Ig-CAMs in cancer. *Nat Rev Cancer*, 4:118-32.

Ceresa, B.P. & Schmid, S.L. (2000). Regulation of signal transduction by endocytosis. *Curr Opin Cell Biol*, 12:204-10.

Chen, C. & Zhuang, X. (2008). Epsin 1 is a cargo-specific adaptor for the clathrin-mediated endocytosis of the influenza virus. *Proc Natl Acad Sci U S A*, 105:11790-5.

Chin, Y.R. & Toker, A. (2009). Function of Akt/PKB signaling to cell motility, invasion and the tumor stroma in cancer. *Cell Signal*, 21:470-6.

Ciardiello, F. & Tortora, G. (2003). Epidermal growth factor receptor (EGFR) as a target in cancer therapy: understanding the role of receptor expression and other molecular determinants that could influence the response to anti-EGFR drugs. *Eur J Cancer*, 39:1348-54.

Citri, A. & Yarden, Y. (2006). EGF-ERBB signalling: towards the systems level. *Nat Rev Mol Cell Biol*, 7:505-16.

Countaway, J.L.; McQuilkin, P.; Girones, N. & Davis, R.J. (1990). Multisite phosphorylation of the epidermal growth factor receptor. Use of site-directed mutagenesis to examine the role of serine/threonine phosphorylation. *J Biol Chem*, 265:3407-16.

Countaway, J.L.; Nairn, A.C. & Davis, R.J. (1992). Mechanism of desensitization of the epidermal growth factor receptor protein-tyrosine kinase. *J Biol Chem*, 267:1129-40.

Craft, N.; Shostak, Y.; Carey, M. & Sawyers, C.L. (1999). A mechanism for hormone-independent prostate cancer through modulation of androgen receptor signaling by the HER-2/neu tyrosine kinase. *Nat Med*, 5:280-5.

Davis, R.J. & Czech, M.P. (1985). Tumor-promoting phorbol diesters cause the phosphorylation of epidermal growth factor receptors in normal human fibroblasts at threonine-654. *Proc Natl Acad Sci U S A*, 82:1974-8.

Davis, R.J. & Czech, M.P. (1987). Stimulation of epidermal growth factor receptor threonine 654 phosphorylation by platelet-derived growth factor in protein kinase C-deficient human fibroblasts. *J Biol Chem*, 262:6832-41.

de Souza, P.L.; Russell, P.J. & Kearsley, J. (2009). Role of the Akt pathway in prostate cancer. *Curr Cancer Drug Targets*, 9:163-75.

DeHaan, A.M.; Wolters, N.M.; Keller, E.T. & Ignatoski, K.M. (2009). EGFR ligand switch in late stage prostate cancer contributes to changes in cell signaling and bone remodeling. *Prostate*, 69:528-37.

Dhillon, A.S.; Hagan, S.; Rath, O. & Kolch, W. (2007). MAP kinase signalling pathways in cancer. *Oncogene*, 26:3279-90.

Di Fiore, P.P. & De Camilli, P. (2001). Endocytosis and signaling. an inseparable partnership. *Cell*, 106:1-4.

Di Guglielmo, G.M.; Baass, P.C.; Ou, W.J.; Posner, B.I. & Bergeron, J.J. (1994). Compartmentalization of SHC, GRB2 and mSOS, and hyperphosphorylation of Raf-1 by EGF but not insulin in liver parenchyma. *Embo J*, 13:4269-77.

Djakiew, D. (2000). Dysregulated expression of growth factors and their receptors in the development of prostate cancer. *Prostate*, 42:150-60.

Douglas, D.A.; Zhong, H.; Ro, J.Y.; Oddoux, C.; Berger, A.D.; Pincus, M.R.; Satagopan, J.M.; Gerald, W.L.; Scher, H.I.; Lee, P. & Osman, I. (2006). Novel mutations of epidermal growth factor receptor in localized prostate cancer. *Front Biosci*, 11:2518-25.

Downward, J. (1996). Control of ras activation. *Cancer Surv*, 27:87-100.

Duan, L.; Miura, Y.; Dimri, M.; Majumder, B.; Dodge, I.L.; Reddi, A.L.; Ghosh, A.; Fernandes, N.; Zhou, P.; Mullane-Robinson, K.; Rao, N.; Donoghue, S.; Rogers, R.A.; Bowtell, D.; Naramura, M.; Gu, H.; Band, V. & Band, H. (2003). Cbl-mediated ubiquitinylation is required for lysosomal sorting of epidermal growth factor receptor but is dispensable for endocytosis. *J Biol Chem*, 278:28950-60.

Dunn, K.L.; Espino, P.S.; Drobic, B.; He, S. & Davie, J.R. (2005). The Ras-MAPK signal transduction pathway, cancer and chromatin remodeling. *Biochem Cell Biol*, 83:1-14.

Elson, S.D.; Browne, C.A. & Thorburn, G.D. (1984). Identification of epidermal growth factor-like activity in human male reproductive tissues and fluids. *J Clin Endocrinol Metab*, 58:589-94.

Epstein, R.J.; Druker, B.J.; Roberts, T.M. & Stiles, C.D. (1990). Modulation of a Mr 175,000 c-neu receptor isoform in G8/DHFR cells by serum starvation. *J Biol Chem*, 265:10746-51.

Feshchenko, E.A.; Langdon, W.Y. & Tsygankov, A.Y. (1998). Fyn, Yes, and Syk phosphorylation sites in c-Cbl map to the same tyrosine residues that become phosphorylated in activated T cells. *J Biol Chem*, 273:8323-31.

Freeman, M.R.; Paul, S.; Kaefer, M.; Ishikawa, M.; Adam, R.M.; Renshaw, A.A.; Elenius, K. & Klagsbrun, M. (1998). Heparin-binding EGF-like growth factor in the human prostate: synthesis predominantly by interstitial and vascular smooth muscle cells and action as a carcinoma cell mitogen. *J Cell Biochem*, 68:328-38.

Gan, Y.; Shi, C.; Inge, L.; Hibner, M.; Balducci, J. & Huang, Y. (2010). Differential roles of ERK and Akt pathways in regulation of EGFR-mediated signaling and motility in prostate cancer cells. *Oncogene*, 29:4947-58.

Gee, J.M.; Robertson, J.F.; Gutteridge, E.; Ellis, I.O.; Pinder, S.E.; Rubini, M. & Nicholson, R.I. (2005). Epidermal growth factor receptor/HER2/insulin-like growth factor receptor signaling and oestrogen receptor activity in clinical breast cancer. *Endocr Relat Cancer*, 12:S99-S111.

Goh, L.K.; Huang, F.; Kim, W.; Gygi, S. & Sorkin, A. (2010). Multiple mechanisms collectively regulate clathrin-mediated endocytosis of the epidermal growth factor receptor. *J Cell Biol*, 189:871-83.

Grandal, M.V. & Madshus, I.H. (2008). Epidermal growth factor receptor and cancer: control of oncogenic signalling by endocytosis. *J Cell Mol Med*, 12:1527-34.

Graus-Porta, D.; Beerli, R.R.; Daly, J.M. & Hynes, N.E. (1997). ErbB-2, the preferred heterodimerization partner of all ErbB receptors, is a mediator of lateral signaling. *Embo J*, 16:1647-55.

Grøvdal, L.M.; Stang, E.; Sorkin, A. & Madshus, I.H. (2004). Direct interaction of Cbl with pTyr 1045 of the EGF receptor (EGFR) is required to sort the EGFR to lysosomes for degradation. *Exp Cell Res*, 300:388-95.

Guy, P.M.; Platko, J.V.; Cantley, L.C.; Cerione, R.A. & Carraway, K.L. (1994). Insect cell-expressed p180erbB3 possesses an impaired tyrosine kinase activity. *Proc Natl Acad Sci U S A*, 91:8132-6.

Harari, D.; Tzahar, E.; Romano, J.; Shelly, M.; Pierce, J.H.; Andrews, G.C. & Yarden, Y. (1999). Neuregulin-4: a novel growth factor that acts through the ErbB-4 receptor tyrosine kinase. *Oncogene*, 18:2681-9.

Harari, P. (2004). Epidermal growth factor receptor inhibition strategies in oncology. *Endocr Relat Cancer*, 11:689-708.

Hatake, K.; Tokudome, N. & Ito, Y. (2007). Next generation molecular targeted agents for breast cancer: focus on EGFR and VEGFR pathways. *Breast Cancer*, 14:132-49.

Haugh, J.M. & Meyer, T. (2002). Active EGF receptors have limited access to PtdIns(4,5)P(2) in endosomes: implications for phospholipase C and PI 3-kinase signaling. *J Cell Sci*, 115:303-10.

He, M. & Young, C.Y. (2009). Mutant epidermal growth factor receptor vIII increases cell motility and clonogenecity in a prostate cell line RWPE1. *J Endocrinol Invest*, 32:272-8.

Heisermann, G.J. & Gill, G.N. (1988). Epidermal growth factor receptor threonine and serine residues phosphorylated in vivo. *J Biol Chem*, 263:13152-8.

Hemavathy, K.; Ashraf, S.I. & Ip, Y.T. (2000). Snail/slug family of repressors: slowly going into the fast lane of development and cancer. *Gene*, 257:1-2.

Hicke, L. (1999). Gettin' down with ubiquitin: turning off cell-surface receptors, transporters and channels. *Trends Cell Biol*, 9:107-12.

Hipp, S.; Walch, A.; Schuster, T.; Losko, S.; Laux, H.; Bolton, T.; Höfler, H. & Becker, K.F. (2009). Activation of epidermal growth factor receptor results in Snail protein but not mRNA over-expression in endometrial cancer. *J Cell Mol Med*:, 13:3858-67.

Hirsch, F.R.; Scagliotti, G.V.; Langer, C.J.; Varella-Garcia, M. & Franklin, W.A. (2003). Epidermal growth factor family of receptors in preneoplasia and lung cancer: perspectives for targeted therapies. *Lung Cancer*, 41:S29-42.

Hofer, D.R.; Sherwood, E.R.; Bromberg, W.D.; Mendelsohn, J.; Lee, C. & Kozlowski, J.M. (1991). Autonomous growth of androgen-independent human prostatic carcinoma cells: role of transforming growth factor alpha. *Cancer Res*, 51:2780-5.

Huang, F.; Goh, L.K. & Sorkin, A. (2007). EGF receptor ubiquitination is not necessary for its internalization. *Proc Natl Acad Sci U S A*, 104:16904-9.

Huang, F.; Khvorova, A.; Marshall, W. & Sorkin, A. (2004). Analysis of clathrin-mediated endocytosis of epidermal growth factor receptor by RNA interference. *J Biol Chem*, 279:16657-61.

Huang, F.; Kirkpatrick, D.; Jiang, X.; Gygi, S. & Sorkin, A. (2006). Differential regulation of EGF receptor internalization and degradation by multiubiquitination within the kinase domain. *Mol Cell*, 21:737-48.

Huang, F. & Sorkin, A. (2005). Growth factor receptor binding protein 2-mediated recruitment of the RING domain of Cbl to the epidermal growth factor receptor is essential and sufficient to support receptor endocytosis. *Mol Biol Cell*, 16:1268-81.

Huang, P.H.; Xu, A.M. & White, F.M. (2009). Oncogenic EGFR signaling networks in glioma. *Sci Signal*, 2:re6.

Huang, Y.; Chang, Y.; Wang, X.; Jiang, J. & Frank, S.J. (2004). Growth hormone alters epidermal growth factor receptor binding affinity via activation of ERKs in 3T3-F442A cells. *Endocrinology*, 145:3297-306.

Huang, Y.; Kim, S.O.; Jiang, J. & Frank, S.J. (2003). Growth hormone-induced phosphorylation of epidermal growth factor (EGF) receptor in 3T3-F442A cells. Modulation of EGF-induced trafficking and signaling. *J Biol Chem*, 278:18902-13.

Huang, Y.; Li, X.; Jiang, J. & Frank, S.J. (2006). Prolactin modulates phosphorylation, signaling and trafficking of epidermal growth factor receptor in human T47D breast cancer cells. *Oncogene*, 25:7565-76.

Hunter, T.; Ling, N. & Cooper, J.A. (1984). Protein kinase C phosphorylation of the EGF receptor at a threonine residue close to the cytoplasmic face of the plasma membrane. *Nature*, 311:480-3.

Jiang, X.; Huang, F.; Marusyk, A. & Sorkin, A. (2003). Grb2 regulates internalization of EGF receptors through clathrin-coated pits. *Mol Biol Cell*, 14:858-70.

Jiang, X. & Sorkin, A. (2003). Epidermal growth factor receptor internalization through clathrin-coated pits requires Cbl RING finger and proline-rich domains but not receptor polyubiquitylation. *Traffic*, 4:529-43.

Johnson, G.L.; Dohlman, H.G. & Graves, L.M. (2005). MAPK kinase kinases (MKKKs) as a target class for small-molecule inhibition to modulate signaling networks and gene expression. *Curr Opin Chem Biol*, 9:325-31.

Jones, P.F.; Jakubowicz, T.; Pitossi, F.J.; Maurer, F. & Hemmings, B.A. (1991). Molecular cloning and identification of a serine/threonine protein kinase of the second-messenger subfamily. *Proc Natl Acad Sci U S A*, 88:4171-5.

Katzmann, D.J.; Odorizzi, G. & Emr, S.D. (2002). Receptor downregulation and multivesicular-body sorting. *Nat Rev Mol Cell Biol*, 3:893-905.

Kim, H.G.; Kassis, J.; Souto, J.C.; Turner, T. & Wells, A. (1999). EGF receptor signaling in prostate morphogenesis and tumorigenesis. *Histol Histopathol*, 14:1175-82.

Kloth, M.T.; Catling, A.D. & Silva, C.M. (2002). Novel activation of STAT5b in response to epidermal growth factor. *J Biol Chem*, 277:8693-701.

Klymkowsky, M.W. & Savagner, P. (2009). Epithelial-mesenchymal transition: a cancer researcher's conceptual friend and foe. *Am J Pathol*, 174:1588-93.

Lai, W.H.; Cameron, P.H.; Doherty, J.J.; Posner, B.I. & Bergeron, J.J. (1989). Ligand-mediated autophosphorylation activity of the epidermal growth factor receptor during internalization. *J Cell Biol*, 109:2751-60.

Laskin, J.J. & Sandler, A.B. (2004). Epidermal growth factor receptor: a promising target in solid tumours. *Cancer Treat Rev*, 30:1-17.

Le Page, C.; Koumakpayi, I.H.; Alam-Fahmy, M.; Mes-Masson, A.M. & Saad, F. (2006). Expression and localisation of Akt-1, Akt-2 and Akt-3 correlate with clinical outcome of prostate cancer patients. *Br J Cancer*, 94:1906-12.

Lee, M.Y.; Chou, C.Y.; Tang, M.J. & Shen, M.R. (2008). Epithelial-mesenchymal transition in cervical cancer: correlation with tumor progression, epidermal growth factor receptor overexpression, and snail up-regulation. *Clin Cancer Res*, 14:4743-50.

Levkowitz, G.; Waterman, H.; Ettenberg, S.A.; Katz, M.; Tsygankov, A.Y.; Alroy, I.; Lavi, S.; Iwai, K.; Reiss, Y.; Ciechanover, A.; Lipkowitz, S. & Yarden, Y. (1999). Ubiquitin ligase activity and tyrosine phosphorylation underlie suppression of growth factor signaling by c-Cbl/Sli-1. *Mol Cell*, 4:1029-40.

Levkowitz, G.; Waterman, H.; Zamir, E.; Kam, Z.; Oved, S.; Langdon, W.Y.; Beguinot, L.; Geiger, B. & Yarden, Y. (1998). c-Cbl/Sli-1 regulates endocytic sorting and ubiquitination of the epidermal growth factor receptor. *Genes Dev*, 12:3663-74.

Li, J.; Yen, C.; Liaw, D.; Podsypanina, K.; Bose, S.; Wang, S.I.; Puc, J.; Miliaresis, C.; Rodgers, L.; McCombie, R.; Bigner, S.H.; Giovanella, B.C.; Ittmann, M.; Tycko, B.; Hibshoosh, H.; Wigler, M.H. & Parsons, R. (1997). PTEN, a putative protein tyrosine phosphatase gene mutated in human brain, breast, and prostate cancer. *Science*, 275:1943-7.

Li, X.; Huang, Y.; Jiang, J. & Frank, S.J. (2008). ERK-dependent threonine phosphorylation of EGF receptor modulates receptor downregulation and signaling. *Cell Signal*, 20:2145-55.

Lichtner, R.B. (2003). Estrogen/EGF receptor interactions in breast cancer: rationale for new therapeutic combination strategies. *Biomedicine Pharmacotherapy*, 57:447-51.

Liu, X.H.; Wiley, H.S. & Meikle, A.W. (1993). Androgens regulate proliferation of human prostate cancer cells in culture by increasing transforming growth factor-alpha (TGF-alpha) and epidermal growth factor (EGF)/TGF-alpha receptor. *J Clin Endocrinol Metab*, 77:1472-8.

Lowenstein, E.J.; Daly, R.J.; Batzer, A.G.; Li, W.; Margolis, B.; Lammers, R.; Ullrich, A.; Skolnik, E.Y.; Bar-Sagi, D. & Schlessinger, J. (1992). The SH2 and SH3 domain-containing protein GRB2 links receptor tyrosine kinases to ras signaling. *Cell*, 70:431-42.

Lu, J.; Guo, H.; Treekitkarnmongkol, W.; Li, P.; Zhang, J.; Shi, B.; Ling, C.; Zhou, X.; Chen, T.; Chiao, P.J.; Feng, X.; Seewaldt, V.L.; Muller, W.J.; Sahin, A.; Hung, M.C. & Yu, D. (2009). 14-3-3zeta Cooperates with ErbB2 to promote ductal carcinoma in situ progression to invasive breast cancer by inducing epithelial-mesenchymal transition. *Cancer Cell*, 16:195-207.

Lu, Q.; Hope, L.W.; Brasch, M.; Reinhard, C. & Cohen, S.N. (2003). TSG101 interaction with HRS mediates endosomal trafficking and receptor down-regulation. *Proc Natl Acad Sci U S A*, 100:7626-31.

Lu, Z.; Ghosh, S.; Wang, Z. & Hunter, T. (2003). Downregulation of caveolin-1 function by EGF leads to the loss of E-cadherin, increased transcriptional activity of beta-catenin, and enhanced tumor cell invasion. *Cancer Cell*, 4:499-515.

Lund, K.A.; Lazar, C.S.; Chen, W.S.; Walsh, B.J.; B., W.J.; Herbst, J.J.; Walton, G.M.; Rosenfeld, M.G.; Gill, G.N. & Wiley, H.S. (1990). Phosphorylation of the epidermal growth factor receptor at threonine 654 inhibits ligand-induced internalization and down-regulation. *J Biol Chem*, 265:20517-23.

Marais, R.; Light, Y.; Paterson, H.F.; Mason, C.S. & Marshall, C.J. (1997). Differential regulation of Raf-1, A-Raf, and B-Raf by oncogenic ras and tyrosine kinases. *J Biol Chem*, 272:4378-83.

Marais, R. & Marshall, C.J. (1996). Control of the ERK MAP kinase cascade by Ras and Raf. *Cancer Surv*, 27:101-25.

Marks, R.A.; Zhang, S.; Montironi, R.; McCarthy, R.P.; MacLennan, G.T.; Lopez-Beltran, A.; Jiang, Z.; Zhou, H.; Zheng, S.; Davidson, D.D.; Baldridge, L.A. & Cheng, L. (2008). Epidermal growth factor receptor (EGFR) expression in prostatic adenocarcinoma after hormonal therapy: a fluorescence in situ hybridization and immunohistochemical analysis. *Prostate*, 68:919-23.

Maroulakou, I.G.; Oemler, W.; Naber, S.P.; Klebba, I.; Kuperwasser, C. & Tsichlis, P.N. (2008). Distinct roles of the three Akt isoforms in lactogenic differentiation and involution. *J Cell Physiol*, 217:468-77.

Massagué, J. & Pandiella, A. (1993). Membrane-anchored growth factors. *Annu Rev Biochem*, 62:515-41.

McKay, M.M. & Morrison, D.K. (2007). Integrating signals from RTKs to ERK/MAPK. *Oncogene*, 26:3113-21.

Mirzoeva, O.K.; Das, D.; Heiser, L.M.; Bhattacharya, S.; Siwak, D.; Gendelman, R.; Bayani, N.; Wang, N.J.; Neve, R.M.; Guan, Y.; Hu, Z.; Knight, Z.; Feiler, H.S.; Gascard, P.; Parvin, B.; Spellman, P.T.; Shokat, K.M.; Wyrobek, A.J.; Bissell, M.J.; McCormick, F.; Kuo, W.L.; Mills, G.B.; Gray, J.W. & Korn, W.M. (2009). Basal subtype and MAPK/ERK kinase (MEK)-phosphoinositide 3-kinase feedback signaling determine susceptibility of breast cancer cells to MEK inhibition. *Cancer Res*, 69:565-72.

Morandell, S.; Stasyk, T.; Skvortsov, S.; Ascher, S. & Huber, L.A. (2008). Quantitative proteomics and phosphoproteomics reveal novel insights into complexity and dynamics of the EGFR signaling network. *Proteomics*, 8:4383-401.

Moreno-Bueno, G.; Portillo, F. & Cano, A. (2008). Transcriptional regulation of cell polarity in EMT and cancer. *Oncogene*, 27:6958-69.

Morgan, T.M.; Koreckij, T.D. & Corey, E. (2009). Targeted therapy for advanced prostate cancer: inhibition of the PI3K/Akt/mTOR pathway. *Curr Cancer Drug Targets*, 9:237-49.

Neto, A.S.; Tobias-Machado, M.; Wroclawski, M.L.; Fonseca, F.L.; Pompeo, A.C. & Del Giglio, A. (2010). Molecular oncogenesis of prostate adenocarcinoma: role of the human epidermal growth factor receptor 2 (HER-2/neu). *Tumori*, 96:645-9.

Nicholson, K.M. & Anderson, N.G. (2002). The protein kinase B/Akt signalling pathway in human malignancy. *Cell Signal*, 14:381-95.

Nicholson, R.I.; Gee, J.M. & Harper, M.E. (2001). EGFR and cancer prognosis. *Eur J Cancer*, 37 Suppl 4:S9-15.

Northwood, I.C.; Gonzalez, F.A.; Wartmann, M.; Raden, D.L. & Davis, R.J. (1991). Isolation and characterization of two growth factor-stimulated protein kinases that phosphorylate the epidermal growth factor receptor at threonine 669. *J Biol Chem*, 266:15266-76.

Olapade-Olaopa, E.O.; Moscatello, D.K.; MacKay, E.H.; Horsburgh, T.; Sandhu, D.P.; Terry, T.R.; Wong, A.J. & Habib, F.K. (2000). Evidence for the differential expression of a variant EGF receptor protein in human prostate cancer. *Br J Cancer*, 82:186-94.

Olayioye, M.A.; Neve, R.M.; Lane, H.A. & Hynes, N.E. (2000). The ErbB signaling network: receptor heterodimerization in development and cancer. *EMBO J*, 19:3159-67.

Orth, J.D.; Krueger, E.W.; Weller, S.G. & McNiven, M.A. (2006). A novel endocytic mechanism of epidermal growth factor receptor sequestration and internalization. *Cancer Res*, 66:3603-10.

Pearson, R.B. & Kemp, B.E. (1991). Protein kinase phosphorylation site sequences and consensus specificity motifs: tabulations. *Methods Enzymol*, 200:62-81.

Peinado, H.; Olmeda, D. & Cano, A. (2007). Snail, Zeb and bHLH factors in tumour progression: an alliance against the epithelial phenotype? *Nat Rev Cancer*, 7:415-28.

Pennock, S. & Wang, Z. (2003). Stimulation of cell proliferation by endosomal epidermal growth factor receptor as revealed through two distinct phases of signaling. *Mol Cell Biol*, 23:5803-15.

Polo, S.; Pece, S. & Di Fiore, P.P. (2004). Endocytosis and cancer. *Curr Opin Cell Biol*, 16:156-61.

Polo, S.; Sigismund, S.; Faretta, M.; Guidi, M.; Capua, M.R.; Bossi, G.; Chen, H.; De Camilli, P. & Di Fiore, P.P. (2002). A single motif responsible for ubiquitin recognition and monoubiquitination in endocytic proteins. *Nature*, 416:451-5.

Prenzel, N.; Zwick, E.; Leserer, M. & Ullrich, A. (2000). Tyrosine kinase signaling in breast cancer: epidermal growth factor receptor: convergence point for signal integration and diversification. *Breast Cancer Res*, 2:184-90.

Qiao, M.; Sheng, S. & Pardee, A.B. (2008). Metastasis and AKT activation. *Cell Cycle*, 7:2991-6.

Quilliam, L.A.; Khosravi-Far, R.; Huff, S.Y. & Der, C.J. (1995). Guanine nucleotide exchange factors: activators of the Ras superfamily of proteins. *Bioessays*, 17:395-404.

Ratan, H.L.; Gescher, A.; Steward, W.P. & Mellon, J.K. (2003). ErbB receptors: possible therapeutic targets in prostate cancer? *BJU Intl*, 92:890-5.

Reutens, A.T. & Begley, C.G. (2002). Endophilin-1: a multifunctional protein. *Int J Biochem Cell Biol*, 34:1173-7.

Rinehart, J.; Adjei, A.A.; Lorusso, P.M.; Waterhouse, D.; Hecht, J.R.; Natale, R.B.; Hamid, O.; Varterasian, M.; Asbury, P.; Kaldjian, E.P.; Gulyas, S.; Mitchell, D.Y.; Herrera, R.; Sebolt-Leopold, J.S. & Meyer, M.B. (2004). Multicenter phase II study of the oral MEK inhibitor, CI-1040, in patients with advanced non-small-cell lung, breast, colon, and pancreatic cancer. *J Clin Oncol*, 22:4456-62.

Roepstorff, K.; Grøvdal, L.; Grandal, M.; Lerdrup, M. & van Deurs, B. (2008). Endocytic downregulation of ErbB receptors: mechanisms and relevance in cancer. *Histochem Cell Biol*, 129:563-78.

Salcini, A.E.; Chen, H.; Iannolo, G.; De Camilli, P. & Di Fiore, P.P. (1999). Epidermal growth factor pathway substrate 15, Eps15. *Int J Biochem Cell Biol*, 31:805-9.

Salomon, D.S.; Brandt, R.; Ciardiello, F. & Normanno, N. (1995). Epidermal growth factor-related peptides and their receptors in human malignancies. *Crit Rev Oncol Hematol*, 19:183-232.

Sansal, I. & Sellers, W.R. (2004). The biology and clinical relevance of the PTEN tumor suppressor pathway. *J Clin Oncol*, 22:2954-63.

Scher, H.I.; Sarkis, A.; Reuter, V.; Cohen, D.; Netto, G.; Petrylak, D.; Lianes, P.; Fuks, Z.; Mendelsohn, J. & Cordon-Cardo, C. (1995). Changing pattern of expression of the epidermal growth factor receptor and transforming growth factor alpha in the progression of prostatic neoplasms. *Clin Cancer Res*, 1:545-50.

Schlomm, T.; Kirstein, P.; Iwers, L.; Daniel, B.; Steuber, T.; Walz, J.; Chun, F.H.; Haese, A.; Kollermann, J.; Graefen, M.; Huland, H.; Sauter, G.; Simon, R. & Erbersdobler, A. (2007). Clinical significance of epidermal growth factor receptor protein overexpression and gene copy number gains in prostate cancer. *Clin Cancer Res*, 13:6579-84.

Sebastian, S.; Settleman, J.; Reshkin, S.; Azzariti, A.; Bellizzi, A. & Paradiso, A. (2006). The complexity of targeting EGFR signalling in cancer: from expression to turnover. *Biochim Biophys Acta*, 1766:120-39.

Sengupta, P.; Bosis, E.; Nachliel, E.; Gutman, M.; Smith, S.O.; Mihályné, G.; Zaitseva, I. & McLaughlin, S. (2009). EGFR juxtamembrane domain, membranes, and calmodulin: kinetics of their interaction. *Biophys J*, 96:4887-95.

Seth, D.; Shaw, K.; Jazayeri, J. & Leedman, P.J. (1999). Complex post-transcriptional regulation of EGF-receptor expression by EGF and TGF-alpha in human prostate cancer cells. *Br J Cancer*, 80:657-69.

Sharma, S.V.; Bell, D.W.; Settleman, J. & Haber, D.A. (2007). Epidermal growth factor receptor mutations in lung cancer. *Nat Rev Cancer*, 7:169-81.

Sherwood, E.R. & Lee, C. (1995). Epidermal growth factor-related peptides and the epidermal growth factor receptor in normal and malignant prostate. *World J Urol*, 13:290-6.

Shoelson, S.E. (1997). SH2 and PTB domain interactions in tyrosine kinase signal transduction. *Curr Opin Chem Biol*, 1:227-34.

Sigismund, S.; Woelk, T.; Puri, C.; Maspero, E.; Tacchetti, C.; Transidico, P.; Di Fiore, P.P. & Polo, S. (2005). Clathrin-independent endocytosis of ubiquitinated cargos. *Proc Natl Acad Sci U S A*, 102:2760-5.

Singh, A.B. & Harris, R.C. (2005). Autocrine, paracrine and juxtacrine signaling by EGFR ligands. *Cell Signal*, 17:1183-93.

Sorkin, A. & von Zastrow, M. (2009). Endocytosis and signalling: intertwining molecular networks. *Nat Rev Mol Cell Biol*, 10:609-22.

Soubeyran, P.; Kowanetz, K.; Szymkiewicz, I.; Langdon, W.Y. & Dikic, I. (2002). Cbl-CIN85-endophilin complex mediates ligand-induced downregulation of EGF receptors. *Nature*, 416:183-7.

Staal, S.P. (1987). Molecular cloning of the akt oncogene and its human homologues AKT1 and AKT2: amplification of AKT1 in a primary human gastric adenocarcinoma. *Proc Natl Acad Sci U S A*, 84:5034-7.

Staal, S.P. & Hartley, J.W. (1998). Thymic lymphoma induction by the AKT8 murine retrovirus. *J Exp Med*, 167:1259-64.

Stang, E.; Blystad, F.D.; Kazazic, M.; Bertelsen, V.; Brodahl, T.; Raiborg, C.; Stenmark, H. & Madshus, I.H. (2004). Cbl-dependent ubiquitination is required for progression of EGF receptors into clathrin-coated pits. *Mol Biol Cell*, 15:3591-604.

Sudol, M. (1998). From Src Homology domains to other signaling modules: proposal of the 'protein recognition code'. *Oncogene*, 17:1469-74.

Takishima, K.; Friedman, B.; Fujiki, H. & Rosner, M.R. (1988). Thapsigargin, a novel promoter, phosphorylates the epidermal growth factor receptor at threonine 669. *Biochem Biophys Res Commun*, 157:740-6.

Takishima, K.; Griswold-Prenner, I.; Ingebritsen, T. & Rosner, M.R. (1991). Epidermal growth factor (EGF) receptor T669 peptide kinase from 3T3-L1 cells is an EGF-stimulated "MAP" kinase. *Proc Natl Acad Sci U S A*, 88:2520-4.

Taub, N.; Teis, D.; Ebner, H.L.; Hess, M.W. & Huber, L.A. (2007). Late endosomal traffic of the epidermal growth factor receptor ensures spatial and temporal fidelity of mitogen-activated protein kinase signaling. *Mol Biol Cell*, 18:4698-710.

Tebar, F.; Sorkina, T.; Sorkin, A.; Ericsson, M. & Kirchhausen, T. (1996). Eps15 is a component of clathrin-coated pits and vesicles and is located at the rim of coated pits. *J Biol Chem*, 271:28727-30.

Teis, D.; Taub, N.; Kurzbauer, R.; Hilber, D.; de Araujo, M.E.; Erlacher, M.; Offterdinger, M.; Villunger, A.; Geley, S.; Bohn, G.; Klein, C.; Hess, M.W. & Huber, L.A. (2006). p14-MP1-MEK1 signaling regulates endosomal traffic and cellular proliferation during tissue homeostasis. *J Cell Biol*, 175:861-8.

Teis, D.; Wunderlich, W. & Huber, L.A. (2002). Localization of the MP1-MAPK scaffold complex to endosomes is mediated by p14 and required for signal transduction. *Dev Cell*, 3:803-14.

Theroux, S.J.; Stanley, K.; Campbell, D.A. & Davis, R.J. (1992a). Mutational removal of the major site of serine phosphorylation of the epidermal growth factor receptor causes potentiation of signal transduction: role of receptor down-regulation. *Mol Endocrinol*, 6:1849-57.

Theroux, S.J.; Taglienti-Sian, C.; Nair, N.; Countaway, J.L.; Robinson, H.L. & Davis, R.J. (1992b). Increased oncogenic potential of ErbB is associated with the loss of a COOH-terminal domain serine phosphorylation site. *J Biol Chem*, 267:7967-70.

Thiery, J.P. (2002). Epithelial-mesenchymal transitions in tumour progression. *Nat Rev Cancer*, 2:442-54.

Thiery, J.P. (2003). Epithelial-mesenchymal transitions in development and pathologies. *Curr Opin Cell Biol*, 15:740-6.

Thiery, J.P. & Sleeman, J.P. (2006). Complex networks orchestrate epithelial-mesenchymal transitions. *Nat Rev Mol Cell Biol*, 7:131-42.

Tzahar, E.; Waterman, H.; Chen, X.; Levkowitz, G.; Karunagaran, D.; Lavi, S.; Ratzkin, B.J. & Yarden, Y. (1996). A hierarchical network of interreceptor interactions determines signal transduction by Neu differentiation factor/neuregulin and epidermal growth factor. *Mol Cell Biol*, 16:5276-87.

Umbas, R.; Isaacs, W.B.; Bringuier, P.P.; Schaafsma, H.E.; Karthaus, H.F.; Oosterhof, G.O.; Debruyne, F.M. & Schalken, J.A. (1994). Decreased E-cadherin expression is associated with poor prognosis in patients with prostate cancer. *Cancer Res*, 54:3929-33.

Umbas, R.; Schalken, J.A.; Aalders, T.W.; Carter, B.S.; Karthaus, H.F.; Schaafsma, H.E.; Debruyne, F.M. & Isaacs, W.B. (1992). Expression of the cellular adhesion molecule E-cadherin is reduced or absent in high-grade prostate cancer. *Cancer Res*, 52:5104-9.

van Bokhoven, A.; Varella-Garcia, M.; Korch, C.; Johannes, W.U.; Smith, E.E.; Miller, H.L.; Nordeen, S.K.; Miller, G.J. & Lucia, M.S. (2003). Molecular characterization of human prostate carcinoma cell lines. *Prostate*, 57:205-25.

Vanden Broeck, D. & De Wolf, M.J. (2006). Selective blocking of clathrin-mediated endocytosis by RNA interference: epsin as target protein. *Biotechniques*, 41:475-84.

Wang, Y.; Pennock, S.; Chen, X. & Wang, Z. (2002a). Endosomal signaling of epidermal growth factor receptor stimulates signal transduction pathways leading to cell survival. *Mol Cell Biol*, 22:7279-90.

Wang, Y.; Pennock, S.; Chen, X. & Wang, Z. (2002b). Internalization of inactive EGF receptor into endosomes and the subsequent activation of endosome-associated EGF receptors. Epidermal growth factor. *Sci STKE*, 2002:pl17.

Ware, J.L. (1999). Growth factor network disruption in prostate cancer progression. *Cancer Metastasis Rev*, 17:443-7.

Waterman, H.; Katz, M.; Rubin, C.; Shtiegman, K.; Lavi, S.; Elson, A.; Jovin, T. & Yarden, Y. (2002). A mutant EGF-receptor defective in ubiquitylation and endocytosis unveils a role for Grb2 in negative signaling. *EMBO J*, 21:303-13.

Waterman, H.; Levkowitz, G.; Alroy, I. & Yarden, Y. (1999). The RING finger of c-Cbl mediates desensitization of the epidermal growth factor receptor. *J Biol Chem*, 274:22151-4.

Wells, A. (1999). EGF receptor. *Intl J Biochem Cell Biol*, 31:637-43.

Wells, A.; Welsh, J.B.; Lazar, C.S.; Wiley, H.S.; Gill, G.N. & Rosenfeld, M.G. (1990). Ligand-induced transformation by a noninternalizing epidermal growth factor receptor. *Science*, 247:962-4.

Wiley, H.S. (2003). Trafficking of the ErbB receptors and its influence on signaling. *Exp Cell Res*, 284:78-88.

Wiley, H.S.; Shvartsman, S.Y. & Lauffenburger, D.A. (2003). Computational modeling of the EGF-receptor system: a paradigm for systems biology. *Trends Cell Biol*, 13:43-50.

Williams, R.L. & Urbé, S. (2007). The emerging shape of the ESCRT machinery. *Nat Rev Mol Cell Biol*, 8:355-68.

Yamazaki, T.; Zaal, K.; Hailey, D.; Presley, J.; Lippincott-Schwartz, J. & Samelson, L.E. (2002). Role of Grb2 in EGF-stimulated EGFR internalization. *J Cell Sci*, 115:1791-802.

Yarden, Y. (2001). The EGFR family and its ligands in human cancer: signaling mechanisms and therapeutic opportunities. *Eur J Cancer*, 37:S3-S8.

Yarden, Y. & Sliwkowski, M.X. (2001). Untangling the ErbB signalling network. *Nat Rev Mol Cell Biol*, 2:127-37.

Yoon, S. & Seger, R. (2006). The extracellular signal-regulated kinase: multiple substrates regulate diverse cellular functions. *Growth Factors*, 24:21-44.

Zhang, D.; Sliwkowski, M.X.; Mark, M.; Frantz, G.; Akita, R.; Sun, Y.; Hillan, K.; Crowley, C.; Brush, J. & Godowski, P.J. (1997). Neuregulin-3 (NRG3): a novel neural tissue-enriched protein that binds and activates ErbB4. *Proc Natl Acad Sci U S A*, 94:9562-7.

Zhou, B.P.; Deng, J.; Xia, W.; Xu, J.; Li, Y.M.; Gunduz, M. & Hung, M.C. (2004). Dual regulation of Snail by GSK-3beta-mediated phosphorylation in control of epithelial-mesenchymal transition. *Nat Cell Biol*, 6:931-40.

10

Integrins as Determinants of Genetic Susceptibility, Tumour Behaviour and Their Potential as Therapeutic Targets

James R. Marthick, Adele F. Holloway and Joanne L. Dickinson
Menzies Research Institute Tasmania
University of Tasmania
Australia

1. Introduction

Metastatic prostate tumours are responsible for the majority of deaths associated with prostate cancer. The most frequent site of prostate cancer metastasis is to bone; over 80% of men who die of the disease have metastatic bony lesions (Bubendorf et al., 2000). Early detection of prostate cancer remains crucial to effective treatment. However, we are still unable to identify with certainty those tumours requiring aggressive and immediate interventions, which are associated with considerable morbidity, from those where a "watchful waiting" approach may be more appropriate. Currently little is known about inherited determinants of an individual's propensity to develop tumours that rapidly progress and metastasise (Hunter, 2006). Experimental evidence investigating the role of integrins in tumourigenesis suggests that they play important roles in tumour progression and metastasis, particularly the development of metastatic lesions in bone. Notably, recent evidence indicates that genetic variants in selected integrins influence risk and/or prostate tumour behaviour.

The integrins represent a large family of cell surface receptors that are responsible for cell to cell adhesion and complex formation with ligands found within the extracellular matrix (ECM). The integrins have important roles in cell proliferation, cell survival, differentiation and cell migration. Thus, these adhesion receptors play important roles in many physiological processes including normal organ development and wound healing. Integrins are obligate, noncovalent, heterodimeric molecules, composed of a larger α subunit and a smaller β subunit. Each of the subunits extends from within the cytoplasm into the ECM. The ECM tail of the α and β subunits are approximately 700-1000 amino acid residues in length, and the cell membrane is spanned by approximately 20-24 residues. Integrin subunits have a short cytoplasmic tail, approximately 15-58 residues in length, with the exception of β₄ which has a cytoplasmic tail approximately 1000 residues (Alghisi and Ruegg, 2006). Within the cytosol they are attached to the cytoskeleton via talin-actin microfilaments. A detailed review on integrin structure can be found in the following publications (Buckley et al., 1999; Humphries et al., 2003; Ivaska and Heino, 2000; Lu et al., 2008). The conservation of integrin structure from more primitive through to higher order organisms highlights their importance to multicellular organisms (Burke, 1999). Upon binding to extracellular ligands, the integrin molecules cluster at the membrane, permitting a focal cellular response and the transduction of signals from the ECM. Further, integrins respond to intracellular signalling resulting in conformational changes to the integrin molecules on the surface of cells, thus permitting modification of interactions with the ECM. Integrin signalling thus permits cells to be exquisitely sensitive to both extracellular ("outside-in") and intracellular ("inside-out") signalling (Burridge et al., 1988).

To date, 24 heterodimers have been identified, derived from 18 α and eight β subunits. Additional variation is provided by subunit 'variants' created by alternate mRNA splicing events. Selected integrins can also form multiple heterodimers; for example, α_v, β_2 and β_1 all form multiple αβ heterodimers (5, 4 and 12 respectively). Most, however, only form one or two heterodimers (Ivaska and Heino, 2000). There is promiscuity in integrin-ligand binding which may reflect the need to initiate different cellular processes using the same available ECM proteins. The ability of integrins to bind to multiple ligands is thought to be an advantage when elicitation of the response is more important than the ECM protein signalling it; for example, in cell migration and wound healing (Alghisi and Ruegg, 2006). The interaction of integrins with these ligands appears to be dependent upon signal transduction via the cytoplasmic tails to the ECM which is evoked by the focal adhesion kinase (FAK) pathway, although the exact mechanism regulating this process remains unclear. It is not surprising, then, that attempts to understand the mechanisms that underlie cell motility and adhesion have implicated the membrane spanning integrins as major regulatory molecules. Cell migration and motility are crucial to maintain and promote healthy cell development, wound healing and immunity. They are complex processes requiring tightly regulated and coordinated intra-cellular signal transduction with the ECM. Instances where uncontrolled cell adhesion and motility remain unchecked can lead to tumourigenesis and metastases (Wehrle-Haller and Imhof, 2003).

Given the physiological functions of integrins, it is not surprising that the role of integrins in neoplasms has been of intense interest over the past decade. Most pertinent to tumour development is the role of integrins in cellular processes, including cell survival and proliferation, cell migration, angiogenesis and lymphangiogenesis. Integrins are now known to play a key role in tumour biology and are implicated in tumour initiation, progression and metastasis. Aberrant expression of integrins also has been demonstrated to play a key role in cancer survival and proliferation. Integrins physically interact with the actin cytoskeleton which provides the traction required for migration to occur (Vicente-Manzanares et al., 2009). Integrin mediated matrix metalloproteinase (MMP) feedback systems control the degradation of ECM proteins. Importantly integrins play an important role in regulation of neovascularisation, required for metastases via the vascular endothelial growth factor (VEGF) pathway.

Much work has focussed on profiling changes in the expression of integrins at different stages of tumour development. In normal prostate tissue, integrins are expressed by normal basal epithelial cells, permitting interaction with the basal lamina comprising collagens, laminins, fibronectin, vitronectin and tenascin. During prostate tumour development, many studies report the overall down-regulation of both α and β integrin subunits. However, prostate tumourigenesis proceeds through defined stages of development from prostatic intraepithelial neoplasia (PIN), high-grade PIN lesions, prostate confined tumour, invasive tumour and finally to androgen-independent tumours. More rigorous examination of the integrin profiles at different stages of tumour development has revealed a more complex expression profile (Goel et al., 2008). Much research effort has focused on the identification of an integrin expression profile as a prognostic marker for prostate cancer. In particular, integrins from the α_v group and in particular $\alpha_v\beta_3$ have been previously identified as a putative prognostic marker for a number of cancers including prostate cancer and its utility as a therapeutic target is under clinical trial (Beekman et al., 2006; Chen et al., 2008; McNeel et al., 2005). It is beyond the scope of this review to provide a detailed analysis of the role of all integrins in prostate tumour development. Overall reviews are available which profile integrin expression in prostate cancer (Alghisi and Ruegg, 2006; Goel et al., 2009; Goel et al., 2008; Lu et al., 2008).

The advent of new high-throughput genotyping technologies has permitted rapid and significant advances in our understanding of the genes contributing to prostate cancer. In particular, genome wide association studies (GWAS) have permitted the identification of common genetic susceptibility variants associated with a significantly increased risk of developing the disease. These discoveries are now providing insight into the biological pathways that determine how disease arises, tumour progression, and the acquired propensity to metastasise. Whilst the role of the vast majority of these variants in prostate cancer remains to be determined, these studies have identified biological pathways important in the development of disease. The integrin family of cell adhesion molecules has recently featured both in the search for prostate cancer susceptibility genes, and in comparative analyses of genetic susceptibility variants and gene expression profiling studies of prostate tumours. Further, studies using a variety of approaches to identify the key drivers of prostate tumour development and progression have identified selected integrins as key molecules in these processes. Indeed, these studies have highlighted integrins as potential therapeutic options against prostate cancer. Here we provide a new perspective on the role of the integrins α_2, α_6 and β_4 in prostate cancer risk and progression. Whilst these receptor subunits have not previously featured prominently in prostate tumour biology, their role in prostate tumour development has more recently come to the fore through the application of next generation molecular techniques to gene discovery in prostate cancer and prostate tumour stem cell studies.

2. Integrin genetic variants and prostate cancer

Family history remains the most frequently identified risk factor for developing prostate cancer, in addition to advancing age. A family history of disease is indicative of an underlying inherited genetic predisposition. Indeed, population studies have repeatedly identified increased risk to relatives of those diagnosed with this cancer. Despite intensive research over more than a decade, the genetic contributors to prostate cancer remained poorly understood. It was not until large scale genome-wide association studies became possible utilising high-throughput genotyping with commercially available arrays that rapid advances in our knowledge of the genetic contributors to prostate cancer and indeed other complex diseases became possible. These advances permitted the genotyping of hundreds of thousands of single nucleotide polymorphisms (SNPs) to test for association with a disease in large numbers of cases and controls. Using this approach, over 30 prostate cancer susceptibility variants have now been identified. These studies have identified genetic variants both in known genes and intergenic regions associated with risk of disease. However, it has become clear that for only for a select few is the role of the variant identified determining prostate cancer risk apparent. For example, the significantly associated variant, rs10993994, in the MSMB1 gene (Eeles et al., 2008) is located within 2bp of transcription initiation site, and has been demonstrated to influence transcriptional activity (Chang et al., 2009). However, to date the functionality of the vast majority of the SNPs identified, many of which are not within or close to known genes, remains unknown. Thus, there are still significant gaps in our understanding of genetic contributors to prostate cancer susceptibility which is impeding translation of these exciting advances into the clinical setting.

Variants within the *ITGA6* gene, which codes for the α_6 integrins, has recently been identified as contributing to the genetic risk of prostate cancer. A large, multi-stage international collaborative GWAS utilising over 30,000 cases and controls has identified seven novel prostate cancer susceptibility loci. One variant identified as significantly associated with disease risk is in intron one of the *ITGA6* gene (Eeles et al., 2009). The SNP identified was rs12621278 on chromosome 2q31 (per allele odds ratio=0.75, confidence interval=95% P=8.7x10[-23]) (Eeles et al., 2009). Most interestingly, Cheng et al., (2010) have since screened 26 SNPs identified by previous GWAS studies (Duggan et al., 2007; Eeles et al., 2009; Eeles et al., 2008; Gudmundsson et al., 2009; Gudmundsson et al., 2007; Gudmundsson et al., 2008; Thomas et al., 2008) in 788 patients that had undergone radical prostatectomies to test for association with aggressive cancer. Five of these SNPs were independently associated with prostate cancer progression; however, the most strongly associated risk variant identified was in *ITGA6* (rs12621278), where a 2.4 fold increase risk of prostate cancer progression (P=0.0003) was reported to be associated with the risk allele. This integrin is also known to play an important role in prostate cancer stem cell biology, vascularisation and metastasis. Thus, given the known role of this integrin in prostate tumour development, this may represent an opportunity for targeted therapy in those cases with *ITGA6* associated genetic susceptibility.

By employing a genome wide linkage approach in the study of familial prostate cancer, we have identified a second integrin as significantly associated with prostate cancer risk (FitzGerald et al., 2009). A region on chromosome 5p13q12 was highlighted by genetic linkage analysis of a large family with multiple, densely aggregated cases of prostate cancer. Two polymorphisms were subsequently found to be significantly associated with prostate cancer risk. The SNP rs3212649 was identified within the three prime untranslated region (3'-UTR), and a second polymorphism, rs1126643 (C807T), located in exon seven. Variant rs3212649 was the most strongly associated with disease in the familial cases (OR=2.43 CI=1.28-4.58) but also in the combined dataset comprising both sporadic and familial cases (OR=1.67 CI=1.07-2.60). This SNP had not been previously reported to be associated with cancer risk. The C807T SNP was also significantly associated with increased prostate cancer risk both in the familial (OR=2.16 CI=1.19-3.92) and combined datasets (OR=1.52 CI=1.01-2.28). Furthermore, the C807T variant has also been previously associated with an increased risk of oral cancers, and also advanced breast cancer (Langsenlehner et al., 2006; Vairaktaris et al., 2006). Whilst presence of the alternate allele at C807T does not alter amino acid sequence, it has been reported to be associated with altered levels of expression of the α_2 receptor on the cell surface (Jacquelin, 2001). It should be noted that there exists significant linkage disequilibrium between rs3212649 and rs1126643 and a number of other SNPs located in the 3'-UTR of the ITGA2 gene. ITGA2 is also known to play an important role in prostate cancer stem cells, angiogenesis and tumour spread and also represents an exciting opportunity for target therapy. The mechanism by which these susceptibility variants influence *ITGA2* gene expression is currently under investigation in our laboratory.

Whilst these GWAS are identifying genetic variants significantly associated with disease risk and progression, the functional implications of many of these variants and their relevance to disease remains to be determined (Manolio, 2010). Thus, the results of GWAS have been examined in combination with microarray gene expression data, providing a systematic approach to the examination of genetic variants associated with disease and observed changes in gene expression. Gorlov et al. (2009) performed a meta-analysis on gene expression data from normal prostate tissue and prostate tumour tissue, and combined it with a GWAS meta-analysis to identify sets of genes over-represented in both types of studies. Cell adhesion genes including α_2, α_6 and β_4 integrins feature prominently amongst the most significantly associated genes and also the most differentially expressed reported in the microarray study (Gorlov et al., 2009). Gorlov and colleagues (2009) also highlight cadherins and integrins as important modulators of prostate cancer development and further argue that whilst GWAS-identified genes are considered to be cancer susceptibility genes associated with tumour initiation, the detection of a tumour requires a minimum tumour size and thus those identified from GWAS are also likely be detecting variants association with tumour progression.

3. Integrin α_2 and α_6 in stem cells

The concept that most solid tumours, including prostate cancer, arise from cancer stem cells possessing the capacity for self-renewal and tumour initiating capacity has led to the search for tumour cell populations with "stem-cell like" properties. Collins et al. (2001) were the first to demonstrate a primary human prostate tumour cell subpopulation with the capacity for self renewal and high clonogenic potential. These cell populations were characterised by high expression of CD44, $\alpha_2\beta_1$, and CD133. Subsequent studies have also identified prostate cancer stem cell populations (Collins, 2005; Guzman-Ramirez et al., 2009; Li, 2008). Guzman-Ramirez et al., (2009) recently isolated cells from surgically excised human prostate tumour tissue and culture of these tumour derived cell populations termed "prostaspheres" resulted in sub-populations expressing high levels of both the α_2 and α_6 integrins. Furthermore, Eaton et al. (2010) have examined the tumour cell stem cell phenotype in 11 matched primary and bone metastasis specimens from prostate cancer patients for the presence of a number of putative stem cell markers. No definitive pattern was observed which established a single marker profile of the metastatic phenotype; integrins α_2 and α_6 were relatively widely expressed across the metastases series in nine of eleven tumours examined. Other groups have since characterised prostate cancer stem cell populations expressing stem cell markers including OCT3/4, BMI1, β-catenin and SMOOTHENED in addition to α_2 and α_6 integrins. Most recently, several studies have identified a link between prostate cancer stem cells and epithelial to mesenchymal transition (EMT) demonstrating the link between the biology of prostate cancer stem cells, EMT and the propensity to metastasise (Kong et al., 2010; Mathews et al., 2010). EMT occurs during normal embryonic development; however, more recently, it has been identified as one of the early stages in the transition from confined tumours to invasive malignancies. The loss of epithelial cell phenotype and the gain of mesenchymal phenotype is accompanied by increased cell motility and invasiveness. This is accompanied by the loss of markers of epithelial phenotype and gain of mesenchymal markers. Profiling of expression of α_2 and α_6 integrin expression and EMT in prostate tumours has only recently been examined (Neal et al., 2011). SNAIL, a key factor promoting EMT decreases cell adhesion and increases α_2 and β_1 expression (Neal et al., 2011). However, there is evidence that known regulators of EMT, for example *ZEB1* influence expression of *ITGB4* (Drake et al., 2010), and down-regulation of $\alpha_6\beta_4$ in the prostate cancer cell line *SNAI2* knockdown studies in PC3 cells (Emadi Baygi et al., 2010) However, EMT in prostate cancer remains controversial.

4. Expression profiles of α_2 and α_6 integrins

Investigations of integrin expression patterns in prostate tumours stratified by tumour stage have produced inconsistent findings. Studies of $\alpha_2\beta_1$ expression in tumours report that expression patterns are abnormal in both primary tumours and lymph node metastases (Pontes-Junior et al., 2009). Whilst there have been several apparently conflicting reports, it appears that normal prostate basal epithelium expresses high levels of α_2 which is down regulated in primary tumours, with conflicting results in metastases. For example, studies of primary and metastatic prostate carcinomas have reported that $\alpha_2\beta_1$ expression is down-regulated in low grade tumours, heterozygous in intermediate grades, and up-regulated in lymph node metastases (Bonkhoff et al., 1993; Knox et al., 1994; Kostenuik et al. 1996). Mirtti et al., (2006) have reported differential expression levels in prostate tumour cell lines, and lower α_2 mRNA and protein expression in higher grade tumours when compared to benign lesions, although the levels of mRNA expression reported by Mirtti et al. (2006) again varied widely in tumours. Moreover, α_6 expression has been shown to be up-regulated in metastases and adenocarcinoma (Bonkhoff et al., 1993; Knox et al., 1994; Nagle et al., 1995; Schmelz et al., 2002), whereas α_2 has been shown to be down-regulated in adenocarcinomas and up-regulated in metastatic tumours (Bonkhoff et al., 1993; Nagle et al., 1995). This variable level of expression observed in prostate tumours is also evident in expression array analyses of $\alpha_2\beta_1$ in prostate tumours, published in the NCBI GEO database (Edgar R, 2002). Ramirez and colleagues (2011) combined previously published microarray studies (Lapointe et al., 2004; Tomlins et al., 2007) to identify that $\alpha_2\beta_1$ expression was markedly reduced or lost with tumour progression in prostate and breast cancer. In normal prostate tissue, α_2 is highly expressed and Ramirez et al., (2011) have shown that α_2 expression decreases progressively as prostate cancer proceeds from PIN lesions, to prostate cancer and then to metastatic prostate cancer where $\alpha_2\beta_1$ expression is completely absent. Ramirez et al. (2011) also suggests that $\alpha_2\beta_1$ may be a prognostic biomarker for identifying patients at risk of metastasis.

Using the profile of overall integrin expression as a predictive tool to measure patient outcomes has received some investigatory attention. Pontes-Junior et al. (2010) measured expression levels of eight integrins ($\alpha_2\beta_1$, $\alpha_v\beta_3$, $\alpha_{IIb}\beta_3$, α_v, $\alpha_3\beta_1$, α_3, β_4 and α_6) in resected tumour tissue from patients with localised prostate cancer, and found that the expression level of integrins α_3 and $\alpha_3\beta_1$ were associated with poor outcomes after a follow up period of ten years (2.5 and 3 fold higher respectively). The majority of integrins were down-regulated in tumour tissue with the exception of α_6, consistent with previous studies (Cress et al., 1995; Edlund et al., 2001; Rabinovitz et al., 1995; Schmelz et al., 2002) where its ability to bind ligands such as laminins and collagens is associated with increased invasiveness and metastases to bone. Down-regulation of $\alpha_2\beta_1$ in the early stages of prostate and breast tumour development has been reported to be associated with poor outcomes, with up-regulation of this integrin in metastasis. Interestingly, increased expression has been reported in colorectal cancer (CRC) and ovarian cancer to be associated with tumour cell spread (Luque-Garcia et al., 2010).

It should perhaps be noted that studies examining integrin expression profiles at different stages of tumour development vary in the integrin subunits targeted for immunohistochemical analysis, some targeting single subunits, others heterodimeric complexes. Edlund et al. (2001) observed a change from normal prostate tissue expressing $\alpha_6\beta_1$ and $\alpha_6\beta_4$ to tumour tissue expressing only $\alpha_6\beta_1$. This loss of the β_4 subunit in carcinomas of the prostate was attributed to differential binding caused by the two different isoforms of α_6 (α_{6A} and α_{6B}). Integrin α_{6A} which is expressed by the prostate cancer cell line LNCaP, preferentially binds to β_1, which is known to have high metastatic ability (Edlund et al., 2001). Therefore, examining changes in heterodimer ratios combined with isoform data may provide a more detailed profile of the α_2 and α_6 contribution to the prostate cancer biomarker model. The variable expression of these integrins in prostate tumour samples is perhaps reflective of the recognised heterogeneous nature of prostate tumours. Further, this observation is supported by the ability to derive sub-population cells expression high levels of α_2 and α_6 and with "stem cell-like" properties from prostate tumours expression. It is also worthwhile noting that examining the integrin expression profiles in tumours may not take into account individual genotype-driven variation in gene expression.

5. Animal models of prostate tumour metastasis and angiogenesis

Animal models have proven useful in the examination of the role of integrins in driving prostate tumour metastasis. In a study aiming to identify the critical molecules regulating prostate tumour metastasis, Hall et al. (2006) utilised LNCaP cells, a cell line of low tumourigenic potential that does not form metastases in mouse models. Selection by growth of LNCaP cells on type I collagen resulted in the generation of the derived LNCaPcol subline with enhanced chemotactic capacity. This subline expressed high levels of $\alpha_2\beta_1$ receptor (in contrast to the parent line) and chemotactic capacity was inhibited by $\alpha_2\beta_1$-specific antibodies. Further, upon injection of the derived LNCaPcol cell line into the tibia of nude mice, 53% of mice developed bony lesions compared with 0% of those injected with parental LNCaP cells. In similar studies, van Slambrouck et al. (2009) have demonstrated that the high bone metastatic potential of the subline, C4-2B, derived from LNCaP cells, is mediated by α_2 signalling. This signalling results in down-stream activation of the critical FAK/src/paxillin/Rac/JNK pathway and activation of metalloproteinases, MMP2 and MMP9, known to play a central role in tumour invasion. Furthermore, van Slambrouck et al. (2009) argue that it is redistribution and clustering of α_2 on the cell surface in their model that activates downstream signalling, rather than altered receptor level as observed by Hall et al. (2006). King et al. (2008) have also utilised a derivative of the prostate cancer cell line PC3 in a mouse xenograft model to demonstrate a role for α_6 in the growth of prostate tumours in bone. PC3N cells were transfected with wild-type and functional mutant α_6 subunits and stable transfectants were injected into femurs of severe combined immuno-deficient (SCID) mice. Whilst both wild-type and mutant transfected PC3N cells established bone tumours, the study showed the PC3N-α_6 mutant transfected cells showed dramatically reduced invasion of bone marrow and less tumour associated bone loss.

The $\alpha_2\beta_1$ receptor also plays a key role in developmental angiogenesis signalling via the VEGF pathway. In a Lewis lung carcinoma (LLC) xenografts model, $\alpha_2\beta_1$ null mice exhibited no response to angiostatic agents targeting $\alpha_2\beta_1$ in contrast to wild-type mice (Woodall et al., 2008). Interestingly, it appears that this effect may be tumour cell dependent, a phenomenon also reported by Zhang et al. (2008), with current evidence suggesting that tumour cell characteristics, such as $\alpha_2\beta_1$ integrin expression, and the interactions with the surrounding tissue environment, under the influence of host genetic factors, determine tumour development and/or metastasis. This is in keeping with the "soil determining the seed" hypothesis of tumour metastasis.

6. Epigenetic regulation of integrins α_2 and α_6

Events causing up-regulation or down-regulation of genes, whether they are DNA based sequence changes or epigenetic events can function to disrupt key genes in cancer development. It is now clear that epigenetic alterations feature prominently in abnormal growth states and there is strong evidence that these alterations can predict tumour behaviour. The apparent paucity of functional loci identified by GWAS and gene expression studies in prostate cancer has also led many research groups to focus on the epigenetic mechanisms influencing gene expression. Evidence that some epigenetic regulatory mechanisms are uniquely sensitive to environmental factors, such as diet and oxidative stress, may be an important mechanism by which environmental factors influence cancer risk (Dobosy et al., 2007). These mechanisms include DNA methylation, histone modification and micro RNAs (miRNA).

Segments of DNA rich in CpG motifs, also known as CpG islands, are the targets for DNA methylation. CpG islands, when present in gene promoters, are an important mechanism by which genes can be regulated by the addition or removal of methyl groups at key CpG motifs. This permits differential expression of genes in different cell types. DNA methylation occurs at cytosine-guanine repeats where a methyl group is attached to a cytosine residue by a DNA methyltransferase or DNMT. DNA methylation can affect gene transcription in two ways: either by preventing the transcriptional machinery from binding or by becoming targets for chromatin remodelling proteins. Global de-methylation or hypo-methylation has been reported in the promoter region of genes causing dysregulation and thus overexpression of genes including oncogenes (Ehrlich, 2009). Dysregulation of the genes that control for normal cellular function, such as integrins, can cause an over proliferation and thus tumour growth.

In disease states such as cancer, disrupted methylation can permit aberrant silencing or re-expression of key genes contributing to tumour development. Epigenetic alterations are a feature of both benign prostatic hyperplasia and prostate tumour development. There is a significant body of evidence highlighting the role of DNA methylation in prostate cancer. However, it is evident from these studies that these changes are complex, with both global loss of methylation across the genome occurring in addition to localised hyper-methylation of gene promoters. Global hypo-methylation is associated with chromosomal instability and activation of proto-oncogenes whilst gene-specific hyper-methylation frequently results in silencing of tumour suppressor genes. In particular, the research has focussed on the identification of a panel of genes that are hyper-methylated in prostate cancer with several key genes identified for example *GSTP1* (Dobosy et al., 2007). As discussed later in this chapter, therapies attempting to reverse silencing of tumour suppressor genes in cancer are of current interest.

However there is also some evidence suggesting that agents promoting de-methylation may actually enhance tumour development, by increasing the expression of genes promoting tumour development (Shukeir et al., 2006).

6.1 DNA methylation and chromatin remodelling

Whilst there has been significant advances in our knowledge of a range those genes altered by epigenetic changes in prostate cancer, at present studies examining epigenetic alteration of integrin gene expression and its role in prostate cancer are limited (Chen et al., 2009; Park et al., 2004; Uhm et al., 2010; Yang et al., 2009). In experiments utilising bisulphite sequencing of cloned DNA derived from prostate cancer cell lines conducted in our laboratory, we have observed that altered methylation of the *ITGA2* promoter is associated with altered gene expression (data not shown). At present, there is no evidence that the α_6 gene promoter is regulated by altered methylation. However, Yang et al. (2009) have reported the β_4 integrin is regulated by both methylation changes and histone modifications. Further, the loss of β_4 expression in mammary gland cells is associated with increased methylation of the β_4 promoter and an increase in repressive histone modifications and EMT (Yang et al., 2009). In addition, enzyme specific assays and bisulphite sequencing reveal that the LNCaP cell lines displayed higher methylation levels than PC3s and this is correlated with gene expression. Our results strongly suggest that *ITGA2* expression may in fact be regulated by epigenetic mechanisms (data not shown).

While yet to be reported in prostate cancer, another mechanism by which integrin epigenetics can regulate gene expression is by chromatin remodelling. Chen et al. (2009) report that integrin $\alpha_6\beta_4$ indirectly affects gene transcription by chromatin remodelling. Several genes including *FST, S100A4, NKx2.2, PDLIM4* and *CAPG* in which expression was previously shown to be controlled by DNA methylation were significantly up-regulated by the expression of $\alpha_6\beta_4$. In addition the inhibition of DNMTs in cells lacking the $\alpha_6\beta_4$ cell line stimulated the expression of these genes. These results suggest that $\alpha_6\beta_4$ can alter the expression of particular genes by stimulating de-methylation at their promoters. Further studies are required to characterise the role of epigenetic mechanisms in the regulation of gene expression of integrins in prostate cancer.

6.2 Micro RNAs

Perhaps the most recent and exciting area of epigenetic regulation in prostate cancer is the field of micro RNAs (miRNA). MiRNAs are small molecules typically 17-22bp in length which binds to the 3'-UTR and either degrade the mRNA directly or prevent it from being translated. This post transcriptional regulation is particularly dependent on the 'seed region' of the miRNA which constitutes the first 7bp-9bp of the miRNA. A number of software programs are available (DIANA, mictoT and PITA), which vary in their predictions depending on the parameters and algorithms used in their design. Polymorphisms within the seed region can alter whether a miRNA will bind or change the energy with which it will bind to the mRNA. These allele specific changes indicate that miRNAs can act as either oncomiRNAs or tumour suppressors, and array studies can contribute to increasing the precision with which tumours are characterised (Zhang et al., 2007). MiRNAs are normally associated with decreased levels of gene expression, as one of the established mechanisms of action is to suppress translation and promote degradation of their target mRNAs. However, up-regulation of genes following transfection of miRNAs predicted to bind to sequences in their 3'-UTRs has been previously reported in a number of studies reviewed by Khan et al. (2009). The potential role of miRNAs in the regulation of integrins in breast cancer was examined by Brendle et al. (2008). In a novel approach, miRNA binding site predictive software was used to predict altered miRNA binding to the 3'-UTRs of several integrins at the location of known genetic variants within these regions. A miRNA binding site was predicted to be altered by the alternate allele at rs743354. Upon subsequent examination it was observed that this SNP within the 3'-UTR of *ITGB4* was significantly associated with oestrogen receptor status and survival in breast cancer patients. In an approach similar to that taken by Brendle et al. (2008), we have determined that several of the SNPs associated with prostate cancer risk in the 3'-UTR of the ITGA2 gene are located in miRNA binding sites. The presence of the alternate allele alters the binding affinity of the miRNA. Our current work is investigating the role of the specific miRNAs in ITGA2 gene regulation.

7. Integrin α_6 and α_2 in prostate cancer therapeutics

Integrins represent ideal therapeutic targets as they are cell surface receptors that interact with extracellular ligands (Lu et al., 2008). The notion of integrins as therapeutic targets has been explored over a number of years, and there are two main mechanisms by which they have been targeted. Integrins are potentially important diagnostic biomarkers for cancer detection and progression, as it has been particularly relevant for prostate cancer which is historically difficult to diagnose with the inherent variability associated with the prostate-specific antigen (PSA) test and associated risks that accompany the collection of biopsy tissue. Secondly, they continue to be targeted directly as a method of preventing oncogenesis. In particular, they have been targeted as therapeutic options for metastases, as they are key mediators of cell dissemination and tumour growth via the angiogenesis pathways. Several of these integrin based therapies have shown promise in late stage cancers, extending life expectancies by several months in some cases. Further, it is often in conjunction with other adjuvant therapies such as chemotherapy and radiotherapy that integrins show the most promise as therapeutic agents. As we move forward into an era of personalised medicines it seems likely that integrins will have a major role to play.

7.1 Antibody based therapies

Integrin-targeted therapies have been of interest for a number of years, however few have targeted α_6 and α_2 heterodimers, and even fewer have been examined in relation to prostate cancer. The majority of studies have focussed on preventing angiogenesis and thus tumour growth, with most examining the α_v heterodimers. However, recently, studies have begun to shift towards the role of α_2 and α_6 in cancer models (Table 1). One of the more promising studies that has undergone human trial utilised α_2 as a platelet biomarker for an anti-integrin drug E7820, a derivative of an aromatic sulphonamide compound (Funahashi et al., 2002). E7820 inhibits angiogenesis via the VEGF or basic fibroblast growth factor (bFGF) pathways, and has been shown to inhibit the α_2 mRNA transcription in human umbilical vein endothelial cell (HUVEC) cultures and, importantly for prostate cancer, it has also been shown to inhibit vascular formation in a type I collagen matrix (Semba et al., 2004). E7820 administered orally twice daily by mice with sub-cutaneous KP-1 tumours displayed a decreasing expression level of α_2 on platelets which was positively correlated with anti-tumour activity (Semba et al., 2004). Stage I trials of E7820 have been completed and stage II trials have commenced, examining the efficacy of E7820 in conjunction with Cetuximab (a monoclonal antibody, targeting the epidermal growth factor receptor EGFR) in metastatic colorectal cancer (mCRC)(ClinicalTrials.gov, 2011b). To date, E7820 combined with Cetuximab, has been well tolerated in patients with advanced metastatic CRC. Integrin α_2 expression levels decreased by 82.1% without significant disruption of platelet function, with median progression-free survival increasing by 1.9 months and median overall survival increasing by 9.6 months (Sawyer, 2010). In addition, stage II trials of E7820 administered in conjunction with FOLFIRI (FOL-folinic acid, F-5-flourouracil and IRI-irinotecan), a traditional chemotherapeutic agent have also commenced in patients with mCRC. This study has begun with the premise of testing the tolerability and efficacy on mCRC for those who have failed first round treatment, before moving on to a larger cohort of patients (ClinicalTrials.gov, 2011a).

Integrins $\alpha_1\beta_1$ and $\alpha_2\beta_1$ play a significant role in driving angiogenesis (Lu et al., 2008) and antibodies targeting the α_2 receptor have shown promising results *in vivo*. Anti α_2 antibody Ha1/29 inhibited endothelial cells in an immobilised collagen gradient assay by approximately 40% (Senger et al., 2002). In addition, Senger et al. (1997; 2002) also applied a combination of anti-$\alpha_1\beta_1$ and $\alpha_2\beta_1$ antibodies to mice harbouring the human A431 squamous cell xenografts which resulted in decreased tumour growth <60% and angiogenesis <40%. The inhibitory effect of anti-α_2 antibodies on endothelial cells in a collagen matrix is likely to be particularly pertinent to prostate cancer where 80% of metastases are to bone; where collagen, the most abundant ligand of α_2, is abundant. Alghisi and Ruegg (2006) suggest that a humanised form of Ha1/29 may be a useful anti-angiogenesis target, and this may be particularly relevant for prostate cancer. Furthermore, antibodies against α_2 have been shown to reduce the invasive capability of mouse mammary carcinoma cells across the basement membrane (Lochter et al., 1999). This was found to be regulated by the expression of the matrix metalloproteinase stromelysin-1. The relationship between MMPs and integrins has been well documented and may represent another avenue for targeted cancer therapy. Murine based anti-α_6 antibodies have also been utilised by Ruiz et al. (1993) who illustrated a lower ability for human melanoma cells to metastasise in nude mice. Metastases were inhibited when the antibody EA-1 was injected in to the mice either before or simultaneously with the melanoma cells (Ruiz et al., 1993).

7.2 RGD peptide / disintegrin based therapies

Integrin $\alpha_2\beta_1$ has been implicated in mediating the effects of peptides designed to target the matrix bound tumour associated protein, angiocidin. Angiocidin is a protein that is found in the sera of patients with melanoma, colon, prostate and breast cancer, in levels that correlate with the progression of the disease, indicating that angiocidin may regulate tumour progression (Gaurnier-Hausser et al., 2008). Disintegrins or RGD based peptides are small, soluble molecules that originate from viper venom toxin and target the RGD (arginine-glycine-aspartate) motif. A 20 amino acid N–terminal peptide disintegrin of angiocidin has been shown to bind to integrin $\alpha_2\beta_1$ in K562 cells (a myelogenous leukaemia cell line) and ligate type I collagen on epithelial and tumour cells in a mouse model (Sabherwal et al., 2006). Soluble peptides that bind to $\alpha_2\beta_1$ integrins at the RGD motif are therefore able to prevent cell attachment and thus induce apoptosis (Buckley et al., 1999). *In vitro* angiocidin-inhibitory peptide trials have been demonstrated to be well tolerated and to reduce cancer burden in murine colon cancer models, with reductions in primary tumour volume and tumour burden (Liebig et al., 2007).

Drug	Type	Target	Tumour/ cell type	Reference
E7820	Peptide	α_2	Broad spectrum anti-tumour activity in seven cell lines and murine models	(Funahashi et al., 2002), (Semba et al., 2004)
E7820 & cetuximab*	Peptide and monoclonal antibody	α_2	Metastatic colorectal cancer	(Sawyer, 2010), (ClinicalTrials.gov, 2011b)
E7820 & FOLFIRI*	Peptide and chemotherapeutic agent	α_2	Metastatic colorectal cancer	(ClinicalTrials.gov, 2011a)
Angiocidin	Disintegrin/ RGD based peptide	$\alpha_2\beta_1$	Myelogenous leukaemia cell line, murine colon cancer models	(Sabherwal et al., 2006), (Liebig et al., 2007)
HYD-1	D-amino acid peptide	$\alpha_6\beta_1$	DU145 prostate carcinoma cell line	(DeRoock et al., 2001), (Cheresh and Spiro, 1987)
Endorepellin	C-terminus of perlecan protein	α_2, $\alpha_2\beta_1$	Lewis lung carcinoma model, HT1080 and A431 cell lines	(Bix et al., 2007), (Woodall et al., 2008)
Perlecan	Heparan sulfate proteoglycan	$\alpha_2\beta_1$	C4-2B and HT1080 cell lines	(Savore et al., 2005), (Mathiak et al., 1997)
HA 1/29	Monoclonal antibody	α_2, $\alpha_2\beta_1$	Human dermal endothelial cells	(Senger et al., 1997, 2002)
EA-1	Monoclonal antibody	α_6	Murine model of melanoma cells	(Ruiz et al., 1993)
SiRNAs	Synthetic oligonucleotides	$\alpha_6\beta_4$	MDA-MB-231 breast carcinoma cell line	(Lipscomb et al., 2003)
Valproic acid (VPA) & RAD001	Histone deacetylase (HDAC) inhibitor and mamallian target of rapamycin (mTOR) inhibitor	α_2, α_6, β_4	PC3 and LNCaP prostate carcinoma cell lines	(Wedel et al., 2011)
Pabinostat & rapamycin	HDAC and mTOR inhibitors	α_2, β_1	PC3 and C2 prostate and renal carcinoma cell lines	(Verheul et al., 2008)

Table 1. A summary of agonists targeting the α_2, α_6 and β_4 integrins. Treatments that have reached phase II of human trial are denoted *. Efforts to reduce tumour progression by targeting angiogenesis with small peptide based molecules have proven promising. The protein fragment endorepellin which is derived from the C-terminus of perlecan a basement membrane and scaffold protein displays remarkable anti-angiogenic properties (Bix et al., 2007). Bix et al. (2007) have reported a significant decrease in vasculature in an LLC mouse model (P=<.001) and interestingly observed that the administration of endorepellin immediately prior to the appearance of the tumours almost completely blocked their growth. Furthermore, Woodall et al. (2008) identified that the anti-angiogenic effects of endorepellin did not occur in the absence of $\alpha_2\beta_1$. The experiment showed that $\alpha_2\beta_1$ knockout mice displayed significantly less vasculature than wild-type mice (P=<.0001). Integrin $\alpha_2\beta_1$ was necessary for the recruitment of endorepellin to the vasculature where it conjugated with the α_2 domain in a cation-independent manner and supressed angiogenesis (Woodall et al., 2008).

Preceding, and contrary, to these findings is that perlecan the precursor molecule from which endorepellin is derived was also found to have anti-angiogenic and tumour suppressing qualities in prostate cancer (Savore et al., 2005). The suppression of perlecan expression with siRNA in the androgen independent bone targeted cell line C4-2B caused a reduction in colony size and the cohesiveness of transfected sub-clones in anchorage-independent growth assays. Further, when injected into athymic mice they showed a reduced growth rate, tumour size, vasculature and a failure to elevate PSA levels (Savore et al. 2005). Similar results have also been reported by Mathiak et al., (1997) in the HT-1080 fibrosarcoma cell line where perlecan cDNA transfected in antisense orientation caused an increased invasiveness through matri-gel coated filters, increased migratory ability through 8μm filters and elevated adhesiveness to type IV collagen substrate. These results are seemingly incongruent with the more recent findings of Bix et al. (2007) and Woodall et al. (2008) that a reduction of perlecan should in theory reduce the endogenous levels of the derivative endorepellin and thus increase tumour growth. Woodall et al., (2008) suggests that is quandary can be reconciled by "the unique dependence" of HT-1080 cell line on integrin $\alpha_2\beta_1$.

While RGD based peptides represent a good target for the collagen binding integrins such as α_2, unfortunately the laminin binding integrins such as α_6 and β_4, which bind in a RGD independent manner, are not clinically useful agonists for RGD mimicking peptides (Cheresh and Spiro, 1987). Therefore, additional therapeutic development is required to target this group of integrins. A D-amino acid peptide KIKMVISWKG (HYD-1) has been shown to bind to integrin $\alpha_6\beta_1$ in the human prostate carcinoma cell line DU-145 (DeRoock et al., 2001). The HYD-1 peptide was illustrated to prevent cellular attachment to ECM proteins and dermal cell fibroblasts (DeRoock et al., 2001). The finding that α_2 and α_6 can be bound by peptides is important and preliminary evidence suggests that they are well tolerated in murine models, intriguingly, DeRoock et al. (2001) also suggests that peptide administration can 'sensitise' cancer cells to radiotherapy, and aid the removal of cancer cells refractory to primary treatment.

7.3 siRNA based therapies

Antisense and siRNA oligonucleotides have enormous potential as therapeutic agents in prostate cancer and cancers in general (Juliano et al., 2011). Currently, siRNA oligonucleotides which target the $\alpha_6\beta_4$ subunit have been shown to reduce migratory and decrease the invasive capability of the breast carcinoma cell line MDA-MB-231 (Lipscomb et al., 2003). It is now clear that targeting one integrin with siRNAs can also lead to increased expression in another integrin. For example Defilles et al. (2009), knocked out $\alpha_v\beta_5$ and $\alpha_v\beta_6$ using several antibodies and disintegrins, which caused the expression of $\alpha_2\beta_1$ to increase. This negative crosstalk between $\alpha_v\beta_5$ and $\alpha_v\beta_6$ integrin also unexpectedly interfered with P13Kinase regulated $\alpha_2\beta_1$ mediated migration (Defilles et al., 2009). This dynamic crosstalk between integrins needs to be considered when administering integrin-targeted therapies. It may be that a suite of different disintegrins will need to be developed to target the numerous different integrins expressed on the cellular surface to effectively combat cell migration and oncogenesis. While the results using siRNAs *in vitro* are extremely promising, difficulties have arisen attempting to deliver these molecules to targeted regions in the animal model. Delivering oligonucleotides into cells in the absence of transfecting reagents is extremely difficult, given their potential as therapeutic agents a suite of mechanisms have been attempted including lipoplexes, polymers and dendrimers (reviewed by Juliano et al., 2011).

Integrins are recycled by endocytotic mechanisms and thus represent a particularly attractive mechanism in which siRNAs and small oligonucleotide delivery and efficacy can be improved. To date, delivery improvement has been made by utilising RGD peptides conjugated to oligonucleotides in the presence of polyethylene glycol (PEG). PEG acts as a protective mechanism against phagocytosis and also allows the peptides to remain functional for a longer period by reducing the interaction with negatively charged cell surface proteoglycans (Juliano et al., 2011). Additional PEG-RGD mediated cellular entry mechanisms have incorporated oligonucleotides into cationic lipoplexes and utilised nano-carrier technology, where upon cellular entry siRNAs are released and transported via cellular pathways (Juliano et al., 2011).

7.4 Epigenetic therapies

Genes altered by epigenetic modification in cancer are of current interest both as diagnostic markers and as targets for epigenetic modifiers as therapeutic agents. Histone modification or altered DNA methylation of α_2 and α_6 integrins as potential targets for such therapies in prostate cancer have not been widely investigated; however, there is preliminary evidence that their activity is targeted by such therapeutic targets. Recently, Wedel and colleagues (2011) have demonstrated in vitro that two drugs, Valproic acid (VPA) and RAD001 reduce tumour cell invasion, migration and adhesion of the prostate cancer cell lines PC3 and LNCaP. Valproic acid is a histone deacetlyase inhibitor and RAD001 is a mammalian target of rapamycin (mTOR) inhibitor. Previous studies have shown that mTOR and Akt phosphorylation is highly correlated with Gleason grade and mTOR has been shown to be a significant prostate cancer biomarker (Dai et al., 2009; Kremer et al., 2006) The separate application of RAD001 or VPA significantly reduced cell adhesion, migration and invasion in PC3 and LNCaP cells, and combination therapy proved to have an additive effect both on migration and invasion but curiously not adhesion. Furthermore, the addition of VPA and RAD001 also changed the cell surface expression of integrins in both cell lines, significantly altering the expression of α_2, α_6 and β_4 integrins. More specifically, the addition of VPA caused a significant down-regulation of α_6 and β_4 integrins in PC3 cells and in LNCaP cells α_2 and α_6 were significantly up-regulated. Given the differential response to the application of VPA to the androgen independent PC3 and androgen dependent LNCaP cell lines, the authors speculate that early and late stage tumours may vary in their response to the application of VPA (Wedel et al., 2011). The simultaneous use of pabinostat (LBH589), also a HDAC inhibitor with rapamycin, also had an additive effect in another prostate cancer model, in particular on the α_2 and β_1 integrins, key drivers of the metastasis (Verheul et al., 2008).

8. Conclusion

Approximately one in seven men are now diagnosed with prostate cancer over their lifetimes; clinicians still lack the ability to identify those tumours that are likely to be aggressive with a propensity to metastasise. There have been significant advances in our understanding of the genetics of prostate cancer, with genetic analyses and gene expression studies highlighting the integrins as key molecules driving prostate cancer and susceptibility and progression. While many early studies have examined the α_v integrins, here we have highlighted the importance of α_2, α_6 and β_4 in prostate cancer. The characterisation of prostate cancer stem cells has identified α_2 and α_6 integrins as important markers in stem cells and may suggest an emerging role for these integrins in EMT, a key event in tumour progression. Further, the integrins α_2 and α_6, which bind to collagen and laminin, have been identified as key drivers of prostate cancer metastasis, particularly to bone. Given that the vast majority of prostate cancer deaths are associated with metastatic disease, with over 80% of these metastases occurring in bone, this represents an exciting avenue for therapeutic development. Advances in technology, such as next generation sequencing, have provided new tools for mapping genetic and epigenetic changes associated with tumour development. Over 30 prostate cancer susceptibility loci have been identified to date, contributing approximately 25% relative risk; however, critical questions remain as to how these genetic changes identified influence gene function and thus prostate cancer. Therefore, there remains a need to address these current gaps in our understanding of genetic susceptibility and how these variants actually influence disease risk and progression, as we are still waiting for the translation of the vast majority of these findings into the clinical setting. Studies of cancer genes have generally focused on elucidation of mutations, deletions or amplification of critical growth promoting or suppressor genes. It is now clear that small molecules that control post transcriptional gene expression such as miRNAs, or aberrant DNA methylation, and chromatin remodelling are also known to contribute to prostate cancer development and progression and are proving attractive targets for future cancer therapies. Knowledge of how therapies targeting DNA methylation and histone modification influence the behaviour of key cancer genes is a key area for future research. Thus, there is the potential for selected integrins such as α_2, α_6 and β_4 to be utilised as therapeutic targets, with several of these having already reached phase II in human clinical trials.

9. Acknowledgements

We thank Annette Banks, Rebekah McWhirter, Kris Hazelwood, Sally Inglis and Annette Edwards for their assistance in performing the genealogical research and/or participant recruitment. We are also greatly indebted to the staff of the Tasmanian Cancer Registry, Tasmanian urologists and pathologists and the wider Tasmanian community. In particular, we wish to acknowledge the participants of the prostate cancer genetics studies conducted at the Menzies Research Institute Tasmania, without whom this research would not be possible. The authors also would like to acknowledge the funding bodies supporting their work including the Australian Cancer Research Foundation, Cancer Australia, Cancer Council Tasmania, the Royal Hobart Hospital Research Foundation, Perpetual Charitable Trusts and the Mazda Foundation.

10. References

Alghisi, G.C., & C. Ruegg. 2006. Vascular integrins in tumor angiogenesis: mediators and therapeutic targets. *Endothelium*. 13:113-135.
Beekman, K.W., A.D. Colevas, K. Cooney, R. Dipaola, R.L. Dunn, M. Gross, E.T. Keller, K.J. Pienta, C.J. Ryan, D. Smith, & M. Hussain. 2006. Phase II evaluations of cilengitide

in asymptomatic patients with androgen-independent prostate cancer: scientific rationale and study design. *Clin Genitourin Cancer.* 4:299-302.

Bix, G., R.A. Iozzo, B. Woodall, M. Burrows, A. McQuillan, S. Campbell, G.B. Fields, & R.V. Iozzo. 2007. Endorepellin, the C-terminal angiostatic module of perlecan, enhances collagen-platelet responses via the alpha2beta1-integrin receptor. *Blood.* 109:3745-3748.

Bonkhoff, H., U. Stein, & K. Remberger. 1993. Differential expression of alpha 6 and alpha 2 very late antigen integrins in the normal, hyperplastic, and neoplastic prostate: simultaneous demonstration of cell surface receptors and their extracellular ligands. *Hum Pathol.* 24:243-248.

Brendle, A., H. Lei, A. Brandt, R. Johansson, K. Enquist, R. Henriksson, K. Hemminki, P. Lenner, & A. Forsti. 2008. Polymorphisms in predicted microRNA-binding sites in integrin genes and breast cancer: ITGB4 as prognostic marker. *Carcinogenesis.* 29:1394-1399.

Bubendorf, L., A. Schopfer, U. Wagner, G. Sauter, H. Moch, N. Willi, T.C. Gasser, & M.J. Mihatsch. 2000. Metastatic patterns of prostate cancer: an autopsy study of 1,589 patients. *Hum Pathol.* 31:578-583.

Buckley, C.D., D. Pilling, N.V. Henriquez, G. Parsonage, K. Threlfall, D. Scheel-Toellner, D.L. Simmons, A.N. Akbar, J.M. Lord, & M. Salmon. 1999. RGD peptides induce apoptosis by direct caspase-3 activation. *Nature.* 397:534-539.

Burke, R. 1999. Invertebrate integrins: structure, function and evolution. *International Review of Cytology* 191:257-284.

Burridge, K., K. Fath, T. Kelly, G. Nuckolls, & C. Turner. 1988. Focal adhesions: transmembrane junctions between the extracellular matrix and the cytoskeleton. *Annu Rev Cell Biol.* 4:487-525.

Chang, B.L., S.D. Cramer, F. Wiklund, S.D. Isaacs, V.L. Stevens, J. Sun, S. Smith, K. Pruett, L.M. Romero, K.E. Wiley, S.T. Kim, Y. Zhu, Z. Zhang, F.C. Hsu, A.R. Turner, J. Adolfsson, W. Liu, J.W. Kim, D. Duggan, J. Carpten, S.L. Zheng, C. Rodriguez, W.B. Isaacs, H. Gronberg, & J. Xu. 2009. Fine mapping association study and functional analysis implicate a SNP in MSMB at 10q11 as a causal variant for prostate cancer risk. *Hum Mol Genet.* 18:1368-1375.

Chen, M., M. Sinha, B.A. Luxon, A.R. Bresnick, & K.L. O'Connor. 2009. Integrin alpha6beta4 controls the expression of genes associated with cell motility, invasion, and metastasis, including S100A4/metastasin. *J Biol Chem.* 284:1484-1494.

Chen, Q., C.D. Manning, H. Millar, F.L. McCabe, C. Ferrante, C. Sharp, L. Shahied-Arruda, P. Doshi, M.T. Nakada, & G.M. Anderson. 2008. CNTO 95, a fully human anti alphav integrin antibody, inhibits cell signaling, migration, invasion, and spontaneous metastasis of human breast cancer cells. *Clin Exp Metastasis.* 25:139-148.

Cheng, I., S.J. Plummer, C. Neslund-Dudas, E.A. Klein, G. Casey, B.A. Rybicki, & J.S. Witte. 2010. Prostate cancer susceptibility variants confer increased risk of disease progression. *Cancer Epidemiol Biomarkers Prev.* 19:2124-2132.

Cheresh, D.A., & R.C. Spiro. 1987. Biosynthetic and functional properties of an Arg-Gly-Asp-directed receptor involved in human melanoma cell attachment to vitronectin, fibrinogen, and von Willebrand factor. *J Biol Chem.* 262:17703-17711.

ClinicalTrials.gov. 2011a. Irinotecan Plus E7820 Versus FOLFIRI in Second-Line Therapy in Patients With Locally Advanced or Metastatic Colon or Rectal Cancer. Vol. 2011. ClinicalTrials.gov a Service of the U.S. National Institutes of Health.

ClinicalTrials.gov. 2011b. A Phase II Study of the Safety and Efficacy of E7820 Plus Cetuximab in Colorectal Cancer, Preceded by a Run-in Study in Advanced Solid Tumors. Vol. 2011. ClinicalTrials.gov A Service of the U.S. National Institutes of Health.

Collins, A.T., Berry, P.A., Hyde, C., Stower, M.J., Maitland, N.J. 2005. Prospective identification of tumorigeneic prostate cancer stem cells. *Cancer Research.* 65:10946-10951.

Collins, A.T., F.K. Habib, N.J. Maitland, & D.E. Neal. 2001. Identification and isolation of human prostate epithelial stem cells based on alpha(2)beta(1)-integrin expression. *J Cell Sci.* 114:3865-3872.

Cress, A.E., I. Rabinovitz, W. Zhu, & R.B. Nagle. 1995. The alpha 6 beta 1 and alpha 6 beta 4 integrins in human prostate cancer progression. *Cancer Metastasis Rev.* 14:219-228.

Dai, B., Y.Y. Kong, D.W. Ye, C.G. Ma, X. Zhou, & X.D. Yao. 2009. Activation of the mammalian target of rapamycin signalling pathway in prostate cancer and its association with patient clinicopathological characteristics. *BJU Int.* 104:1009-1016.

Defilles, C., J.C. Lissitzky, M.P. Montero, F. Andre, C. Prevot, E. Delamarre, N. Marrakchi, J. Luis, & V. Rigot. 2009. alphavbeta5/beta6 integrin suppression leads to a stimulation of alpha2beta1 dependent cell migration resistant to PI3K/Akt inhibition. *Exp Cell Res.* 315:1840-1849.

DeRoock, I.B., M.E. Pennington, T.C. Sroka, K.S. Lam, G.T. Bowden, E.L. Bair, & A.E. Cress. 2001. Synthetic peptides inhibit adhesion of human tumor cells to extracellular matrix proteins. *Cancer Res.* 61:3308-3313.

Dobosy, J.R., J.L. Roberts, V.X. Fu, & D.F. Jarrard. 2007. The expanding role of epigenetics in the development, diagnosis and treatment of prostate cancer and benign prostatic hyperplasia. *J Urol.* 177:822-831.

Drake, J.M., J.M. Barnes, J.M. Madsen, F.E. Domann, C.S. Stipp, & M.D. Henry. 2010. ZEB1 coordinately regulates laminin-332 and {beta}4 integrin expression altering the invasive phenotype of prostate cancer cells. *J Biol Chem.* 285:33940-33948.

Duggan, D., S.L. Zheng, M. Knowlton, D. Benitez, L. Dimitrov, F. Wiklund, C. Robbins, S.D. Isaacs, Y. Cheng, G. Li, J. Sun, B.L. Chang, L. Marovich, K.E. Wiley, K. Balter, P. Stattin, H.O. Adami, M. Gielzak, G. Yan, J. Sauvageot, W. Liu, J.W. Kim, E.R. Bleecker, D.A. Meyers, B.J. Trock, A.W. Partin, P.C. Walsh, W.B. Isaacs, H. Gronberg, J. Xu, & J.D. Carpten. 2007. Two genome-wide association studies of aggressive prostate cancer implicate putative prostate tumor suppressor gene DAB2IP. *J Natl Cancer Inst.* 99:1836-1844.

Eaton, C.L., M. Colombel, G. van der Pluijm, M. Cecchini, A. Wetterwald, J. Lippitt, I. Rehman, F. Hamdy, & G. Thalman. 2010. Evaluation of the frequency of putative prostate cancer stem cells in primary and metastatic prostate cancer. *Prostate.* 70:875-882.

Edgar R, D.M., Lash A. 2002. Gene Expression Omnibus: NCBI gene expression hybridization array data repository. *Nucleic Acids Res.* 30:207-210.

Edlund, M., T. Miyamoto, R.A. Sikes, R. Ogle, G.W. Laurie, M.C. Farach-Carson, C.A. Otey, H.E. Zhau, & L.W. Chung. 2001. Integrin expression and usage by prostate cancer cell lines on laminin substrata. *Cell Growth Differ.* 12:99-107.

Eeles, R.A., Z. Kote-Jarai, A.A. Al Olama, G.G. Giles, M. Guy, G. Severi, K. Muir, J.L. Hopper, B.E. Henderson, C.A. Haiman, J. Schleutker, F.C. Hamdy, D.E. Neal, J.L. Donovan, J.L. Stanford, E.A. Ostrander, S.A. Ingles, E.M. John, S.N. Thibodeau, D. Schaid, J.Y. Park, A. Spurdle, J. Clements, J.L. Dickinson, C. Maier, W. Vogel, T. Dork, T.R. Rebbeck, K.A. Cooney, L. Cannon-Albright, P.O. Chappuis, P. Hutter, M. Zeegers, R. Kaneva, H.W. Zhang, Y.J. Lu, W.D. Foulkes, D.R. English, D.A. Leongamornlert, M. Tymrakiewicz, J. Morrison, A.T. Ardern-Jones, A.L. Hall, L.T. O'Brien, R.A. Wilkinson, E.J. Saunders, E.C. Page, E.J. Sawyer, S.M. Edwards, D.P. Dearnaley, A. Horwich, R.A. Huddart, V.S. Khoo, C.C. Parker, N. Van As, C.J. Woodhouse, A. Thompson, T. Christmas, C. Ogden, C.S. Cooper, M.C. Southey, A. Lophatananon, J.F. Liu, L.N. Kolonel, L. Le Marchand, T. Wahlfors, T.L. Tammela, A. Auvinen, S.J. Lewis, A. Cox, L.M. FitzGerald, J.S. Koopmeiners, D.M. Karyadi, E.M. Kwon, M.C. Stern, R. Corral, A.D. Joshi, A. Shahabi, S.K. McDonnell, T.A. Sellers, J. Pow-Sang, S. Chambers, J. Aitken, R.A. Gardiner, J. Batra, M.A. Kedda, F. Lose, A. Polanowski, B. Patterson, J. Serth, A. Meyer, M. Luedeke, K. Stefflova, A.M. Ray, E.M. Lange, J. Farnham, H. Khan, C. Slavov, A. Mitkova, G. Cao, et al. 2009. Identification of seven new prostate cancer susceptibility loci through a genome-wide association study. *Nat Genet.* 41:1116-1121.

Eeles, R.A., Z. Kote-Jarai, G.G. Giles, A.A. Olama, M. Guy, S.K. Jugurnauth, S. Mulholland, D.A. Leongamornlert, S.M. Edwards, J. Morrison, H.I. Field, M.C. Southey, G. Severi, J.L. Donovan, F.C. Hamdy, D.P. Dearnaley, K.R. Muir, C. Smith, M. Bagnato, A.T. Ardern-Jones, A.L. Hall, L.T. O'Brien, B.N. Gehr-Swain, R.A. Wilkinson, A. Cox, S. Lewis, P.M. Brown, S.G. Jhavar, M. Tymrakiewicz, A. Lophatananon, S.L. Bryant, A. Horwich, R.A. Huddart, V.S. Khoo, C.C. Parker, C.J. Woodhouse, A. Thompson, T. Christmas, C. Ogden, C. Fisher, C. Jamieson, C.S. Cooper, D.R. English, J.L. Hopper, D.E. Neal, & D.F. Easton. 2008. Multiple newly identified loci associated with prostate cancer susceptibility. *Nat Genet.* 40:316-321.

Ehrlich, M. 2009. DNA hypomethylation in cancer cells. *Epigenomics.* 1:239-259.

Emadi Baygi, M., Z.S. Soheili, F. Essmann, A. Deezagi, R. Engers, W. Goering, & W.A. Schulz. 2010. Slug/SNAI2 regulates cell proliferation and invasiveness of metastatic prostate cancer cell lines. *Tumour Biol.* 31:297-307.

FitzGerald, L.M., B. Patterson, R. Thomson, A. Polanowski, S. Quinn, J. Brohede, T. Thornton, D. Challis, D.A. Mackey, T. Dwyer, S. Foote, G.N. Hannan, J. Stankovich, J.D. McKay, & J.L. Dickinson. 2009. Identification of a prostate cancer susceptibility gene on chromosome 5p13q12 associated with risk of both familial and sporadic disease. *Eur J Hum Genet.* 17:368-377.

Funahashi, Y., N.H. Sugi, T. Semba, Y. Yamamoto, S. Hamaoka, N. Tsukahara-Tamai, Y. Ozawa, A. Tsuruoka, K. Nara, K. Takahashi, T. Okabe, J. Kamata, T. Owa, N. Ueda, T. Haneda, M. Yonaga, K. Yoshimatsu, & T. Wakabayashi. 2002. Sulfonamide derivative, E7820, is a unique angiogenesis inhibitor suppressing an expression of integrin alpha2 subunit on endothelium. *Cancer Res.* 62:6116-6123.

Gaurnier-Hausser, A., V.L. Rothman, S. Dimitrov, & G.P. Tuszynski. 2008. The novel angiogenic inhibitor, angiocidin, induces differentiation of monocytes to macrophages. *Cancer Res.* 68:5905-5914.

Goel, H.L., N. Alam, I.N. Johnson, & L.R. Languino. 2009. Integrin signaling aberrations in prostate cancer. *Am J Transl Res.* 1:211-220.

Goel, H.L., J. Li, S. Kogan, & L.R. Languino. 2008. Integrins in prostate cancer progression. *Endocr Relat Cancer.* 15:657-664.

Gorlov, I.P., G.E. Gallick, O.Y. Gorlova, C. Amos, & C.J. Logothetis. 2009. GWAS meets microarray: are the results of genome-wide association studies and gene-expression profiling consistent? Prostate cancer as an example. *PLoS One.* 4:e6511.

Gudmundsson, J., P. Sulem, D.F. Gudbjartsson, T. Blondal, A. Gylfason, B.A. Agnarsson, K.R. Benediktsdottir, D.N. Magnusdottir, G. Orlygsdottir, M. Jakobsdottir, S.N. Stacey, A. Sigurdsson, T. Wahlfors, T. Tammela, J.P. Breyer, K.M. McReynolds, K.M. Bradley, B. Saez, J. Godino, S. Navarrete, F. Fuertes, L. Murillo, E. Polo, K.K. Aben, I.M. van Oort, B.K. Suarez, B.T. Helfand, D. Kan, C. Zanon, M.L. Frigge, K. Kristjansson, J.R. Gulcher, G.V. Einarsson, E. Jonsson, W.J. Catalona, J.I. Mayordomo, L.A. Kiemeney, J.R. Smith, J. Schleutker, R.B. Barkardottir, A. Kong, U. Thorsteinsdottir, T. Rafnar, & K. Stefansson. 2009. Genome-wide association and replication studies identify four variants associated with prostate cancer susceptibility. *Nat Genet.* 41:1122-1126.

Gudmundsson, J., P. Sulem, A. Manolescu, L.T. Amundadottir, D. Gudbjartsson, A. Helgason, T. Rafnar, J.T. Bergthorsson, B.A. Agnarsson, A. Baker, A. Sigurdsson, K.R. Benediktsdottir, M. Jakobsdottir, J. Xu, T. Blondal, J. Kostic, J. Sun, S. Ghosh, S.N. Stacey, M. Mouy, J. Saemundsdottir, V.M. Backman, K. Kristjansson, A. Tres, A.W. Partin, M.T. Albers-Akkers, J. Godino-Ivan Marcos, P.C. Walsh, D.W. Swinkels, S. Navarrete, S.D. Isaacs, K.K. Aben, T. Graif, J. Cashy, M. Ruiz-Echarri, K.E. Wiley, B.K. Suarez, J.A. Witjes, M. Frigge, C. Ober, E. Jonsson, G.V. Einarsson, J.I. Mayordomo, L.A. Kiemeney, W.B. Isaacs, W.J. Catalona, R.B. Barkardottir, J.R. Gulcher, U. Thorsteinsdottir, A. Kong, & K. Stefansson. 2007. Genome-wide association study identifies a second prostate cancer susceptibility variant at 8q24. *Nat Genet.* 39:631-637.

Gudmundsson, J., P. Sulem, T. Rafnar, J.T. Bergthorsson, A. Manolescu, D. Gudbjartsson, B.A. Agnarsson, A. Sigurdsson, K.R. Benediktsdottir, T. Blondal, M. Jakobsdottir, S.N. Stacey, J. Kostic, K.T. Kristinsson, B. Birgisdottir, S. Ghosh, D.N. Magnusdottir, S. Thorlacius, G. Thorleifsson, S.L. Zheng, J. Sun, B.L. Chang, J.B. Elmore, J.P. Breyer, K.M. McReynolds, K.M. Bradley, B.L. Yaspan, F. Wiklund, P. Stattin, S. Lindstrom, H.O. Adami, S.K. McDonnell, D.J. Schaid, J.M. Cunningham, L. Wang, J.R. Cerhan, J.L. St Sauver, S.D. Isaacs, K.E. Wiley, A.W. Partin, P.C. Walsh, S. Polo, M. Ruiz-Echarri, S. Navarrete, F. Fuertes, B. Saez, J. Godino, P.C. Weijerman, D.W. Swinkels, K.K. Aben, J.A. Witjes, B.K. Suarez, B.T. Helfand, M.L. Frigge, K. Kristjansson, C. Ober, E. Jonsson, G.V. Einarsson, J. Xu, H. Gronberg, J.R. Smith, S.N. Thibodeau, W.B. Isaacs, W.J. Catalona, J.I. Mayordomo, L.A. Kiemeney, R.B.

Barkardottir, J.R. Gulcher, U. Thorsteinsdottir, A. Kong, & K. Stefansson. 2008. Common sequence variants on 2p15 and Xp11.22 confer susceptibility to prostate cancer. *Nat Genet.* 40:281-283.

Guzman-Ramirez, N., M. Voller, A. Wetterwald, M. Germann, N.A. Cross, C.A. Rentsch, J. Schalken, G.N. Thalmann, & M.G. Cecchini. 2009. In vitro propagation and characterization of neoplastic stem/progenitor-like cells from human prostate cancer tissue. *Prostate.* 69:1683-1693.

Hall, C.L., J. Dai, K.L. van Golen, E.T. Keller, & M.W. Long. 2006. Type I collagen receptor (alpha 2 beta 1) signaling promotes the growth of human prostate cancer cells within the bone. *Cancer Res.* 66:8648-8654.

Humphries, M.J., P.A. McEwan, S.J. Barton, P.A. Buckley, J. Bella, & A.P. Mould. 2003. Integrin structure: heady advances in ligand binding, but activation still makes the knees wobble. *Trends Biochem Sci.* 28:313-320.

Hunter, K. 2006. Host genetics influence tumour metastasis. *Nat Rev Cancer.* 6:141-146.

Ivaska, J., & J. Heino. 2000. Adhesion receptors and cell invasion: mechanisms of integrin-guided degradation of extracellular matrix. *Cell Mol Life Sci.* 57:16-24.

Jacquelin, B., Tarantino, M., Kritzik, . 2001. Allele-dependent transcriptional regulation of the human integrin alpha2 gene. *Blood.* 97:1721-1726.

Juliano, R.L., X. Ming, O. Nakagawa, R. Xu, & H. Yoo. 2011. Integrin targeted delivery of gene therapeutics. *Theranostics.* 1:211-219.

Khan, A.A., D. Betel, M.L. Miller, C. Sander, C.S. Leslie, & D.S. Marks. 2009. Transfection of small RNAs globally perturbs gene regulation by endogenous microRNAs. *Nat Biotechnol.* 27:549-555.

King, T.E., S.C. Pawar, L. Majuta, I.C. Sroka, D. Wynn, M.C. Demetriou, R.B. Nagle, F. Porreca, & A.E. Cress. 2008. The role of alpha 6 integrin in prostate cancer migration and bone pain in a novel xenograft model. *PLoS One.* 3:e3535.

Knox, J.D., A.E. Cress, V. Clark, L. Manriquez, K.S. Affinito, B.L. Dalkin, & R.B. Nagle. 1994. Differential expression of extracellular matrix molecules and the alpha 6-integrins in the normal and neoplastic prostate. *Am J Pathol.* 145:167-174.

Kong, D., S. Banerjee, A. Ahmad, Y. Li, Z. Wang, S. Sethi, & F.H. Sarkar. 2010. Epithelial to mesenchymal transition is mechanistically linked with stem cell signatures in prostate cancer cells. *PLoS One.* 5:e12445.

Kostenuik, P.J., O. Sanchez-Sweatman, F.W. Orr, & G. Singh. 1996. Bone cell matrix promotes the adhesion of human prostatic carcinoma cells via the alpha 2 beta 1 integrin. *Clin Exp Metastasis.* 14:19-26.

Kremer, C.L., R.R. Klein, J. Mendelson, W. Browne, L.K. Samadzedeh, K. Vanpatten, L. Highstrom, G.A. Pestano, & R.B. Nagle. 2006. Expression of mTOR signaling pathway markers in prostate cancer progression. *Prostate.* 66:1203-1212.

Langsenlehner, U., W. Renner, B. Yazdani-Biuki, T. Eder, T.C. Wascher, B. Paulweber, H. Clar, G. Hofmann, H. Samonigg, & P. Krippl. 2006. Integrin alpha-2 and beta-3 gene polymorphisms and breast cancer risk. *Breast Cancer Res Treat.* 97:67-72.

Lapointe, J., C. Li, J.P. Higgins, M. van de Rijn, E. Bair, K. Montgomery, M. Ferrari, L. Egevad, W. Rayford, U. Bergerheim, P. Ekman, A.M. DeMarzo, R. Tibshirani, D. Botstein, P.O. Brown, J.D. Brooks, & J.R. Pollack. 2004. Gene expression profiling identifies clinically relevant subtypes of prostate cancer. *Proc Natl Acad Sci U S A.* 101:811-816.

Li, H., Calhoun-Davis, T., Claypool, K., Tang D.G. 2008. PC3 human prostate carcinoma cell holoclones contain self-renewing tumour inititating cells. *Cancer Research.* 68:1820-1825.

Liebig, C., N. Agarwal, G.E. Ayala, G. Verstovsek, G.P. Tuszynski, & D. Albo. 2007. Angiocidin inhibitory peptides decrease tumor burden in a murine colon cancer model. *J Surg Res.* 142:320-326.

Lipscomb, E.A., A.S. Dugan, I. Rabinovitz, & A.M. Mercurio. 2003. Use of RNA interference to inhibit integrin (alpha6beta4)-mediated invasion and migration of breast carcinoma cells. *Clin Exp Metastasis.* 20:569-576.

Lochter, A., M. Navre, Z. Werb, & M.J. Bissell. 1999. alpha1 and alpha2 integrins mediate invasive activity of mouse mammary carcinoma cells through regulation of stromelysin-1 expression. *Mol Biol Cell.* 10:271-282.

Lu, X., D. Lu, M. Scully, & V. Kakkar. 2008. The role of integrins in cancer and the development of anti-integrin therapeutic agents for cancer therapy. *Perspect Medicin Chem.* 2:57-73.

Luque-Garcia, J.L., J.L. Martinez-Torrecuadrada, C. Epifano, M. Canamero, I. Babel, & J.I. Casal. 2010. Differential protein expression on the cell surface of colorectal cancer cells associated to tumor metastasis. *Proteomics.* 10:940-952.

Manolio, T.A. 2010. Genomewide association studies and assessment of the risk of disease. *N Engl J Med.* 363:166-176.

Mathews, L.A., E.M. Hurt, X. Zhang, & W.L. Farrar. 2010. Epigenetic regulation of CpG promoter methylation in invasive prostate cancer cells. *Mol Cancer.* 9:267.

Mathiak, M., C. Yenisey, D.S. Grant, B. Sharma, & R.V. Iozzo. 1997. A role for perlecan in the suppression of growth and invasion in fibrosarcoma cells. *Cancer Res.* 57:2130-2136.

McNeel, D.G., J. Eickhoff, F.T. Lee, D.M. King, D. Alberti, J.P. Thomas, A. Friedl, J. Kolesar, R. Marnocha, J. Volkman, J. Zhang, L. Hammershaimb, J.A. Zwiebel, & G. Wilding. 2005. Phase I trial of a monoclonal antibody specific for alphavbeta3 integrin (MEDI-522) in patients with advanced malignancies, including an assessment of effect on tumor perfusion. *Clin Cancer Res.* 11:7851-7860.

Mirtti, T., C. Nylund, J. Lehtonen, H. Hiekkanen, L. Nissinen, M. Kallajoki, K. Alanen, D. Gullberg, & J. Heino. 2006. Regulation of prostate cell collagen receptors by malignant transformation. *Int J Cancer.* 118:889-898.

Nagle, R.B., J. Hao, J.D. Knox, B.L. Dalkin, V. Clark, & A.E. Cress. 1995. Expression of hemidesmosomal and extracellular matrix proteins by normal and malignant human prostate tissue. *Am J Pathol.* 146:1498-1507.

Neal, C.L., D. McKeithen, & V.A. Odero-Marah. 2011. Snail negatively regulates cell adhesion to extracellular matrix and integrin expression via the MAPK pathway in prostate cancer cells. *Cell Adh Migr.* 5.

Park, J., S.H. Song, T.Y. Kim, M.C. Choi, H.S. Jong, J.W. Lee, N.K. Kim, W.H. Kim, & Y.J. Bang. 2004. Aberrant methylation of integrin alpha4 gene in human gastric cancer cells. *Oncogene.* 23:3474-3480.

Pontes-Junior, J., S.T. Reis, M. Dall'oglio, L.C. Neves de Oliveira, J. Cury, P.A. Carvalho, L.A. Ribeiro-Filho, K.R. Moreira Leite, & M. Srougi. 2009. Evaluation of the expression of integrins and cell adhesion molecules through tissue microarray in lymph node metastases of prostate cancer. *J Carcinog*. 8:3.

Pontes-Junior, J., S.T. Reis, L.C. de Oliveira, A.C. Sant'anna, M.F. Dall'oglio, A.A. Antunes, L.A. Ribeiro-Filho, P.A. Carvalho, J. Cury, M. Srougi, & K.R. Leite. 2010. Association between integrin expression and prognosis in localized prostate cancer. *Prostate*. 70:1189-1195.

Rabinovitz, I., R.B. Nagle, & A.E. Cress. 1995. Integrin alpha 6 expression in human prostate carcinoma cells is associated with a migratory and invasive phenotype in vitro and in vivo. *Clin Exp Metastasis*. 13:481-491.

Ramirez, N.E., Z. Zhang, A. Madamanchi, K.L. Boyd, L.D. O'Rear, A. Nashabi, Z. Li, W.D. Dupont, A. Zijlstra, & M.M. Zutter. 2011. The alphabeta integrin is a metastasis suppressor in mouse models and human cancer. *J Clin Invest*. 121:226-237.

Ruiz, P., D. Dunon, A. Sonnenberg, & B.A. Imhof. 1993. Suppression of mouse melanoma metastasis by EA-1, a monoclonal antibody specific for alpha 6 integrins. *Cell Adhes Commun*. 1:67-81.

Sabherwal, Y., V.L. Rothman, S. Dimitrov, D.Z. L'Heureux, C. Marcinkiewicz, M. Sharma, & G.P. Tuszynski. 2006. Integrin alpha2beta1 mediates the anti-angiogenic and anti-tumor activities of angiocidin, a novel tumor-associated protein. *Exp Cell Res*. 312:2443-2453.

Savore, C., C. Zhang, C. Muir, R. Liu, J. Wyrwa, J. Shu, H.E. Zhau, L.W. Chung, D.D. Carson, & M.C. Farach-Carson. 2005. Perlecan knockdown in metastatic prostate cancer cells reduces heparin-binding growth factor responses in vitro and tumor growth in vivo. *Clin Exp Metastasis*. 22:377-390.

Sawyer, M.B., Iqbal, S., Lenz, H., Rocha Lima, C. S., Rossignol, D. P., Krivelevich, I., Fan, J., El-Khoueiry, A. B. 2010. Phase II study of E7820 in combination with cetuximab in subjects (pts) with metastatic and refractory colorectal cancer (CRC). Cross Cancer Institute, Edmonton, AB, Canada; University of Southern California Norris Comprehensive Cancer Center, Los Angeles, CA; University of Miami Sylvester Comprehensive Cancer Center, Miami, FL; Eisai, Inc., Woodcliff Lake, NJ Edmonton.

Schmelz, M., A.E. Cress, K.M. Scott, F. Burger, H. Cui, K. Sallam, K.M. McDaniel, B.L. Dalkin, & R.B. Nagle. 2002. Different phenotypes in human prostate cancer: alpha6 or alpha3 integrin in cell-extracellular adhesion sites. *Neoplasia*. 4:243-254.

Semba, T., Y. Funahashi, N. Ono, Y. Yamamoto, N.H. Sugi, M. Asada, K. Yoshimatsu, & T. Wakabayashi. 2004. An angiogenesis inhibitor E7820 shows broad-spectrum tumor growth inhibition in a xenograft model: possible value of integrin alpha2 on platelets as a biological marker. *Clin Cancer Res*. 10:1430-1438.

Senger, D.R., K.P. Claffey, J.E. Benes, C.A. Perruzzi, A.P. Sergiou, & M. Detmar. 1997. Angiogenesis promoted by vascular endothelial growth factor: regulation through alpha1beta1 and alpha2beta1 integrins. *Proc Natl Acad Sci U S A*. 94:13612-13617.

Senger, D.R., C.A. Perruzzi, M. Streit, V.E. Koteliansky, A.R. de Fougerolles, & M. Detmar. 2002. The alpha(1)beta(1) and alpha(2)beta(1) integrins provide critical support for vascular endothelial growth factor signaling, endothelial cell migration, and tumor angiogenesis. *Am J Pathol*. 160:195-204.

Shukeir, N., P. Pakneshan, G. Chen, M. Szyf, & S.A. Rabbani. 2006. Alteration of the methylation status of tumor-promoting genes decreases prostate cancer cell invasiveness and tumorigenesis in vitro and in vivo. *Cancer Res*. 66:9202-9210.

Thomas, G., K.B. Jacobs, M. Yeager, P. Kraft, S. Wacholder, N. Orr, K. Yu, N. Chatterjee, R. Welch, A. Hutchinson, A. Crenshaw, G. Cancel-Tassin, B.J. Staats, Z. Wang, J. Gonzalez-Bosquet, J. Fang, X. Deng, S.I. Berndt, E.E. Calle, H.S. Feigelson, M.J. Thun, C. Rodriguez, D. Albanes, J. Virtamo, S. Weinstein, F.R. Schumacher, E. Giovannucci, W.C. Willett, O. Cussenot, A. Valeri, G.L. Andriole, E.D. Crawford, M. Tucker, D.S. Gerhard, J.F. Fraumeni, Jr., R. Hoover, R.B. Hayes, D.J. Hunter, & S.J. Chanock. 2008. Multiple loci identified in a genome-wide association study of prostate cancer. *Nat Genet*. 40:310-315.

Tomlins, S.A., R. Mehra, D.R. Rhodes, X. Cao, L. Wang, S.M. Dhanasekaran, S. Kalyana-Sundaram, J.T. Wei, M.A. Rubin, K.J. Pienta, R.B. Shah, & A.M. Chinnaiyan. 2007. Integrative molecular concept modeling of prostate cancer progression. *Nat Genet*. 39:41-51.

Uhm, K.O., J.O. Lee, Y.M. Lee, E.S. Lee, H.S. Kim, & S.H. Park. 2010. Aberrant DNA methylation of integrin alpha4: a potential novel role for metastasis of cholangiocarcinoma. *J Cancer Res Clin Oncol*. 136:187-194.

Vairaktaris, E., C. Yapijakis, S. Derka, S. Vassiliou, Z. Serefoglou, A. Vylliotis, J. Wiltfang, I. Springer, E. Nkenke, P. Kessler, & F.W. Neukam. 2006. Association of platelet glycoprotein Ia polymorphism with minor increase of risk for oral cancer. *Eur J Surg Oncol*. 32:455-457.

Van Slambrouck, S., A.R. Jenkins, A.E. Romero, & W.F. Steelant. 2009. Reorganization of the integrin alpha2 subunit controls cell adhesion and cancer cell invasion in prostate cancer. *Int J Oncol*. 34:1717-1726.

Verheul, H.M., B. Salumbides, K. Van Erp, H. Hammers, D.Z. Qian, T. Sanni, P. Atadja, & R. Pili. 2008. Combination strategy targeting the hypoxia inducible factor-1 alpha with mammalian target of rapamycin and histone deacetylase inhibitors. *Clin Cancer Res*. 14:3589-3597.

Vicente-Manzanares, M., C.K. Choi, & A.R. Horwitz. 2009. Integrins in cell migration--the actin connection. *J Cell Sci*. 122:199-206.

Wedel, S., L. Hudak, J.M. Seibel, J. Makarevic, E. Juengel, I. Tsaur, C. Wiesner, A. Haferkamp, & R.A. Blaheta. 2011. Impact of combined HDAC and mTOR inhibition on adhesion, migration and invasion of prostate cancer cells. *Clin Exp Metastasis*. 28:479-491.

Wehrle-Haller, B., & B.A. Imhof. 2003. Integrin-dependent pathologies. *J Pathol*. 200:481-487.

Woodall, B.P., A. Nystrom, R.A. Iozzo, J.A. Eble, S. Niland, T. Krieg, B. Eckes, A. Pozzi, & R.V. Iozzo. 2008. Integrin alpha2beta1 is the required receptor for endorepellin angiostatic activity. *J Biol Chem*. 283:2335-2343.

Yang, X., B. Pursell, S. Lu, T.K. Chang, & A.M. Mercurio. 2009. Regulation of beta 4-integrin expression by epigenetic modifications in the mammary gland and during the epithelial-to-mesenchymal transition. *J Cell Sci*. 122:2473-2480.

Zhang, B., X. Pan, G.P. Cobb, & T.A. Anderson. 2007. microRNAs as oncogenes and tumor suppressors. *Dev Biol*. 302:1-12.

Zhang, Z., N.E. Ramirez, T.E. Yankeelov, Z. Li, L.E. Ford, Y. Qi, A. Pozzi, & M.M. Zutter. 2008. alpha2beta1 integrin expression in the tumor microenvironment enhances tumor angiogenesis in a tumor cell-specific manner. *Blood*. 111:1980-1988.

11

Cytotoxic Endonucleases: New Targets for Prostate Cancer Chemotherapy

Xiaoying Wang, Marina V. Mikhailova and Alexei G. Basnakian
University of Arkansas for Medical Sciences
and Central Arkansas Veterans Healthcare System
Little Rock, Arkansas
USA

1. Introduction

Prostate cancer is one of the most common malignancies in Western countries and the world (Baade et al., 2009). It is the third most common cause of death from cancer in men of all ages and the most common cause of death from cancer in men over age 75. The current standard therapies for prostate cancer include radiation, surgery, hormonal therapy and chemotherapy (Debruyne, 2002; Freytag et al., 2007; Nelius et al., 2009; Rozkova et al., 2009). Chemotherapy is almost always a salvage therapy for advanced prostate cancer, and chemoresistance is emerging problem in prostate cancer therapy. Strategies to overcome the chemoresistance of prostate cancer cells have not been developed partially because mechanisms of it are unknown and likely to be numerous. Chemoresistance has a tendency to occur both to clinically established therapeutic agents and novel targeted therapeutics implicating both intrinsic and acquired mechanisms of drug resistance (Djeu & Wei, 2009). Most likely, these are the mechanisms which are universal for cytoprotection from cell death induced by various factors.

Cell death by apoptosis is one of the most universal mechanisms of cell response to injury. It plays the major role in carcinogenesis and prostate tumor progression. Suppression of apoptosis was proposed to cause inappropriate survival of genetically aberrant cells during carcinogenesis (Vineis, 2003). Cancer cells seem to be designed to propagate and survive in a new and hostile environment by suppressing their natural mechanisms of cell death. The neoplastic transformation of prostate epithelial cells is known to be associated with decreased apoptotic cell death (Inokuchi et al., 2009; Shilkaitis et al., 2000). The progression of prostate cancer, in particular, androgen-independent prostate cancer or prostate adenocarcinomas, was also shown to be associated with decreased apoptosis (Raffo et al., 1995; Singh & Lokeshwar, 2009). The latter is the predominant form of tumor cell demise caused by chemotherapeutic agents and it plays an important role in cancer chemosensitivity and radiosensitivity (Arnold & Isaacs, 2002; Debes & Tindall, 2004). Targeting various mechanisms of apoptosis to cure prostate cancer has been suggested in many studies, naming potential molecular targets and key apoptotic regulators such as upstream and downstream caspases, p53, Phosphatase and tensin homolog (PTEN), prostate apoptosis response gene-4 (Par-4), Bcl-2 (B-cell lymphoma 2) protein, transcription factor

NF-kappa B, serine/threonine protein kinase and others (Uzzo et al., 2008; Wang et al., 2004). Precisely, manipulating with sensitivity to cytotoxic agents to alter cancer progression has been suggested as a therapeutic approach for prostate cancer in some reports (McKenzie & Kyprianou, 2006; Watson & Fitzpatrick, 2005). However, for some reason, almost no attention was paid to apoptotic/cytotoxic endonucleases as potential targets.

2. Cytotoxic endonucleases in normal prostate and prostate cancer cells

Cytotoxic endonucleases, also called "apoptotic endonucleases," are the initially recognized group of enzymes responsible for premortem and postmortem DNA fragmentation associated with cell death by apoptosis (Hengartner, 2001; Samejima & Earnshaw, 2005). Importantly, the same enzymes were later shown to provide DNA fragmentation that accompanies necrosis, autophagy, mitotic catastrophe and all other types of cell death. Therefore the term "apoptotic endonucleases" should be considered outdated.

Major representatives of cytotoxic endonucleases include: deoxyribonuclease I (DNase I) (Polzar et al., 1993), deoxyribonuclease II (DNase II) (Krieser & Eastman, 1998), Endonuclease G (EndoG) (Li et al., 2001), caspase-activated DNase (CAD) (Enari et al., 1998), and DNase gamma (Shiokawa et al., 1997). Some of these enzymes, for example DNases I and II had been known before 1960s. However the actual role of the cytotoxic endonucleases was clarified much later. Cytotoxic endonucleases were found in all studied cells and tissues, including the prostate (Koizumi, 1995; Napirei et al., 2004). The enzymes belong to the family of hydrolyses that cleave phosphodiether bonds in DNA. They differ in certain catalytic characteristics and DNA sequence specificity, and yet produce very similar type of DNA damage consisting of single-stranded or double-strand DNA breaks. Most harmful and hard to repair DNA breaks and double-stranded. They can be produced by so called "single hit" or "double hit" mechanism. In a "single hit" mode, both DNA strands are cut simultaneously at the same site. This mechanism is mainly characteristic of DNase II. The much more common mechanism is "double hit," in which strands are cleaved independently to result in a double-strand DNA break if the single-stranded breaks coincide with a 2-base or less shift between them. This mechanism is characteristic of DNase I and all other endonucleases, except DNase II.

Independently from the mechanism, endonuclease-generated breaks have been shown to strongly interfere with DNA synthesis in both normal and cancer cells (Nagata, 2000). That is why, while sometimes considered downstream effectors of apoptotic cascades, the endonucleases can cause DNA fragmentation and imminent and irreversible cell death when acting alone after overexpression or introduction into the cell (Enari et al., 1998; Krieser & Eastman, 1998; Polzar et al., 1993). The endonucleases are commonly found active during cell death; however, the overall link between these enzymes and apoptosis is weak. Some of the endonucleases seem to be dispensable in normal apoptosis (Davidson & Harper, 2005; Irvine et al., 2005; Napirei et al., 2000). On the other hand, their participation in cell death in general after tissue injury seems crucial and evidence of this is overwhelming. Recent studies demonstrated that inactivation of the endonucleases causes protection of normal and cancer cells against a variety of injuries *in vitro* and *in vivo* (Basnakian et al., 2006; Basnakian et al., 2005; Napirei et al., 2006; Yin et al., 2007), suggesting that the endonucleases are essential for and mechanistically linked to injury-related cell death. In addition to causing cell death itself, the endonuclease are certainly essential for clean up after cell death, removal of DNA from blood plasma, and destroying "foreign" DNA from bacteria and viruses consumed by cells (Buzder et al., 2009). These roles of cytotoxic endonucleases are less relevant to prostate cancer and thus will not be considered in this review.

Although all cells and tissues seem to express all endonucleases, the spectrum of them differs between the tissues. The reason for such redundancy of the cytotoxic endonucleases is not known, which allows speculation about the importance of DNA destruction from immediately prior to long after cell death.

The most expressed and active endonuclease in normal prostate is DNase I, previously also known as Ca/Mg-dependent endonuclease (Kyprianou et al., 1988; Kyprianou & Isaacs, 1988). Ca/Mg-dependent endonuclease-mediated DNA fragmentation is used as a marker of apoptosis in prostate cancer. The degradation of genomic DNA into nucleosome-sized fragments is an early event in castration-induced androgen withdrawal that involves death of the androgen-dependent epithelial cells following an increase of endonuclease activity (Banerjee et al., 2000; Brandstrom et al., 1994; Kyprianou et al., 1988).

DNase I is found in all studied species and tissues (Lacks, 1981). It is expressed mainly in tissues of the digestive system, though the specific activity of the enzyme varies between the organs (Gonzalez et al., 2001; Jacob et al., 2002; Lacks, 1981). In digestive tissues (intestine, pancreas, salivary glands), it is a secreted enzyme intended to hydrolyze DNA in the alimentary tract. In non-digestive tissues (including prostate), the role of DNase I is not known. Bovine or mouse DNase I bind specifically to G-actin and blocks its polymerization (Lacks, 1981). The enzyme from all sources endonucleolytically cleaves double- or single-stranded DNA to $3'OH/5'P$-end oligonucleotides, requires divalent cations, particularly Ca^{2+} and Mg^{2+}, is inhibited by Zn^{2+}, and has a neutral pH optimum. Inside the cell, the enzyme is located in the cytoplasm (Peitsch et al., 1993). It has also been shown inside nuclei, but the mechanism of its introduction into nuclei has not been studied. Inhibition of DNase I by internalized nuclear anti-DNA antibodies was shown to provide protection of cells against apoptotic stimuli (Madaio et al., 1996). No known nuclear localization signal was identified in DNase I, and "leakage" through nuclear pores was suggested (Polzar et al., 1993). Among various organs and tissues, prostate, pancreas, salivatory glands and kidney tubular epithelium have the highest levels of DNase I activity (Lacks, 1981; Polzar et al., 1993). Little is known about DNase I regulation *in vivo*. An alternative pre-mRNA splicing both in 5'UTR and in coding region was shown to be a mechanism of DNase I regulation (Basnakian et al., 1998; Basnakian et al., 2002). It is known that some DNase I isoforms can be generated by post-translational modification, namely mannose-type glycosylation of the protein (Lacks, 1981).

Studies of endonucleases associated with prostate cancer are very limited. Usually neoplastic transformation is associated with the decrease of endonuclease expression and activity in various cancers, thus making them "immortal" (Banfalvi et al., 2007; Basnakian et al., 2006; Basnakian et al., 1991; Wang et al., 2008). The most profound decrease of endonuclease activity was observed in malignant invasive prostate and breast cancer cells (Basnakian et al., 2006; Wang et al., 2008). The decrease of endonuclease activity had been also observed in other cancers and models of carcinogenesis (Basnak'ian et al., 1989; Basnakian et al., 1991). Immortalization of rat fibroblasts with the S1A segment of SA7 adenovirus also led to a significant decrease of endonuclease activity (Basnak'ian et al.,

1989). Another report indicated that an endonuclease activity is decreased in diethylnitrosamine (DEN)-induced hepatomas in rats compared to normal liver tissue (Basnakian et al., 1991). The decrease was proportional to the degree of dedifferentiation and the activity was the lowest in poorly differentiated tumors.

With the decrease of main prostate endonuclease, DNase I, the endonuclease activity in human prostate cancer cells is provided by EndoG. This endonuclease has a unique site-selectivity, initially attacking poly(dG).poly(dC) sequences in double-stranded DNA, as denoted by this enzyme's name. The enzyme also has RNase activity. EndoG predominantly resides in the intermembrane space of mitochondrion (Ohsato et al., 2002). Mammalian EndoG is synthesized as a 32 kDa propeptide in the cytoplasm and imported into mitochondria through a process mediated by its amino-terminal mitochondrion-targeting sequence (Cote & Ruiz-Carrillo, 1993; Ruiz-Carrillo & Renaud, 1987). The EndoG protein precursor is inactive (Ikeda & Kawasaki, 2001). The signal peptide is cleaved off after entering the mitochondria and the mature active 27 kDa EndoG is released from mitochondria during apoptosis, moves to the nuclei and cleaves nuclear DNA without sequence specificity (Li et al., 2001). EndoG expression varies in different tissues and in embryonic tissues the expression of EndoG is very low (Apostolov et al., 2007b). As opposed to DNase I, the enzyme has a greater activity on single-stranded nucleic acid substrates, single-stranded DNA and RNA. It preferentially cleaves non-canonical structures of DNA, damaged DNA, triplex DNA, and R-loops that appear non-specifically during transcription (Masse & Drolet, 1999). Cisplatin-treated DNA was shown to be preferentially cleaved by EndoG (Ikeda & Ozaki, 1997). EndoG requires either Mn^{2+} or Mg^{2+} ions, and is inhibited 15-fold at physiological ionic strengths (Widlak et al., 2001). Fe^{2+} and Zn^{2+} inhibit the enzyme activity. The EndoG gene in mice is a single copy gene, which consists of 3 exons (Prats et al., 1997). The loss of EndoG activity in C.elegans resulted in increased cell survival (Hengartner, 2001). However, EndoG knockout mouse is viable (Irvine et al., 2005). Reduction of EndoG in C.elegans using siRNA or genetic mutation affected normal DNA degradation, as revealed by staining with TUNEL assay, and resulted in the delayed appearance of cell corpses during development in C.elegans (Parrish et al., 2001). Thus in comparison to other endonucleases, EndoG is uniquely compartmentalized in mitochondria and it does not have known intracellular inhibitors (like DNase I or CAD). The EndoG location site may indicate that this enzyme is not an instrument of immediate response to cell injury.

EndoG seems to be particularly important in cancer cells because it regulates their sensitivity to chemotherapeutic agents (Basnakian et al., 2006). This report suggests the presence of EndoG in non-invasive breast cancer cells determines their sensitivity to apoptosis, which may be taken into consideration for developing the chemotherapeutic strategy for cancer treatment. In other cells, EndoG has been recognized as a key endonuclease in the caspase-independent apoptosis (Abbott et al., 2001; Bahi et al., 2006), mitotic catastrophe (Diener et al., ; Wang et al., 2008), and necrosis (Apostolov et al., 2007a; Jiang et al., 2006).

Because anticancer drugs induce apoptosis in cancer cells through endonuclease-mediated DNA fragmentation (Ploski & Aplan, 2001; Shrivastava et al., 2000), and the inhibition of endonucleases has a protective effect (Shrivastava et al., 2000), endonuclease should be considered as important mediators of cancer cell death and potential therapeutic targets for the anticancer therapy. However, delivery of endonucleases or modulation of endonuclease activity are not currently used for cancer therapy, in particular, for prostate cancer therapy.

3. Modulation of EndoG by DNA methylation and histone deacetylation

Epigenetic changes are believed to be the most common alteration at the DNA level in prostate cancer (Schulz & Hatina, 2006; Walton et al., 2008). Two types of DNA epigenetic changes that are known to occur in prostate cancer include regional DNA hypermethylation and regional/global DNA hypomethylation. Hypermethylation of the promoter region that contains CpG island occurs in a large number of genes and is usually associated with gene silencing in the vast majority of prostate cancer cases (Li et al., 2005; Perry et al., 2006; Rennie & Nelson, 1998). Studies have shown that hypermethylation of this region may be eventually used as a tumor biomarker for early diagnosis and risk assessment of prostate cancer. Furthermore, the prevalence of epigenetic changes in prostate cancer and the potential reversibility of DNA methylation alterations by DNA methylation inhibitors suggest that these changes are a viable target for cancer chemotherapy and chemoprevention strategies (Egger et al., 2004; Kopelovich et al., 2003; Yoo & Jones, 2006).

Mammalian genome contains patterns of methylated cytosines for normal function, but until recently the structural organization of the methylation landscape of the human genome was unclear (Rollins et al., 2006). It has been reported that the human genome consists of short (<4 kb) unmethylated domains enriched in promoters, CpG islands, and first exons, embedded in a matrix of long methylated domains (Rollins et al., 2006). Analysis of promoter sequences of all known human cytotoxic endonucleases – described below - showed that EndoG is the only cytotoxic endonuclease that contains a CpG island, a segment of DNA with high G+C content and a site for methylation, in the promoter region (Wang et al., 2008).

A large number of studies have shown that methylation of promoter CpG islands plays an important role in gene silencing (Ruchusatsawat et al., 2006; Taghavi & van Lohuizen, 2006). The broadly accepted definition of a CpG island as a 200-bp fragment of DNA with G + C content greater than 50% and observed CpG/expected CpG ratio higher than 0.6 failed to exclude many sequences (such as *Alu* repeats and unknown sequences) that are not associated with regulatory regions of genes (Takai & Jones, 2002). Recent studies indicate that the usage of a modified algorithm to search for CpG islands using a more stringent definition (G + C content higher than 55% and a length greater than 500 bp with observed CpG/expected CpG ratio 0.65) resulted in the exclusion of the majority of *Alu* repetitive and unknown sequences associated with the 5′ region of genes (Takai & Jones, 2002). In view of these considerations, we applied this algorithm to the analysis of endonuclease genes, which could be regulated by DNA methylation. All known human cell death endonucleases and their sequence variants were analyzed using the CpG Island Searcher program (available at http://www.cpgislands.com (Takai & Jones, 2003)): DNase 1, DNase 1L1 variants 1, 2, 3 and 4; DNase 1L2, DNase 1L3 (DNase gamma), DNase 2α, DNase 2β variants 1 and 2, L-DNase II (LEI), CAD and EndoG. Surprisingly, this analysis showed that EndoG is the only gene that satisfied the criteria of containing a long CpG island in the promoter and exon 1 of the gene.

The methylation status of the EndoG promoter/exon 1 in prostate cancer cells was then determined by using the methylation-sensitive McrBC-PCR method. McrBC is a bacterial endonuclease, that does not act on unmethylated DNA, but cleaves DNA containing 5-methylcytosine in one or both strands and thus nullifies PCR amplification (Nakayama et al., 2004). This experiment showed that in three studied prostate cancer cell lines, LNCaP, 22Rv1 and PC3, EndoG promoter methylation was the lowest in 22Rv1 cells and highest in PC3 cells. Further comparison of the three prostate cancer cell lines showed that EndoG is highly expressed in 22Rv1 and LNCaP cells. In PC3 cells, EndoG was not expressed and the EndoG gene CpG island was hypermethylated (Wang et al., 2008).

The expression of EndoG correlated positively with sensitivity to docetaxel, cisplatin and etoposide, and the silencing of EndoG by siRNA decreased the sensitivity of the cells to the chemotherapeutic agents in the two EndoG-expressing cell lines. To determine whether the level of EndoG expression affects the sensitivity of prostate cancer cells to chemotherapeutic drugs, we exposed the three cell lines to two anticancer agents, cisplatin (0-100 μM) and etoposide (0-300 μM), which are known to induce cell death *in vitro* (Fang et al., 2004; Lee et al., 2006). As expected, the two cell lines that expressed EndoG, 22Rv1 and LNCaP, were highly sensitive to both chemotherapeutic agents. EndoG-deficient PC3 cells, in contrast, were insensitive to these drugs in the range of concentrations used.

Further study determined that cisplatin-induced death of prostate cancer cells can be prevented by EndoG silencing. Although EndoG is known to participate in cell death, it was necessary to determine whether the role of EndoG was the same in prostate cancer cells subjected to injury by cytotoxic agents as has been described in other cells. To test a causal relationship, EndoG was silenced in 22Rv1 cells by applying siRNA. To show that siRNA was delivered to the cells, fluorescent DY547-labeled siRNA was used. After DY547-siRNA transfection, 22Rv1 cells were exposed to 80 μM cisplatin, a concentration that had induced significant cell death in the above experiments. Next, TUNEL assay was conducted to measure DNA fragmentation. The assay showed the DNA fragmentation was decreased, indicating that silencing of EndoG leads to significant decrease of EndoG expression and protects cells from DNA fragmentation. As expected, EndoG silencing resulted in the increased viability of cisplatin-treated 22Rv1 cells as measured using clonogenic assay. The results suggest EndoG is responsible for cisplatin-induced death in prostate cancer cells.

It is interesting that inhibition of DNA methylation induced EndoG and increased sensitivity of PC3 cells to cisplatin and etoposide. 5-aza-2'-deoxycytidine (decitabine), which is a DNA methylation inhibitor, caused hypomethylation of the EndoG promoter in PC3 cells, induced EndoG mRNA and protein expression, and made the cells sensitive to the chemotherapy agents. Using McrBC-PCR method, we determined that the treatment of PC3 cells with decitabine inhibited methylation of the CpG island in the EndoG gene. The same concentration of decitabine also increased EndoG expression as determined by real-time RT-PCR and Western blotting. These data clearly suggested EndoG expression is regulated by DNA methylation. Importantly, the induction of EndoG by demethylation caused a significant increase in sensitivity to cisplatin and etoposide.

Finally, the acetylation of histones by trichostatin A (TSA), a histone deacetylase inhibitor, induced EndoG expression in 22Rv1 cells, while it had no such effect in PC3 cells. These data indicated EndoG may be regulated by methylation of its gene promoter, and partially by histone acetylation, and that EndoG is essential for prostate cancer cell death in the used models. Histone modification, in particular, histone acetylation, is another epigenetic mechanism that is important in regulation of genes in prostate cancer (Das et al., 2006; Egger et al., 2004; Wang et al., 2008; Yoo & Jones, 2006). To determine whether and how histone acetylation regulates EndoG expression, two prostate cancer cell lines were treated with TSA, and EndoG protein expression was studied using Western blotting. The exposure of the cells to TSA induced high levels of EndoG expression in EndoG-positive 22Rv1 cells, whereas in EndoG-deficient PC3 cells, EndoG was not induced. Again, EndoG induction by TSA caused increased sensitivity to cisplatin. These data demonstrated that chromatin acetylation is important for EndoG expression. Taken together with the above methylation experiments, these data indicate that DNA methylation plays a primary role in EndoG regulation as compared to histone acetylation. In other words, the CpG island of the EndoG gene has to be hypomethylated in order to allow regulation of EndoG expression by histone acetylation.

4. Endonuclease delivery to prostate cancer cells and tumors

Although these are attractive and potentially therapeutically useful approaches, modulations of endonuclease expression by DNA methylation or histone acetylation may not be a realistic approach because the specificity of epigenetic regulation is notoriously low. An alternative to these methods may be a gene delivery and overexpression in the target cancer cells. To determine whether overexpression of EndoG would make PC3 cells sensitive to the chemotherapy agents, the cells were transfected with human mature EndoG gene. To model chemotherapy in vitro, we used docetaxel, which is an FDA-approved the first line chemotherapeutic agent in castration-refractory prostate cancer (Oudard et al., 2007; Ryan et al., 2001). Despite survival benefits with docetaxel based chemotherapy, prognosis for castration-refractory prostate cancer patients usually is poor and patients typically show rapid progression (Oudard et al., 2005; Wang et al., 2008). Progressive prostate cancer is associated with the development, and subsequent expansion of tumor cells that are resistant to apoptotic triggers and dysregulation of apoptosis is often characterized by insufficient apoptosis (Kruslin, 2009; Mori et al., 1996). Therefore a delivery of EndoG gene was expected to increase sensitivity of prostate cancer cells to docetaxel.

As described below, this genetic manipulation resulted in significant increase of PC3 cells sensitivity to docetaxel and cisplatin in vitro. Similar results were obtained when PC3 cells were transfected with EndoG precursor gene suggesting that the drugs induce speedy processing of the protein to mature endonuclease.

PC3 cells were chosen because they have very low expression of EndoG (Wang et al., 2008). Human EndoG gene (NM 004435.2) was cloned in the mammalian expression vector pECFP.N1 to result in an expression of EndoG protein fused with the enhanced cyan fluorescence protein (CFP). The expression of the chimeric protein was confirmed by fluorescent microscopy. Cells were then treated with docetaxel and cell death was measured using lactate dehydrogenase (LDH) release assay. This experiment showed the sensitivity of the PC3 cells expressing EndoG-CFP to docetaxel was much higher than the cells expressing CFP alone (Figure 1). The same result was also observed in cisplatin-induced cells death:

EndoG overexpression resulted in an over 4-folds elevation of cisplatin-induced cell death (data not shown). We also have compared mature EndoG gene and precursor EndoG gene overexpression cytotoxicity and their effects on cisplatin-induced cell death, and found that both types of EndoG had familiar effect (data not shown).

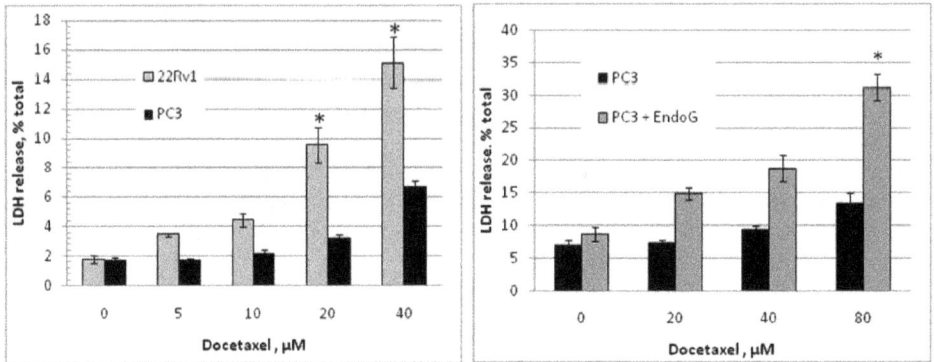

Fig. 1. EndoG expression enhances prostate cancer cells' sensitivity to docetaxel in vitro. Left panel: Cell death measured by LDH release assay in EndoG-expressing 22Rv1 and EndoG-negative PC3 cells, which were exposed to varying concentrations of docetaxel for 24h (n=4, *p<0.05). Right panel: Cell death measured by LDH release assay in PC3 cells with or without EndoG precursor overexpression 24 hrs after exposure to varying concentrations of docetaxel (n=4, *p<0.05).

Finally, parental PC3 cells and PC3 cells overexpressing human EndoG precursor were implanted in prostates of SCID mice to produce orthotopic tumors. The animals with xenografts were subjected to the docetaxel chemotherapy and the tumor size progression was monitored by high frequency ultrasound visualization. This experiment showed that EndoG-expressing tumors shrink in response to chemotherapy, while control tumors made of EndoG-negative parental PC3 cells were chemoresistant. To produce orthotopic xenografts, 8-weeks old male SCID mice were injected with human prostate cancer PC3 cells or EndoG gene-transfected PC3 cells by surgical orthotopic implantation. $2x10^5$ cells were mixed with matrigel at 1:1 ratio (v/v) in a total volume of 20µl were injected in the left ventral prostate lobes after surgical opening of the lower abdomen skin and peritoneal membrane. Ultrasound image could identify prostate tumor as early for 6 days after implantation. Monitoring of the tumor growth showed that the prostate lobe eventually was occupied by the tumor and lost its original shape. At the 12th day, the mice received docetaxel (10mg/kg) via peritoneal cavity injection while the control mice received saline injection. Ultrasound images were taken at the 6, 12, and 18 days after orthotopic implantation. By day 18, PC3 xenograft tumors significantly grew up regardless of the docetaxel treatment; EndoG-PC3 xenografts without docetaxel treatment grew up less, while the docetaxel-treated EndoG-PC3 xenografts did not grow in size and instead shrunk (Figure 2). Histology analysis confirmed the EndoG overexpression in tumors, which coincided with positive TUNEL staining, thus confirming EndoG overexpression made xenografts sensitive to the docetaxel treatment.

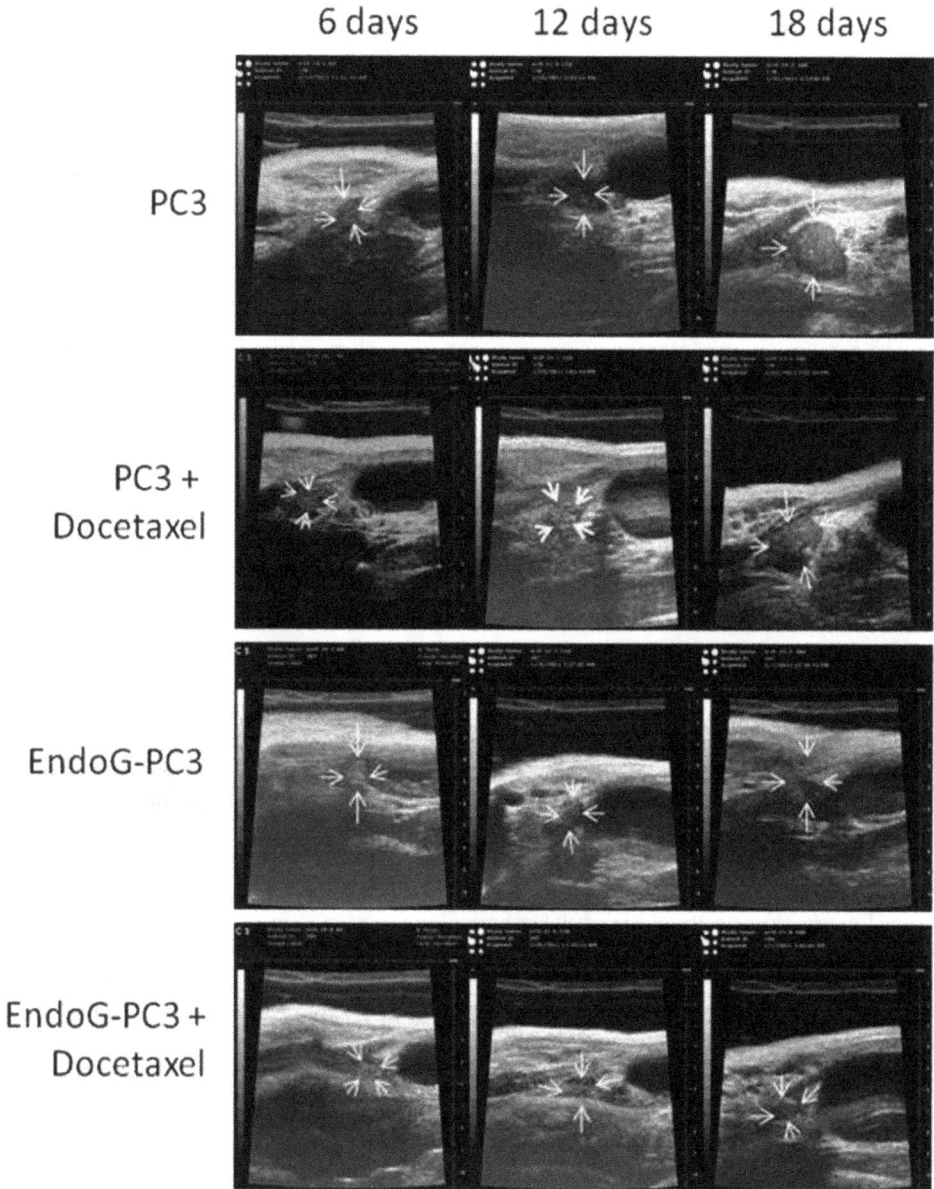

Fig. 2. EndoG expression facilitates docetaxel sensitivity of orthotopic PC3 xenograft tumors. Human prostate cancer PC3 cells were transfected with EndoG precursor gene. Parental EndoG-deficient cells or EndoG-expressing PC3 cells were implanted in ventral prostate. Docetaxel (10 mg/kg) was administrated at the 12th day after implantation. Tumor sizes were monitored by intravital ultrasound sonography using VisualSonics Vevo 770 instrument. Arrows indicate tumor edges.

5. Conclusive remarks

Overall, our studies demonstrated that the expression and activity of the cytotoxic endonucleases are decreased in prostate cancer cells that are resistant to chemotherapy (Wang et al., 2008). This is consistent with previous studies of breast cancer, which also showed disappearance of DNase I in immortalized breast epithelial cells, and decrease of EndoG that coincided with dedifferentiation and invasiveness of breast cancer (Basnakian et al., 2006). EndoG is shown essential for prostate cancer cell death induced by chemotherapy. Expression of EndoG positively correlated with the sensitivity to chemotherapeutic agents cisplatin and etoposide, while the silencing of EndoG by siRNA in two cancer lines, 22Rv1 and LNCaP, decreased the sensitivity of the cells to the chemotherapeutic agents. In PC3 cell line, which does not express EndoG, the chemotherapeutic agent 5-aza-2′-deoxycytidine caused hypomethylation of the EndoG promoter, induced EndoG expression, and made the cells sensitive to both cisplatin and etoposide. In our latest studies described above, the overexpression of EndoG in PC3 cells made them also sensitive to docetaxel *in vitro* and *in vivo*. Therefore these studies demonstrate the first application of endonucleases as a helper drug for the chemotherapy of prostate cancer.

Because the mechanisms of chemo- and radiosensitivity of cells are very similar, these observations may be easily extrapolated to the radiotherapy of prostate cancer. Future studies may be necessary to determine the role of other epigenetic mechanisms in regulation of EndoG and their role in chemoresistance to prostate cancer and cancers of other organs. Chemotherapy is currently one of the frequently used therapeutic strategies for prostate cancer (Dyrstad et al., 2006; Kaku et al., 2006; Nakabayashi & Oh, 2006), and measurement of EndoG may be a potentially useful approach to evaluate chemosensitivity of cancer cells to determine optimal conditions for chemotherapy prior to the therapy.

If further *in vivo* studies confirm our observation that EndoG is a potential key mediator of prostate cancer cell death regulated by the methylation of *EndoG* gene promoter, future epigenetic therapeutics will need to be targeted to EndoG. A development of this approach may lead to similar therapeutic strategies for cancer of other organs.

Recent study determined that DNase I and EndoG, which represent most of DNase activity in prostate epithelial and many other cells and are linked in a single pathway, in which DNase I expression positively modulates EndoG expression (Yin et al., 2007). DNase I has the highest specific activity (per mg protein) among all known endonucleases, and it is the only endonuclease that can be directly incorporated into cells. The mechanisms of DNA destruction and the role in cell death are same between the two endonucleases. Therefore, it may not be necessary to deliver EndoG gene to prostate tumors and instead deliver DNase I protein packed in liposomes, which are attractive as vehicles because they have low toxicity. The only example of an endonuclease being applied for a therapy is human recombinant DNase I is used in complex therapy of cystic fibrosis. Future studies may lead to the first application of endonucleases as a helper drug for chemotherapy of prostate cancer.

6. References

Abbott, D. W., Ivanova, V. S., Wang, X., Bonner, W. M., and Ausio, J., 2001, Characterization of the stability and folding of H2A.Z chromatin particles: implications for transcriptional activation: J Biol Chem, v. 276, p. 41945-9.

Apostolov, E. O., Shah, S. V., Ok, E., and Basnakian, A. G., 2007a, Carbamylated Low-Density Lipoprotein Induces Monocyte Adhesion to Endothelial Cells Through Intercellular Adhesion Molecule-1 and Vascular Cell Adhesion Molecule-1: Arterioscler Thromb Vasc Biol.

Apostolov, E. O., Wang, X., Shah, S. V., and Basnakian, A. G., 2007b, Role of EndoG in development and cell injury: Cell Death Differ, v. 14, p. 1971-4.

Arnold, J. T., and Isaacs, J. T., 2002, Mechanisms involved in the progression of androgen-independent prostate cancers: it is not only the cancer cell's fault: Endocr Relat Cancer, v. 9, p. 61-73.

Baade, P. D., Youlden, D. R., and Krnjacki, L. J., 2009, International epidemiology of prostate cancer: geographical distribution and secular trends: Mol Nutr Food Res, v. 53, p. 171-84.

Bahi, N., Zhang, J., Llovera, M., Ballester, M., Comella, J. X., and Sanchis, D., 2006, Switch from caspase-dependent to caspase-independent death during heart development: essential role of endonuclease G in ischemia-induced DNA processing of differentiated cardiomyocytes: J Biol Chem, v. 281, p. 22943-52.

Banerjee, S., Banerjee, P. P., and Brown, T. R., 2000, Castration-induced apoptotic cell death in the Brown Norway rat prostate decreases as a function of age: Endocrinology, v. 141, p. 821-32.

Banfalvi, G., Trencsenyi, G., Ujvarosi, K., Nagy, G., Ombodi, T., Bedei, M., Somogyi, C., and Basnakian, A. G., 2007, Supranucleosomal organization of chromatin fibers in nuclei of Drosophila S2 cells: DNA Cell Biol, v. 26, p. 55-62.

Basnak'ian, A. G., Topol, L. Z., Kirsanova, I. D., Votrin, II, and Kiselev, F. L., 1989, [Activity of topoisomerase I and endonucleases in cells transfected by a ras oncogene]: Mol Biol (Mosk), v. 23, p. 750-7.

Basnakian, A. G., Apostolov, E. O., Yin, X., Abiri, S. O., Stewart, A. G., Singh, A. B., and Shah, S. V., 2006, Endonuclease G promotes cell death of non-invasive human breast cancer cells: Exp Cell Res, v. 312, p. 4139-49.

Basnakian, A. G., Apostolov, E. O., Yin, X., Napirei, M., Mannherz, H. G., and Shah, S. V., 2005, Cisplatin nephrotoxicity is mediated by deoxyribonuclease I: J Am Soc Nephrol, v. 16, p. 697-702.

Basnakian, A. G., Boubnov, N. V., Kirsanova, I. D., and Votrin, II, 1991, Nuclear topoisomerase I and DNase activities in rat diethylnitrosamine-induced hepatoma, in regenerating and fetal liver: Biochem Int, v. 24, p. 429-37.

Basnakian, A. G., Singh, A. B., and Shah, S. V., 1998, Rat kidney DNase I pre-mRNA is alternatively spliced both in 5'-untranslated region and in coding region. Proceedings of the ASN 31st Annual Meeting, Oct 25-28, 1998, Philadelphia, PA: J Am Soc Nephrol, v. 9, p. 573A.

Basnakian, A. G., Singh, A. B., and Shah, S. V., 2002, Identification and expression of deoxyribonuclease (DNase) I alternative transcripts in the rat: Gene, v. 289, p. 87-96.

Brandstrom, A., Westin, P., Bergh, A., Cajander, S., and Damber, J. E., 1994, Castration induces apoptosis in the ventral prostate but not in an androgen-sensitive prostatic adenocarcinoma in the rat: Cancer Res, v. 54, p. 3594-601.

Buzder, T., Yin, X., Wang, X., Banfalvi, G., and Basnakian, A. G., 2009, Uptake of Foreign Nucleic Acids in Kidney Tubular Epithelial Cells Deficient in Proapoptotic Endonucleases: DNA Cell Biol.

Cote, J., and Ruiz-Carrillo, A., 1993, Primers for mitochondrial DNA replication generated by endonuclease G: Science, v. 261, p. 765-9.

Das, P. M., Ramachandran, K., Vanwert, J., Ferdinand, L., Gopisetty, G., Reis, I. M., and Singal, R., 2006, Methylation mediated silencing of TMS1/ASC gene in prostate cancer: Mol Cancer, v. 5, p. 28.

Davidson, B. L., and Harper, S. Q., 2005, Viral delivery of recombinant short hairpin RNAs: Methods Enzymol, v. 392, p. 145-73.

Debes, J. D., and Tindall, D. J., 2004, Mechanisms of androgen-refractory prostate cancer: N Engl J Med, v. 351, p. 1488-90.

Debruyne, F., 2002, Hormonal therapy of prostate cancer: Semin Urol Oncol, v. 20, p. 4-9.

Diener, T., Neuhaus, M., Koziel, R., Micutkova, L., and Jansen-Durr, P., Role of endonuclease G in senescence-associated cell death of human endothelial cells: Exp Gerontol.

Djeu, J. Y., and Wei, S., 2009, Clusterin and chemoresistance: Adv Cancer Res, v. 105, p. 77-92.

Dyrstad, S. W., Shah, P., and Rao, K., 2006, Chemotherapy for prostate cancer: Curr Pharm Des, v. 12, p. 819-37.

Egger, G., Liang, G., Aparicio, A., and Jones, P. A., 2004, Epigenetics in human disease and prospects for epigenetic therapy: Nature, v. 429, p. 457-63.

Enari, M., Sakahira, H., Yokoyama, H., Okawa, K., Iwamatsu, A., and Nagata, S., 1998, A caspase-activated DNase that degrades DNA during apoptosis, and its inhibitor ICAD: Nature, v. 391, p. 43-50.

Fang, X., Zheng, C., Liu, Z., Ekman, P., and Xu, D., 2004, Enhanced sensitivity of prostate cancer DU145 cells to cisplatinum by 5-aza-2'-deoxycytidine: Oncol Rep, v. 12, p. 523-6.

Freytag, S. O., Stricker, H., Peabody, J., Pegg, J., Paielli, D., Movsas, B., Barton, K. N., Brown, S. L., Lu, M., and Kim, J. H., 2007, Five-year follow-up of trial of replication-competent adenovirus-mediated suicide gene therapy for treatment of prostate cancer: Mol Ther, v. 15, p. 636-42.

Gonzalez, V. M., Fuertes, M. A., Alonso, C., and Perez, J. M., 2001, Is cisplatin-induced cell death always produced by apoptosis?: Mol Pharmacol, v. 59, p. 657-63.

Hengartner, M. O., 2001, Apoptosis. DNA destroyers: Nature, v. 412, p. 27, 29.

Ikeda, S., and Kawasaki, N., 2001, Isolation and characterization of the Schizosaccharomyces pombe cDNA encoding the mitochondrial endonuclease(1): Biochim Biophys Acta, v. 1519, p. 111-6.

Ikeda, S., and Ozaki, K., 1997, Action of mitochondrial endonuclease G on DNA damaged by L-ascorbic acid, peplomycin, and cis-diamminedichloroplatinum (II): Biochem Biophys Res Commun, v. 235, p. 291-4.

Inokuchi, J., Lau, A., Tyson, D. R., and Ornstein, D. K., 2009, Loss of annexin A1 disrupts normal prostate glandular structure by inducing autocrine IL-6 signaling: Carcinogenesis, v. 30, p. 1082-8.

Irvine, R. A., Adachi, N., Shibata, D. K., Cassell, G. D., Yu, K., Karanjawala, Z. E., Hsieh, C. L., and Lieber, M. R., 2005, Generation and characterization of endonuclease G null mice: Mol Cell Biol, v. 25, p. 294-302.

Jacob, M., Napirei, M., Ricken, A., Dixkens, C., and Mannherz, H. G., 2002, Histopathology of lupus-like nephritis in Dnase1-deficient mice in comparison to NZB/W F1 mice: Lupus, v. 11, p. 514-27.

Jiang, H., Sha, S. H., Forge, A., and Schacht, J., 2006, Caspase-independent pathways of hair cell death induced by kanamycin in vivo: Cell Death Differ, v. 13, p. 20-30.

Kaku, H., Saika, T., Tsushima, T., Nagai, A., Yokoyama, T., Abarzua, F., Ebara, S., Manabe, D., Nasu, Y., and Kumon, H., 2006, Combination chemotherapy with estramustine phosphate, ifosfamide and cisplatin for hormone-refractory prostate cancer: Acta Med Okayama, v. 60, p. 43-9.

Koizumi, T., 1995, Deoxyribonuclease II (DNase II) activity in mouse tissues and body fluids: Exp Anim, v. 44, p. 169-71.

Kopelovich, L., Crowell, J. A., and Fay, J. R., 2003, The epigenome as a target for cancer chemoprevention: J Natl Cancer Inst, v. 95, p. 1747-57.

Krieser, R. J., and Eastman, A., 1998, The cloning and expression of human deoxyribonuclease II. A possible role in apoptosis: J Biol Chem, v. 273, p. 30909-14.

Kruslin, B., 2009, [Apoptosis in pathologic prostatic processes]: Acta Med Croatica, v. 63 Suppl 2, p. 49-52.

Kyprianou, N., English, H. F., and Isaacs, J. T., 1988, Activation of a Ca2+-Mg2+-dependent endonuclease as an early event in castration-induced prostatic cell death: Prostate, v. 13, p. 103-17.

Kyprianou, N., and Isaacs, J. T., 1988, Activation of programmed cell death in the rat ventral prostate after castration: Endocrinology, v. 122, p. 552-62.

Lacks, S. A., 1981, Deoxyribonuclease I in mammalian tissues. Specificity of inhibition by actin: J Biol Chem, v. 256, p. 2644-8.

Lee, M. G., Huh, J. S., Chung, S. K., Lee, J. H., Byun, D. S., Ryu, B. K., Kang, M. J., Chae, K. S., Lee, S. J., Lee, C. H., Kim, J. I., Chang, S. G., and Chi, S. G., 2006, Promoter CpG hypermethylation and downregulation of XAF1 expression in human urogenital malignancies: implication for attenuated p53 response to apoptotic stresses: Oncogene, v. 25, p. 5807-22.

Li, L. C., Carroll, P. R., and Dahiya, R., 2005, Epigenetic changes in prostate cancer: implication for diagnosis and treatment: J Natl Cancer Inst, v. 97, p. 103-15.

Li, L. Y., Luo, X., and Wang, X., 2001, Endonuclease G is an apoptotic DNase when released from mitochondria: Nature, v. 412, p. 95-9.

Madaio, M. P., Fabbi, M., Tiso, M., Daga, A., and Puccetti, A., 1996, Spontaneously produced anti-DNA/DNase I autoantibodies modulate nuclear apoptosis in living cells: Eur J Immunol, v. 26, p. 3035-41.

Masse, E., and Drolet, M., 1999, R-loop-dependent hypernegative supercoiling in Escherichia coli topA mutants preferentially occurs at low temperatures and correlates with growth inhibition: J Mol Biol, v. 294, p. 321-32.

McKenzie, S., and Kyprianou, N., 2006, Apoptosis evasion: the role of survival pathways in prostate cancer progression and therapeutic resistance: J Cell Biochem, v. 97, p. 18-32.

Mori, O., Hachisuka, H., Morita, M., Kiyokawa, C., and Sasai, Y., 1996, Apoptosis identified with DNA fragmentation in basal cell carcinomas: Arch Dermatol Res, v. 288, p. 258-61.

Nagata, S., 2000, Apoptotic DNA fragmentation: Exp Cell Res, v. 256, p. 12-8.

Nakabayashi, M., and Oh, W. K., 2006, Chemotherapy for high-risk localized prostate cancer: BJU Int, v. 97, p. 679-83.

Nakayama, M., Gonzalgo, M. L., Yegnasubramanian, S., Lin, X., De Marzo, A. M., and Nelson, W. G., 2004, GSTP1 CpG island hypermethylation as a molecular biomarker for prostate cancer: J Cell Biochem, v. 91, p. 540-52.

Napirei, M., Basnakian, A. G., Apostolov, E. O., and Mannherz, H. G., 2006, Deoxyribonuclease 1 aggravates acetaminophen-induced liver necrosis in male CD-1 mice: Hepatology, v. 43, p. 297-305.

Napirei, M., Karsunky, H., Zevnik, B., Stephan, H., Mannherz, H. G., and Moroy, T., 2000, Features of systemic lupus erythematosus in Dnase1-deficient mice: Nat Genet, v. 25, p. 177-81.

Napirei, M., Ricken, A., Eulitz, D., Knoop, H., and Mannherz, H. G., 2004, Expression pattern of the deoxyribonuclease 1 gene: lessons from the Dnase1 knockout mouse: Biochem J, v. 380, p. 929-37.

Nelius, T., Klatte, T., de Riese, W., Haynes, A., and Filleur, S., 2009, Clinical outcome of patients with docetaxel-resistant hormone-refractory prostate cancer treated with second-line cyclophosphamide-based metronomic chemotherapy: Med Oncol.

Ohsato, T., Ishihara, N., Muta, T., Umeda, S., Ikeda, S., Mihara, K., Hamasaki, N., and Kang, D., 2002, Mammalian mitochondrial endonuclease G. Digestion of R-loops and localization in intermembrane space: Eur J Biochem, v. 269, p. 5765-70.

Oudard, S., Banu, E., Beuzeboc, P., Voog, E., Dourthe, L. M., Hardy-Bessard, A. C., Linassier, C., Scotte, F., Banu, A., Coscas, Y., Guinet, F., Poupon, M. F., and Andrieu, J. M., 2005, Multicenter randomized phase II study of two schedules of docetaxel, estramustine, and prednisone versus mitoxantrone plus prednisone in patients with metastatic hormone-refractory prostate cancer: J Clin Oncol, v. 23, p. 3343-51.

Oudard, S., Banu, E., Scotte, F., Beuzeboc, P., Guyader, C., and Medioni, J., 2007, [New targeted therapies in hormone-refractory prostate cancer]: Bull Cancer, v. 94, p. F62-8.

Parrish, J., Li, L., Klotz, K., Ledwich, D., Wang, X., and Xue, D., 2001, Mitochondrial endonuclease G is important for apoptosis in C. elegans: Nature, v. 412, p. 90-4.

Peitsch, M. C., Polzar, B., Stephan, H., Crompton, T., MacDonald, H. R., Mannherz, H. G., and Tschopp, J., 1993, Characterization of the endogenous deoxyribonuclease involved in nuclear DNA degradation during apoptosis (programmed cell death): Embo J, v. 12, p. 371-7.

Perry, A. S., Foley, R., Woodson, K., and Lawler, M., 2006, The emerging roles of DNA methylation in the clinical management of prostate cancer: Endocr Relat Cancer, v. 13, p. 357-77.

Ploski, J. E., and Aplan, P. D., 2001, Characterization of DNA fragmentation events caused by genotoxic and non-genotoxic agents: Mutat Res, v. 473, p. 169-80.

Polzar, B., Peitsch, M. C., Loos, R., Tschopp, J., and Mannherz, H. G., 1993, Overexpression of deoxyribonuclease I (DNase I) transfected into COS-cells: its distribution during apoptotic cell death: Eur J Cell Biol, v. 62, p. 397-405.

Prats, E., Noel, M., Letourneau, J., Tiranti, V., Vaque, J., Debon, R., Zeviani, M., Cornudella, L., and Ruiz-Carrillo, A., 1997, Characterization and expression of the mouse endonuclease G gene: DNA Cell Biol, v. 16, p. 1111-22.

Raffo, A. J., Perlman, H., Chen, M. W., Day, M. L., Streitman, J. S., and Buttyan, R., 1995, Overexpression of bcl-2 protects prostate cancer cells from apoptosis in vitro and confers resistance to androgen depletion in vivo: Cancer Res, v. 55, p. 4438-45.

Rennie, P. S., and Nelson, C. C., 1998, Epigenetic mechanisms for progression of prostate cancer: Cancer Metastasis Rev, v. 17, p. 401-9.

Rollins, R. A., Haghighi, F., Edwards, J. R., Das, R., Zhang, M. Q., Ju, J., and Bestor, T. H., 2006, Large-scale structure of genomic methylation patterns: Genome Res, v. 16, p. 157-63.

Rozkova, D., Tiserova, H., Fucikova, J., Last'ovicka, J., Podrazil, M., Ulcova, H., Budinsky, V., Prausova, J., Linke, Z., Minarik, I., Sediva, A., Spisek, R., and Bartunkova, J., 2009, FOCUS on FOCIS: combined chemo-immunotherapy for the treatment of hormone-refractory metastatic prostate cancer: Clin Immunol, v. 131, p. 1-10.

Ruchusatsawat, K., Wongpiyabovorn, J., Shuangshoti, S., Hirankarn, N., and Mutirangura, A., 2006, SHP-1 promoter 2 methylation in normal epithelial tissues and demethylation in psoriasis: J Mol Med, v. 84, p. 175-82.

Ruiz-Carrillo, A., and Renaud, J., 1987, Endonuclease G: a (dG)n X (dC)n-specific DNase from higher eukaryotes: Embo J, v. 6, p. 401-7.

Ryan, C. W., Stadler, W. M., and Vogelzang, N. J., 2001, Docetaxel and exisulind in hormone-refractory prostate cancer: Semin Oncol, v. 28, p. 56-61.

Samejima, K., and Earnshaw, W. C., 2005, Trashing the genome: the role of nucleases during apoptosis: Nat Rev Mol Cell Biol.

Schulz, W. A., and Hatina, J., 2006, Epigenetics of prostate cancer: beyond DNA methylation: J Cell Mol Med, v. 10, p. 100-25.

Shilkaitis, A., Green, A., Steele, V., Lubet, R., Kelloff, G., and Christov, K., 2000, Neoplastic transformation of mammary epithelial cells in rats is associated with decreased apoptotic cell death: Carcinogenesis, v. 21, p. 227-33.

Shiokawa, D., Ohyama, H., Yamada, T., and Tanuma, S., 1997, Purification and properties of DNase gamma from apoptotic rat thymocytes: Biochem J, v. 326 (Pt 3), p. 675-81.

Shrivastava, P., Sodhi, A., and Ranjan, P., 2000, Anticancer drug-induced apoptosis in human monocytic leukemic cell line U937 requires activation of endonuclease(s): Anticancer Drugs, v. 11, p. 39-48.

Singh, R. K., and Lokeshwar, B. L., 2009, Depletion of intrinsic expression of Interleukin-8 in prostate cancer cells causes cell cycle arrest, spontaneous apoptosis and increases the efficacy of chemotherapeutic drugs: Mol Cancer, v. 8, p. 57.

Taghavi, P., and van Lohuizen, M., 2006, Developmental biology: two paths to silence merge: Nature, v. 439, p. 794-5.

Takai, D., and Jones, P. A., 2002, Comprehensive analysis of CpG islands in human chromosomes 21 and 22: Proc Natl Acad Sci U S A, v. 99, p. 3740-5.

Takai, D., and Jones, P. A., 2003, The CpG island searcher: a new WWW resource: In Silico Biol, v. 3, p. 235-40.

Uzzo, R. G., Haas, N. B., Crispen, P. L., and Kolenko, V. M., 2008, Mechanisms of apoptosis resistance and treatment strategies to overcome them in hormone-refractory prostate cancer: Cancer, v. 112, p. 1660-71.

Vineis, P., 2003, Cancer as an evolutionary process at the cell level: an epidemiological perspective: Carcinogenesis, v. 24, p. 1-6.

Walton, T. J., Li, G., Seth, R., McArdle, S. E., Bishop, M. C., and Rees, R. C., 2008, DNA demethylation and histone deacetylation inhibition co-operate to re-express estrogen receptor beta and induce apoptosis in prostate cancer cell-lines: Prostate, v. 68, p. 210-22.

Wang, G., Reed, E., and Li, Q. Q., 2004, Apoptosis in prostate cancer: progressive and therapeutic implications (Review): Int J Mol Med, v. 14, p. 23-34.

Wang, Q. F., Tilly, K. I., Tilly, J. L., Preffer, F., Schneyer, A. L., Crowley, W. F., Jr., and Sluss, P. M., 1996, Activin inhibits basal and androgen-stimulated proliferation and induces apoptosis in the human prostatic cancer cell line, LNCaP: Endocrinology, v. 137, p. 5476-83.

Wang, X., Tryndyak, V., Apostolov, E. O., Yin, X., Shah, S. V., Pogribny, I. P., and Basnakian, A. G., 2008, Sensitivity of human prostate cancer cells to chemotherapeutic drugs depends on EndoG expression regulated by promoter methylation: Cancer Lett, v. 270, p. 132-43.

Watson, R. W., and Fitzpatrick, J. M., 2005, Targeting apoptosis in prostate cancer: focus on caspases and inhibitors of apoptosis proteins: BJU Int, v. 96 Suppl 2, p. 30-4.

Widlak, P., Li, L. Y., Wang, X., and Garrard, W. T., 2001, Action of recombinant human apoptotic endonuclease G on naked DNA and chromatin substrates: cooperation with exonuclease and DNase I: J Biol Chem, v. 276, p. 48404-9.

Yin, X., Apostolov, E. O., Shah, S. V., Wang, X., Bogdanov, K. V., Buzder, T., Stewart, A. G., and Basnakian, A. G., 2007, Induction of Renal Endonuclease G by Cisplatin Is Reduced in DNase I-Deficient Mice: J Am Soc Nephrol, v. 18, p. 2544-53.

Yoo, C. B., and Jones, P. A., 2006, Epigenetic therapy of cancer: past, present and future: Nat Rev Drug Discov, v. 5, p. 37-50.

12

Modulation of One-Carbon Metabolism by B Vitamins: Implications for Transformation and Progression of Prostate Cancer

Glenn Tisman
Cancer Research Building, Whittier, CA
USA

1. Introduction

Extensive laboratory, epidemiological and clinical investigations suggest that prostate cancer might be affected by enhanced folate or B12 ingestion and or other perturbations of one-carbon (CH3−) metabolism. Over the last decade, largely due to government mandated dietary fortification with folic acid (FA), our clinic patients experienced a 4-6-fold increase in the median level of serum folate (5 ng/ml → 24 ng/ml). The National Health and Nutrition Examination Surveys (NHANES) confirm similar elevated levels Figure 1 (Dietrich et al, 2005; McDowell et al, 2008; Yang et al, 2010).

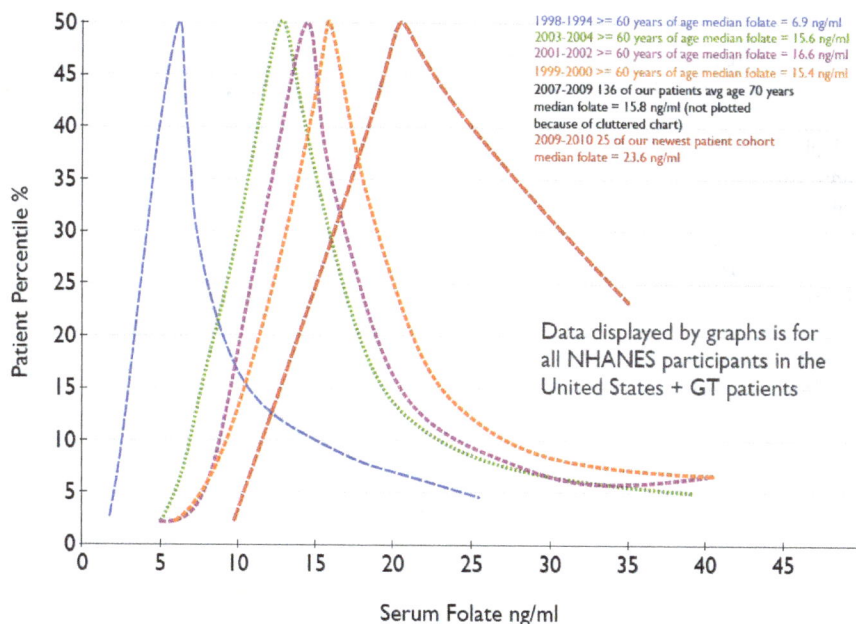

Fig. 1. Median serum/plasma blood folate levels NHANES and GT data.

Exposure to varying concentrations of FA and other B vitamins may transform benign cells to malignant and/or accelerate tumor growth. This review explores clinical observations and biochemistry of B vitamin mediated one-carbon metabolism with general emphasis on neoplasia and particular focus on prostate cancer.

2. Folic acid found to enhance tumor growth: Historical note

Sidney Farber, a pediatric pathologist practicing in Boston's Children Hospital in the mid 1940s, is generally given credit for establishing that FA stimulates human leukemia cell proliferation; however, a careful review of the literature does not confirm that assessment. In fact, Sidney Farber's clinical research group's seminal paper did not include treatment with FA (Farber et al, 1947). This manuscript, published in 1947 in the popular journal Science, reported on Farber's experience with the di- and triglutamate derivatives of oxidized folic acid (diopterin and teropterin, both supplied by Lederle Laboratories of Pearl River, NY under the direction of Yellapragada Subba Row, PhD). The fact is that Farber's landmark paper, routinely referenced in the literature, never stated FA could accelerate leukemia or any other malignancy.

Dr. Richard Lewisohn, famous for his excellence in surgery and his 1917 research on citrated blood as the preferred anticoagulant for transfusion was semiretired in the early 1940's and working in a trivial basement laboratory at Mount Sinai Hospital in NYC. At that time, he was given two folate compounds that were isolated at the Lederle Laboratories: liver L. casei factor (folic acid) and fermentation L. casei factor. The mislabeling of these compounds was the source of confusion for his initial paper mistakenly stating that folic acid was an inhibitor of spontaneous mouse mammary cancer (Leuchtenberger et al, 1945). The compound he thought was FA was in fact pteroyltriglutamate or teropterin.

Later, Hutchings and Stokstad of Lederle informed Lewisohn's group that the correct tentative designation of liver L. casei factor as used in Lewisohn's first report was actually fermentation L. casei factor (the triglutamate of pteroylglutamic acid or teropterin (Angier et al, 1946).

In Lewisohn's subsequent paper (Lewisohn et al, 1946) he confirmed that the mislabeled folic acid (liver L. casei factor) was actually fermentation L. casei factor or teropterin. Clarifying this confusing issue, the initial study revealed that teropterin injection inhibited spontaneous mouse mammary cancer while folic acid (liver L. casei factor), as confirmed in subsequent experiments, stimulated mouse mammary primary tumor growth and its pulmonary metastases while shortening overall survival (Lewisohn et al, 1946). To our knowledge, this is the first literature-documented study revealing FA stimulation of cancer cells (mouse mammary cancer) and their metastasis.

Next, in 1948, the hematologist Robert Heinle (Heinle & Welch, 1948) and later in 1950 the laboratory researcher Howard Skipper (Skipper et al, 1950) were first to document in the clinic and laboratory respectively that FA stimulated chronic myelogenous leukemia in man and acute leukemia in the rat.

The first mention that Farber was aware of what he termed an "acceleration phenomenon" appeared in his work published in 1948 in the NEJM (Farber et al, 1948). In that paper, he referred back to the Science 1947 manuscript stating that the reported children with leukemia displayed acceleration of the leukemic process within the marrow in response to diopterin or teropterin therapy. However, that finding had never been mentioned in the 1947 landmark Science report.

The idea that B12 could accelerate chronic myelogenous leukemia in a patient with pernicious anemia and B12 deficiency was first demonstrated by Jose Corcino in 1971 while working in Dr. Victor Herbert's lab in the Bronx, NY (Corcino et al, 1971). In 1994, Dr. Ralph Green confirmed that observation in other patients with pernicious anemia (Green, 1994). Finally, in 2009, Tisman first demonstrated that B12 administration accelerated the growth of the epithelial prostate tumor in a patient with pernicious anemia and untreated prostate cancer, while at the same time correcting his anemia (Tisman et al, 2009).

3. Contemporary observations spur interest in folate, B12 and prostate neoplasia

In 1998 the US government mandated that the US diet be fortified with FA in an attempt to prevent birth defects such as spina bifida and anencephaly. Subsequent to government-mandated fortification of US, Canadian and Chilean diets with FA, numerous reports appeared documenting a higher incidence of certain cancers (colon, rectum, breast, prostate), reviewed by Young-In Kim and others (Hirsch et al, 2009; Kim, 2007; Kim, 2007; Kim, 2008; Smith et al, 2008).

The newest data relate elevated serum and prostate tissue folate to increased Gleason's grade and proliferation of prostate tumors compared to normal donor prostate tissue (Tomaszewski et al, 2011). FA supplementation was associated with a 2.6 fold increase in incidence (Figueiredo et al, 2009) and stage (Lawson et al, 2007) of prostate tumors. Collin noted serum folate-related increase in PSA velocity (Collin et al, 2010) enough to advance low-risk prostate cancer to higher risk with decreased survival (D'Amico et al, 2005) Figure 2.

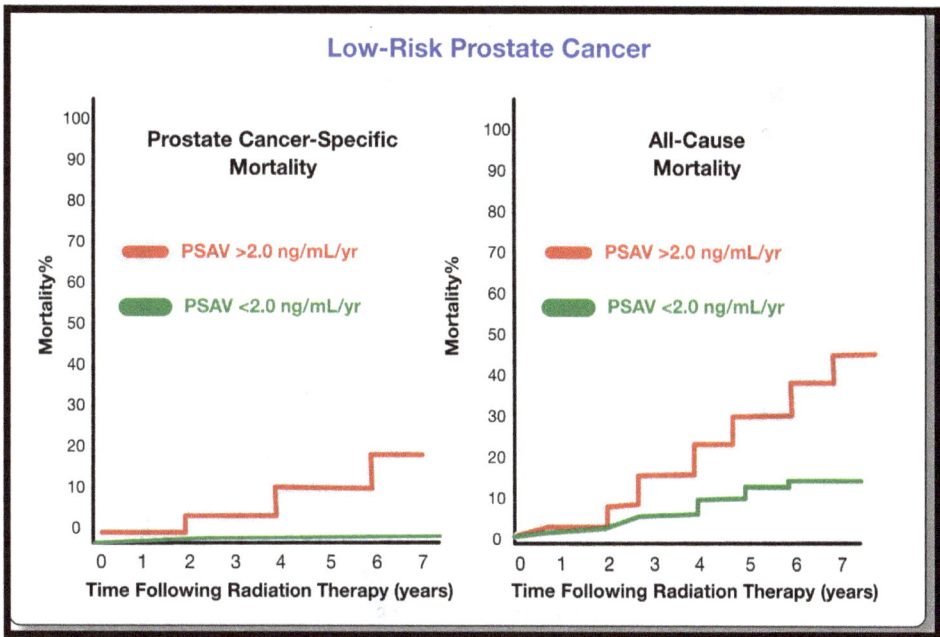

Fig. 2. Higher serum/plasma folate, associated with PSA velocity > 2.0 may increase mortality.

Others related high B12 levels to prostate cancer (Hultdin et al, 2005; Johansson et al, 2009; Weinstein et al, 2006; Vlajinac et al, 1997). We reported direct stimulation of prostate cancer by administration of B12 to a B12 deficient patient (Tisman et al, 2009) and by a supplement containing a combination of B12 and mixed folates Figures 3 and 4 (Tisman & Garcia, 2011).

Patients with prostate cancer frequently ingest a variety of B vitamin-containing supplements (Velicer & Ulrich, 2008; Bailey et al, 2010) including FA and B12. We confirmed this almost universal finding in our clinic. Many are oblivious that their supplements contain larger than needed doses of vitamins. Others take comfort in supplement ingestion immediately after a cancer diagnosis while some use them in an attempt at prophylaxis (Holmes et al, 2010). Holmes' group noted folic acid supplement use before a colorectal cancer diagnosis was 35.4%. This statistic increased to 55.1% after receiving a diagnosis.

We start our review by briefly presenting two of our patients with prostate cancer whose clinical course was adversely impacted by the administration of B12 and mixed folates. This is to be followed by a rather in depth review of B vitamin metabolism as relates to biochemistry that could affect the prostate and its malignant transformation.

3.1 Patient 1

A 75 year-old man presented with prostate cancer and was later found to have pernicious anemia. After a period of 10 months of expectant surveillance it was noted that he was anemic; serum vitamin B_{12} level was 32 pg/ml (300-900 pg/ml) and holotranscobalamin 0 pg/ml (>70 pg/ml). There was an unexpected rapid progression of Gleason's score during watchful waiting. Therapeutic injection of vitamin B12 was accompanied by acceleration of PSA and prostatic acid phosphatase with shortening of prostate-specific antigen doubling time (Tisman et al, 2009) Figure 3.

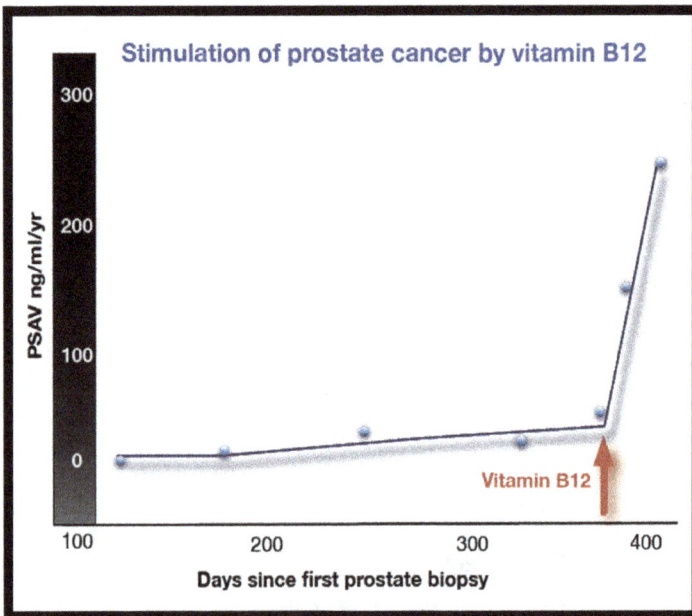

Fig. 3. Patient 1,PSA velocity in response to B12

3.2 Patient 2

A 71 year-old man was diagnosed in 1997 with Stage T1c prostate cancer, Gleason's score = 3+4 = 7. Primary therapy included intermittent androgen deprivation to resistance. While receiving docetaxel chemotherapy for 18 weeks with a continually increasing PSA, withdrawal of ingestion of 10 daily doses of a supplement composed of (500 mcg of vitamin B12 as cyanocobalamin, and 400 mcg each of folic acid as pteroylglutamic acid and 400 mcg of L-5-methyltetrahydrofolate = 800 mcg of mixed folates) was associated with a return to normal of serum prostate specific antigen Figure 4 (in press JMCR).

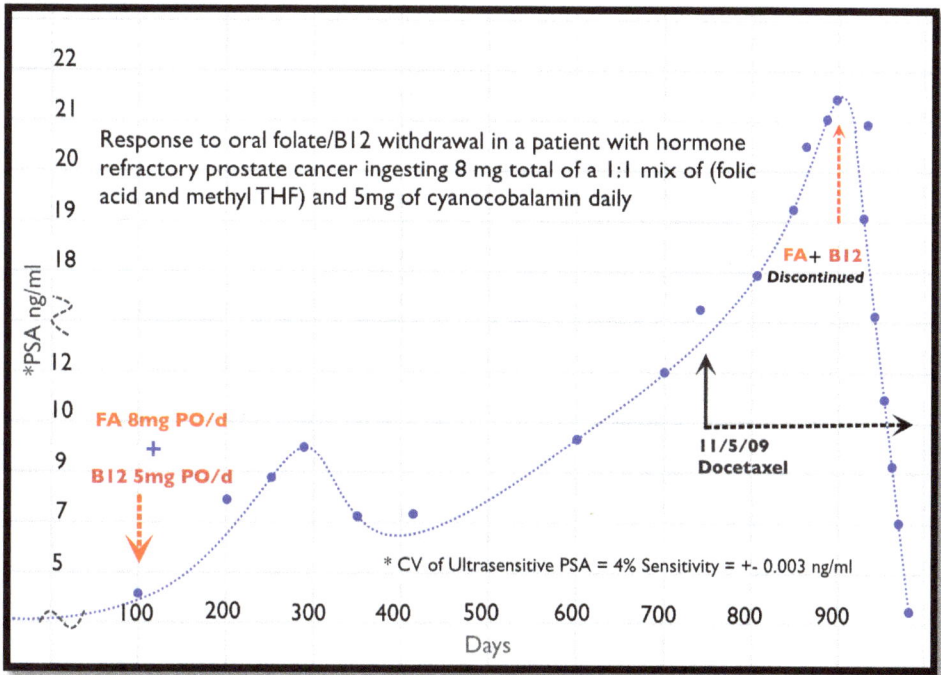

Fig. 4. Patient 2, PSA & withdrawal of B12 and folates

4. Mechanisms of modulation of one-carbon metabolism associated with B vitamin nutrition

Figures 5 and 6 help visualization of the nomenclature and structure of folate vitamers of the "one-carbon" pool. A normal diet supplies methyl groups through methionine and choline, however physiological needs exceed dietary intake. Man makes up the difference by *de novo* synthesis of methyl groups (CH3−). As illustrated in Figure 7, both dietary methionine and choline supply CH3− groups. Note the re-methylation of homocysteine generating methionine, later to be metabolized to S-adenosylmethionine (SAM).

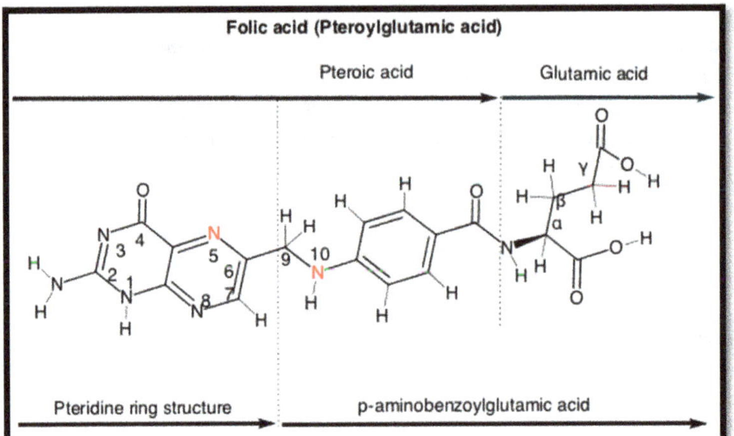

Coenzyme	Substitutent N5		N10
5-Formyltetrahydrofolate	-HCO		-H
5,10-Methenyltetrahydrofolate		=CH-	
5,10-Methylenetetrahydrofolate		-CH2-	
5-Methyltetrahydrofolate	-CH3		-H
Tetrahydrofolate	-H		-H
10-Formyltetrahydrofolate	-H		-HCO
10-Formiminotetrahydrofolic	-H		-HCNH

Fig. 5. Folate(s) nomenclature

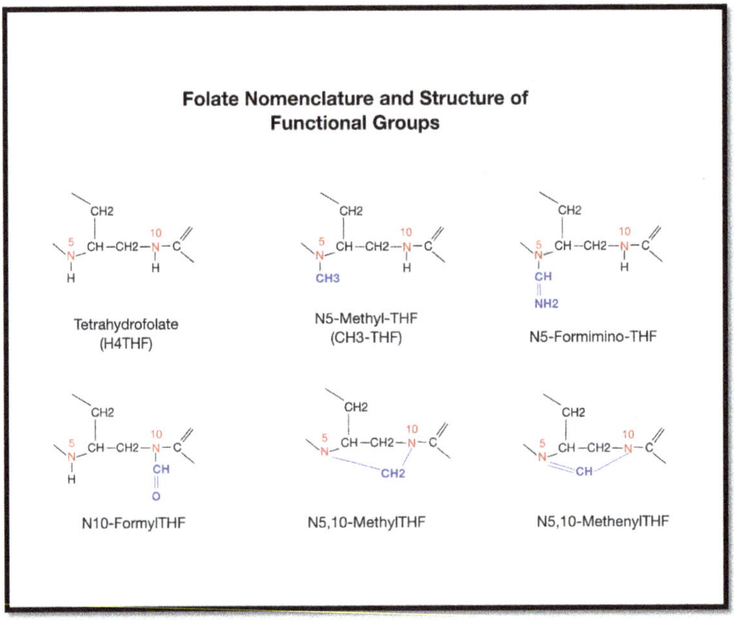

Fig. 6. Folate nomenclature and structure

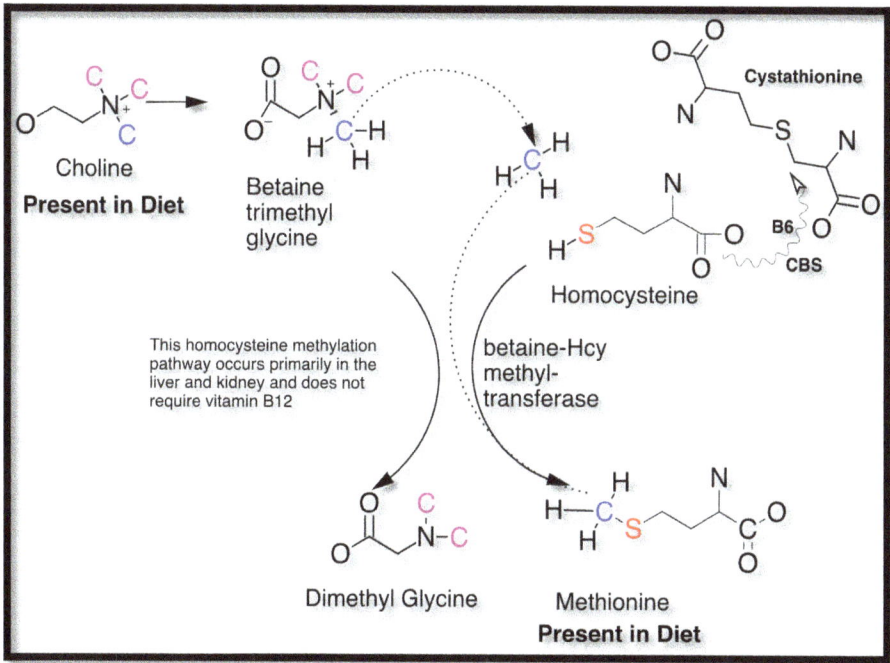

Fig. 7. Sources of dietary CH3— groups

Six fully reduced folate coenzymes, 5-formyl-THF, 5-formamino-THF, 10-formyl-THF, 5,10-methenyl-THF, 5,10-methylene-THF, and 5-methyl-THF (Figures) transfer methyl groups through folate-dependent enzymes. One-carbon fragments in various states of oxidation, when bound to reduced folate coenzymes, are referred to as the one-carbon pool Figures 5, 6 and 8 and are involved in multiple trans methylation reactions. These include the re-methylation of homocysteine leading to methionine and S-adenosylmethionine (SAM) (Figures 7 and 8). SAM is termed the universal methylator, and is involved in more than 100 methylation reactions either directly as in DNA epimethylation or indirectly in the synthesis of DNA-thymine from dUMP, purines (adenine and guanine) and for methylation of protein, RNA, histones etc.

5. Folate fortification, some adverse effects

For purposes of this review, B9 refers to folic acid (FA), the pharmaceutically synthesized, oxidized folic acid (FA) and folate(s) refers to the naturally occurring, usually reduced vitamers found in green leafy vegetables. Man is incapable of self-synthesis of folates and is fully dependent on folates provided by bowel flora, diet and supplements. FA is not normally found in nature, is inexpensive, water-soluble, and an artificial provitamin to reduced folates. Natural forms of the vitamin exist in nature with appended peptide tails of gamma linked glutamate amino acids (usually 5-8 in length). Polyglutamate forms are based mainly on 5-methytetrahydrofolate (CH3—THF) and account for approximately 90% of the folates in fresh foods, the majority of the remainder is based on 10-formyltetrahydrofolate (10-formylTHF) (Butterworth & Santini, 1963; Santini et al, 1964).

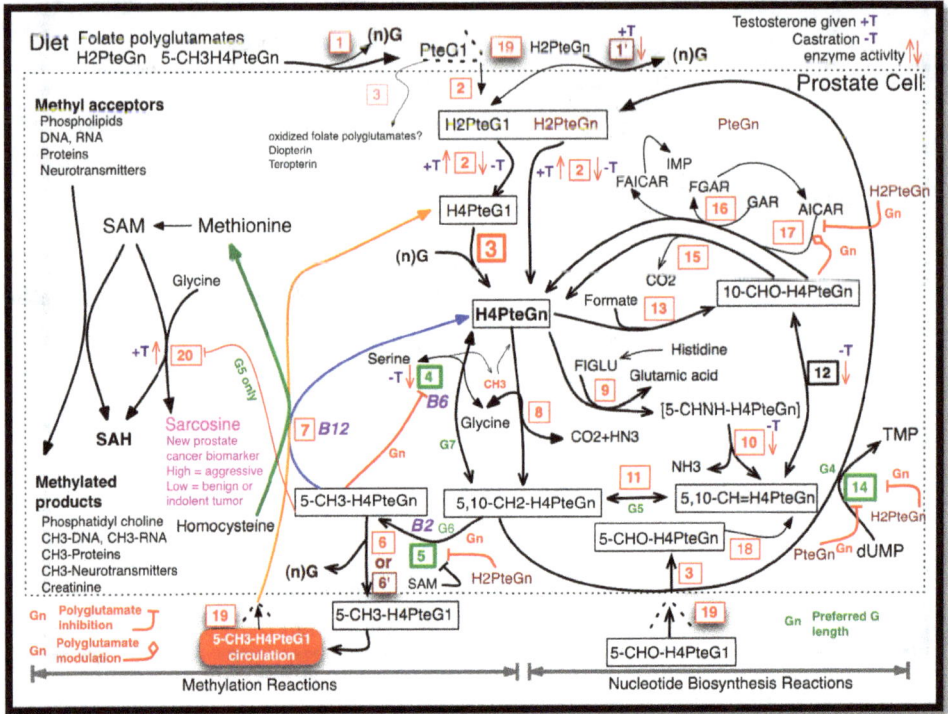

Fig. 8. Folate coenzyme forms, folate-requiring enzymes, important polyglutamates (Gn) and testosterone effects. 1) gamma-glutamyl hydrolase (enterocyte brush border) 1') PSMA prostate specific membrane antigen (2) dihydrofolate reductase 3) folylpolygamma-glutamate synthetase 4) Serinehydroxymethyl transferase 5) methylenetetrahydrofolate reductase 6) gammaglutamyl hydrolase (possibly lysosomal) 6') PSM' Prostate Membrane Antigen splice variant 7) cobalamin dependent methionine synthase 8) glycine cleavage enzyme system 9) glutamate ormimino-transferase 10) formiminotetrahydrofolate cyclodeaminase 11) methylenetetrahydrofolate dehydrogenase 12) methenyltetrahydrofolate cyclohydrolase* 13) formyl tetrahydrofolate synthetase 14) thymidylate synthase 15) formyltetrahydrofolate dehydrogenase 16) phosphoribosyl glycinamide (GAR) formyl transferase 17) phosphoribosylaminoimidazolecarboxamide (AICAR) formyl transferase 18) 5-formyl etrahydrofolate cycloligase 19) folate/methotrexate transport system 20)** glycinemethyl transferase. Dihydrofolate monoglutamate is a weak inhibitor with a Kt = 50 µM, while the pentaglutamate is a potent competitive inhibitor with a Ki of 3.8 µM (Bertrand et al, 1987). Only 5-Me-THFG5 inhibits this enzyme.

Prior to 1998, folate was primarily delivered by diet while FA was added to multivitamin products furnished by health food stores. After 1998, because neural tube defects were related to folate deficiency, US law mandated that FA be added to the food supply. Fortification has proven 19% effective (Honein et al, 2001) in rescuing approximately ~1500-2000 live births a year from neural tube anomalies (spina bifida and anencephaly). However, fortification was followed by reports of reversal of the declining incidence of colorectal cancer in the US, Canada and Chile (Mason et al, 2007; Hirsch et al, 2009). After FA supplementation in the US, there were approximately 15,000 additional cases of colorectal cancer per year (Mason et al, 2007). In the following years, larger amounts of FA were ingested to metabolically lower serum levels of the vasculotoxic amino acid, homocysteine. It was thought that lowering homocysteine would decrease the incidence of arteriosclerotic cardiovascular disease. However, studies thus far have been inconsistent and not confirmed this assumption save for a possible benefit in stroke prevention (Chen, J (J), Xu, X (X), et al., 2010; Wang et al, 2007; Robinson et al, 1998) and thrombophilia.

Alarmingly, there are now laboratory animal (Lindzon et al, 2009; Ly et al, 2011) and epidemiological reports pointing to excessive malignancy, including prostate (Figueiredo et al, 2009), breast ({Campbell 2002); Chen et al, 2005; Ericson et al, 2009; Stevens et al, 2010) colorectal and other cancers (Kim, 2005) associated with both hyper and hypo-sufficiency of folate and folate enzyme polymorphisms, reviewed by Young-In Kim and others (Kim, 2007; Kim, 2008; Kim, 2005; Smith et al, 2008) see Table 1.

Study	B2	B6	B12	Folate
Kasperzyk et al, 2009		Hi B6 less risk of death from CaP		
Key et al, 1997		Hi B6 Less risk of CaP		
Collin et al, 2010			Hi B12 Hi CaP	
Hultdin et al, 2005			Hi B12 Hi risk for CaP	Hi Fol Hi risk for CaP
Johansson et al, 2008			Hi B12 Hi risk for CaP	
Vlajinac et al, 1997			Hi B12 Hi risk for CaP	
Collin et al, 2010			Hi B12 Hi risk for CaP	Hi Fol Hi risk for CaP
Pelucchi et al, 2005				Hi Fol protects against CaP
Collin et al, 2010				Hi Fol Hi risk PSAV > 2
Figueiredo et al, 2009				Hi Fol Hi risk for CaP 2.7-fold higher
Johansson et al, 2009	Hi B2 Hiher risk for CaP			

Table 1. Significant epidemiological studies relating B vitamins with prostate cancer (CaP)

5.1 Folate fortification: Effects on chemotherapy

5-fluorouracil and capecitabine (a prodrug metabolized to fluoropyrimidines) are active in breast and colon cancer. In the presence of high serum levels of folate and or in the presence of certain folate-metabolizing enzyme polymorphisms (Kim, 2009; Maring et al, 2005; Sharma et al, 2008), their toxicity is greatly magnified (Midgley & Kerr, 2009). This requires lowering of the recommended dose of folate in the US (Hennessy et al, 2005). This appears to be due to strengthening of the ternary complex between 5,10 methyleneTHF, F-dUMP and thymidylate synthase with enhanced inhibition of DNA-thymine synthesis.

5.2 B vitamin metabolism, malignant transformation and effects of enzyme polymorphisms on neoplasia

Impaired *de novo* DNA-thymine synthesis associated with absolute, relative or functional deficiency of folate coenzymes or folate-metabolizing enzyme concentration shifts may result in uracil misincorporation into DNA, defective DNA base excision repair, double strand chromosome breaks, and DNA point mutations resulting in malignant transformation (Blount et al, 1997; Milic et al, 2010) Figure 9. The resulting chromosomal breaks are identical to specific breaks found in common cancers (Yunis & Soreng, 1984).

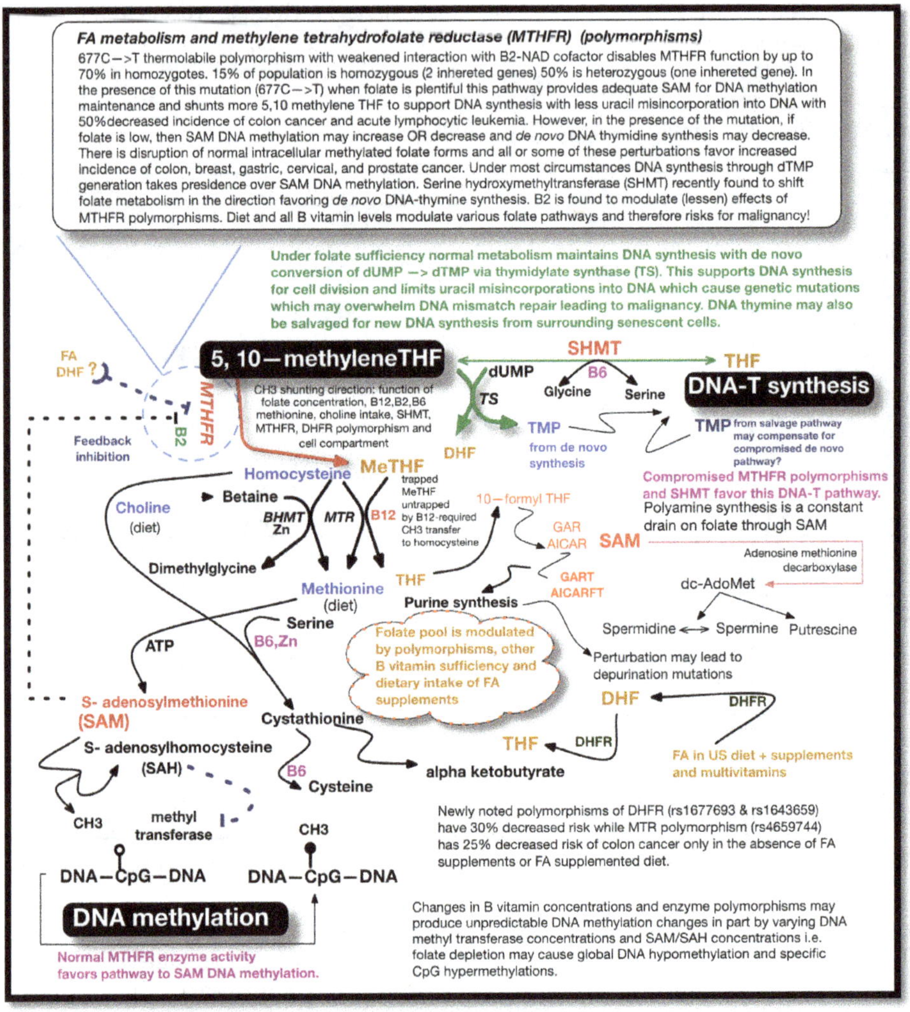

FA metabolism and methylene tetrahydrofolate reductase (MTHFR) (polymorphisms)

677C—>T thermolabile polymorphism with weakened interaction with B2-NAD cofactor disables MTHFR function by up to 70% in homozygotes. 15% of population is homozygous (2 inherited genes) 50% is heterozygous (one inhereted gene). In the presence of this mutation (677C—>T) when folate is plentiful this pathway provides adequate SAM for DNA methylation maintenance and shunts more 5,10 methylene THF to support DNA synthesis with less uracil misincorporation into DNA with 50%decreased incidence of colon cancer and acute lymphocytic leukemia. However, in the presence of the mutation, if folate is low, then SAM DNA methylation may increase OR decrease and *de novo* DNA thymidine synthesis may decrease. There is disruption of normal intracellular methylated folate forms and all or some of these perturbations favor increased incidence of colon, breast, gastric, cervical, and prostate cancer. Under most circumstances DNA synthesis through dTMP generation takes presidence over SAM DNA methylation. Serine hydroxymethyltransferase (SHMT) recently found to shift folate metabolism in the direction favoring *de novo* DNA-thymine synthesis. B2 is found to modulate (lessen) effects of MTHFR polymorphisms. Diet and all B vitamin levels modulate various folate pathways and therefore risks for malignancy!

Fig. 9. *De novo* and salvage pathways to DNA-thymine synthesis, SAM methylation of DNA, polyamine synthesis and MTHFR polymorphisms

S-adenosylmethionine (SAM) is regulated by multiple factors including the enzyme glycine N-methyltransferase (GNMT) (Luka et al, 2009; Wang et al, 2011) and is governed in part by testosterone, vitamin A and specifically the potent inhibitory folatepentaglutamate, 5-CH3 – THFG5 see Figure 10. The effects of altered SAM production may result in DNA hypo- and or hypermethylation thereby changing gene expression, which may result in malignant transformation (Davis & Uthus, 2004; De Cabo et al, 1995; Duthie, 1999; Duthie et al, 2002; Duthie, 2010; Esteller et al, 2002; Esteller, 2003; Esteller, 2007; Jones & Baylin, 2002; Ulrey et al, 2005; Wainfan et al, 1989) Compromised DNA-thymine synthesis (dUMP → TMP) results in uracil misincorporation into DNA and hastens malignant transformation, tumor proliferation and aggressiveness (Chango et al, 2009; Choi et al, 2004; James et al, 2003; Jang et al, 2005; Liu et al, 2006) Figures 9 and 10.

Additional studies show examples of change due to large doses of dietary FA. Rats fed 40 mg/kg compared to 2 mg/kg FA induced more hepatic SAM in Dams phenotypically resulting in fetuses of less weight and shortened vertex-coccyx length (Achón et al, 2000). High FA given to rats worsened experimentally induced liver fibrosis (Marsillach et al, 2008). Alternatively, folate insufficiency and/or B12 insufficiency slows cell metabolism and division. This is manifest in the clinic as macroovalocytic anemia with bone marrow megaloblastic change, and if severe, pancytopenia, as reviewed by Tisman (Tisman, 2005). Abnormal histones, targets for SAM-mediated epimethylation, are thought responsible for the clock-face

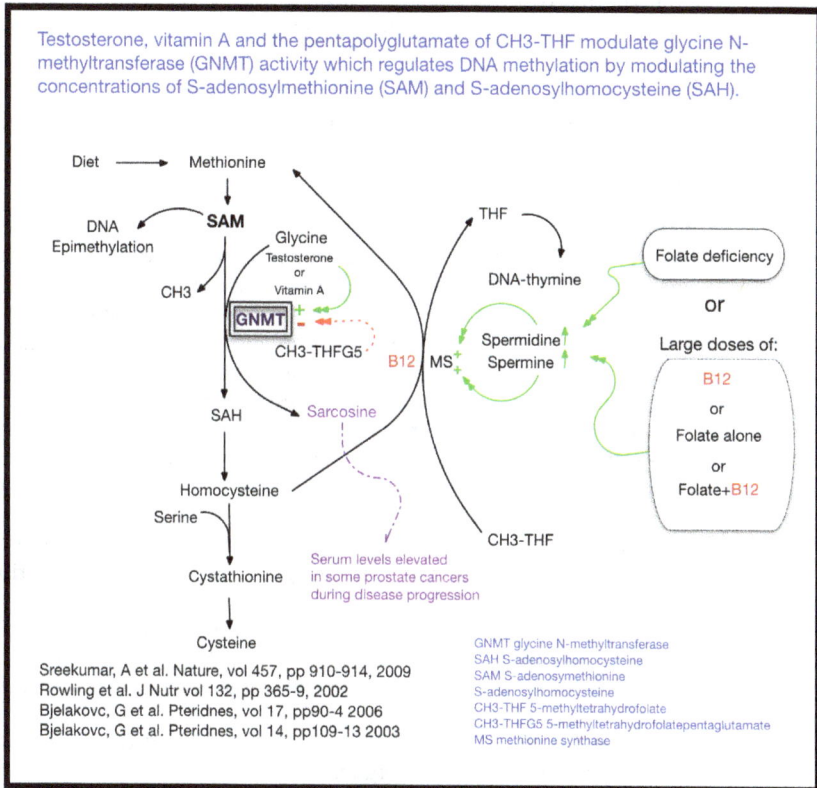

Fig. 10. GNMT modulation by Testosterone, CH3 – THFG5 **polyglutamate** and vitamin A, effects of folates and B12 on polyamines and spermidine and spermine on methionine synthetase.

appearance of chromatin within basophilic megaloblasts (Das et al, 2005). Though megaloblastic change is characteristic of blood cells, similar morphology is noted in other cells undergoing cell division during B12 and or folate insufficiency. These include enterocytes, oral and glossal mucosa cells, bronchial mucosa and the uterine cervix (Herbert, 1959).

Exciting work in Young-In Kim's lab disclosed that high intrauterine and post-weaning dietary exposure to FA increased the risk of mammary tumors of offspring. They conjecture the tumor-promoting effect could have been mediated by altered DNA methylation and DNA methyl transferase activity during pregnancy (Ly et al, 2011). However, other experiments with rats by this group disclosed that maternal, but not post-weaning, FA supplementation reduced the odds of colorectal adenocarcinoma by 64% in carcinogen challenged offspring. It was proposed that the protective effect may have been due to increased global DNA methylation and decreased epithelial proliferation (Sie et al, 2011). They hint that there may be tissue-specific and divergent responses to both high and low FA exposure.

Historically, B12 and folate deficiency is associated with malignancy. B12 deficiency of pernicious anemia is accompanied by a 3-18 fold increase in gastric cancer (Kuster et al, 1972). Approximately 10% of those suffering from celiac disease, which is almost always associated with folate deficiency, were noted to develop malignancy (Chanarin, 1969; Dormandy et al, 1963;). Though B12 and folate may lead to pancytopenia in the short term, chronic insufficiency or gestational exposure to folate lack or hypersufficiency may lead to latent neoplastic change.

6. Newer concepts of nutrition: Compartmentalization, organ-specific nutrient deficiency, nutrient-nutrient interaction and cell kinetic modulation of nutrient adequacy

Epidemiological analyses measure nutrient consumption through questionnaires, serum levels of vitamins and metabolites and simultaneous analysis of clinical correlations with hypothesized relationships. Unfortunately, these studies frequently ignore micronutrient variation over long periods, presence of one or many interacting enzyme polymorphisms which vary with different populations, simultaneous variations of multiple interacting vitamers i.e. B12, B9, B2, B6, Figures 9 and 11 and the kinetic state of cellular metabolism at the time of the study.

As an example of simultaneous B vitamin variation, we present our data from our untreated cancer patient population as we studied serum levels of B vitamins, Figure 11. Forty-four percent of patients were found to have at least one of six measured parameters of B vitamin sufficiency in the abnormal range. Many were simultaneously deficient and or hypersufficient of several metabolically interacting B vitamins.

To understand how a specific organ such as the prostate may manifest vitamin deficiency while simultaneously others do not, we review relevant principles of nutrient distribution and utilization:

1. Clement Finch (Finch et al, 1950) taught that total body cellular iron deficiency appears gradually. There occurs an orderly decline in body iron starting with loss of plasma iron, followed by depletion of hepatic and marrow stores, decrease in red cell size finally culminating in anemia.

2. Victor Herbert expanded Finch's work demonstrating micronutrient distribution varied simultaneously from cell to cell and organ-to-organ. Nutrient sufficiency for folate and B12, he claimed, was compartmentalized and progressed in an orderly fashion (Herbert, 1987) (see Figures 12 and 13). One cell type could be nutritionally satisfied and in apparent equilibrium with hepatic, red cell and serum folate. Simultaneously, other more kinetically active cells could struggle with deficiency. Work in Herbert's lab by Das showed that the

adequacy of a cell's folate and or B12 stores reflected the folate/B12 status at the time the cell was metabolically active (Das et al, 1980), which is the time that intracellular vitamin transport is active. Susan Duthie confirmed simultaneous discordance of folate stores between red blood and buccal mucosal cells (Basten et al, 2004).

3. Bruce Ames' theory of "micronutrient triage" (Ames, 2006) dovetails with that of Herbert. He teaches that through allocation and distribution, scarce micronutrients are triaged to the most metabolically acute process required for cell survival.

4. Finally, Heaney (Heaney, 2003) presented his view of "long-latency disease" whereby a minimal level of chronic nutrient deficiency would take years before tissue damage became apparent. As examples, he points to stroke due to folate-related hyperhomocysteinemia (Wang et al, 2007) and thrombophilia from folate and B6 lack (Remacha et al, 2002) resulting in thrombosis (Hron et al, 2007).

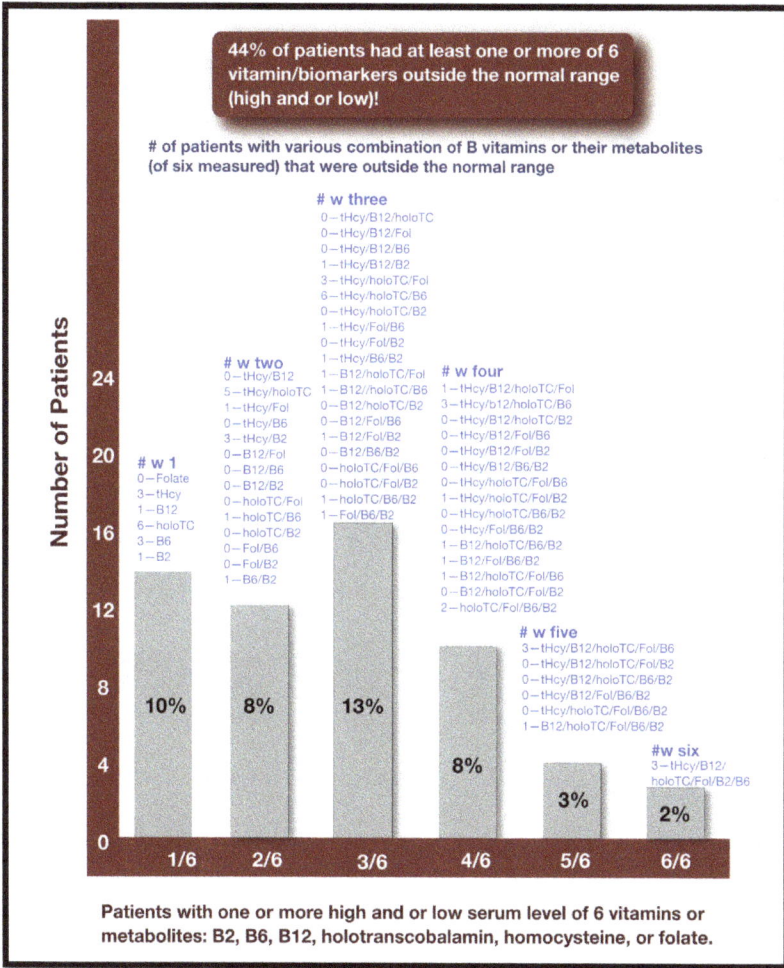

Fig. 11. Frequency of multiple simultaneous vitamin abnormalities among untreated cancer patients.

Awareness of these concepts helps in understanding how seemingly unrelated vitamin metabolism, cellular kinetics and nutrition might simultaneously starve select organs while others thrive.

7. Cell-specific metabolic preferences in one-carbon metabolism

Herbert demonstrated that patients' tumors and their own normal bone marrow cells more often than not differed in degree and preference for *de novo* and salvage pathways for DNA-thymine synthesis (Tisman et al, 1973) Figure 9. These inherent metabolic differences dictated sensitivity to vitamin deficiency and drugs such as fluorinated pyrimidines, methotrexate and other anti-fols.

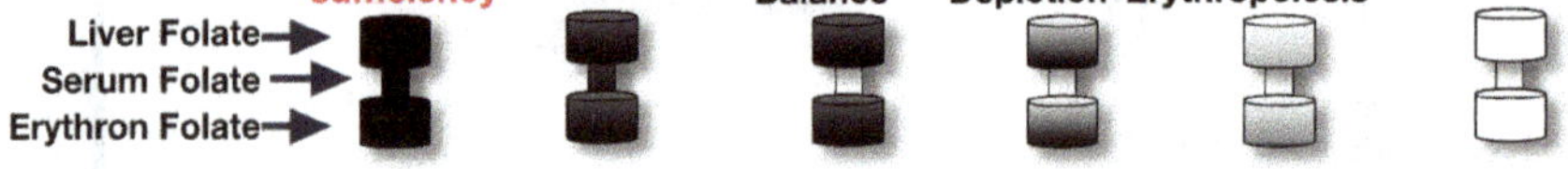

Stage:	Hyper-sufficiency	Normal	Negative Folate Balance	Folate Depletion	Folate-deficient Erythropoiesis	Anemia
Liver Folate→ Serum Folate → Erythron Folate→						
Serum Folate	>35 ng/ml	>5 ng/ml	<3-4 ng/ml	<3ng/ml	<3 ng/ml	<3ng/ml
RBC Folate	>200 ng/ml	>200 ng/ml	>200 ng/ml		<160 ng/ml	<120 ng/ml	<100 ng/ml
dU suppression	Normal	Normal	Normal	Normal	Abnormal	Abnormal
Hypersegmentation	Normal <3.5	Normal <3.5	Normal <3.5	Normal <3.5	Abnormal >3.5	Abnormal >3.5
Liver Folate	>3 mcg/g	>3 mcg/g	>3 mcg/g	<1.6 mcg/g	<1.2 mcg/g	<1.0 mcg/g
Erythrocytes	Normal	Normal	Normal	Normal	Normal	Macro-ovalocytes
MCV	Normal	Normal	Normal	Normal	Normal	Elevated
Hemoglobin	Normal	Normal	Normal	Normal	Normal	Low
Plasma clearance of intravenous folate	Normal	Normal	Normal	Normal	Increased	Increased
Homocysteine	7-10 microM/L	10-12 microM/L	10-12 microM/L	Elevated	Elevated	Elevated
Elevated cancer risk	Likely	No	Unlikely	Possibly	Probably	Likely
Acceleration of pre- and malignant tissue	Likely	No	Unlikely	Unlikely	No	Possible deceleration

Fig. 12. Sequential stages of folate deficiency

Young-In Kim's group studied two colon cancer cell lines, HCT 116 and Caco2 (Hayashi et al, 2007), both grown in folate-limiting medium. They reported that the Caco2 line preserved *de novo* DNA-thymine synthesis while HCT 116 cells preserved SAM and DNA methylation pathways.

Bistulfi's lab (Bistulfi et al, 2009) studied an example of cell-specific nutrition in prostate cells. They presented evidence of high folate requirements by prostate cells to maintain SAM to support extraordinarily large amounts of polyamine synthesis (Figure 14). Folate insufficiency resulted in increased gene promoter CpG island and DNA-histone methylation Figure 14. The cell DNA methylome changed to produce the more aggressive phenotype *in vitro*; cells became anchorage-independent and showed reduced sensitivity to folate depletion.

Stage:	Normal	Negative B12 Balance	B12 Depletion	B12-deficient Erythropoiesis	Anemia
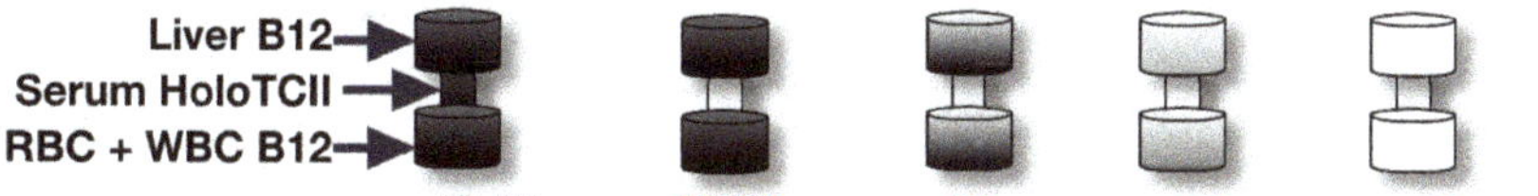 Liver B12 → Serum HoloTCII → RBC + WBC B12 →					
HoloTCII	>50-70 pg/ml	<50-70 pg/ml	<20 pg/ml	<12 pg/ml	<12 pg/ml
TC II % sat	>5%	<5%	<2%	<1%	<1%
Holohap	>150pg/ml	>150pg/ml	<150pg/ml	<100pg/ml	<100pg/ml
dU suppression	Normal	Normal	Normal	Abnormal	Abnormal
Hypersegmentation	No	No	No	Yes	Yes
TBBC*% sat	>15%	>15%	>15%	<15%	<10%
Hap % sat	>20%	>20%	>20%	<20%	<10%
RBC Folate	>160ng/ml	>160ng/ml	>160ng/ml	<140ng/ml	<140ng/ml
Erythrocytes	Normal	Normal	Normal	Normal	Macro-ovalocytosis
MCV	Normal	Normal	Normal	Normal	Elevated
Hemoglobin	Normal	Normal	Normal	Normal	Low
TC II	Normal	Normal	Normal	Elevated	Elevated
Methylmalonate	No	No	No	?	Yes
Myelin damage	No	No	No	?	?
Homocysteine	8-12 microM/L	8-12 microM/L	Elevated	Elevated	Elevated

Fig. 13. Sequential stages for B12 deficiency

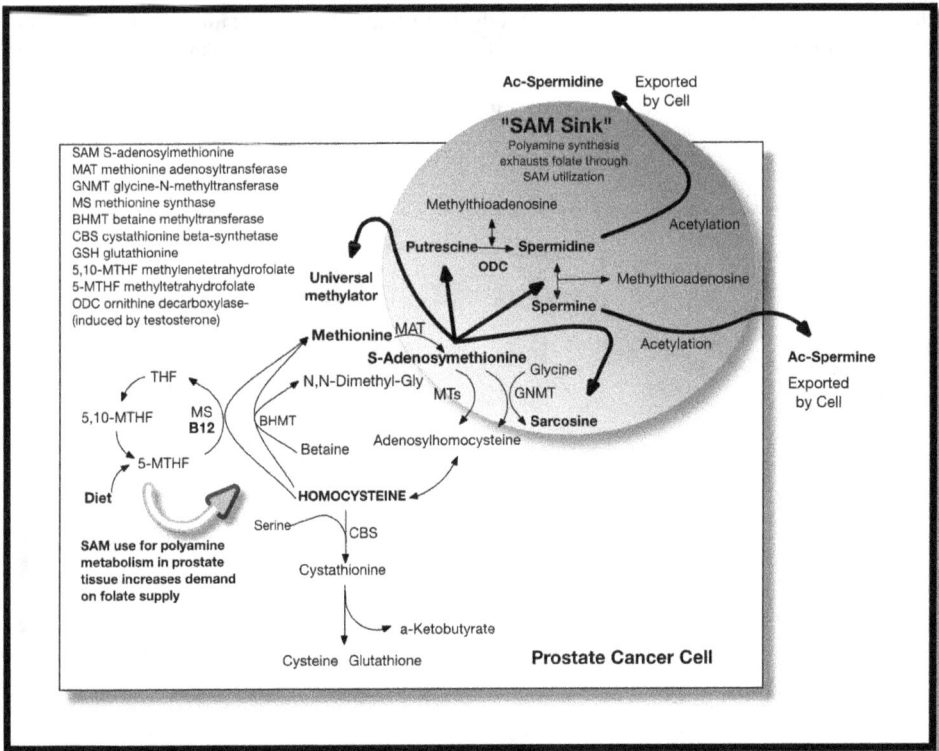

Fig. 14. Prostate cells draw heavily of their SAM supply to maintain disproportionate polyamine synthesis

There is mounting biochemical and epidemiological support that cancers of the prostate may result in part from micronutrient imbalance leading to mutations and the aberrant epimethylome triggering abnormal gene expression (van Engeland et al, 2003; Cooper & Foster, 2009; Diaw et al, 2007; Ernst et al, 2002; Esteller, 2007; Esteller, 2008; Li et al, 2005; Li & Dahiya, 2007; Maruyama et al, 2002; Perry et al, 2006; Sasaki et al, 2002; Shukeir et al, 2006; Yegnasubramanian et al, 2008). Folate metabolizing enzyme polymorphisms complicate the overall picture (Cai et al, 2010) (Figure 9) through interaction with B vitamin metabolism causing results of epidemiological studies to be inconsistent; this has been extensively reviewed (Kim, 2007; Kim, 2004; Kim, 2005; Kim, 2009; Sanderson et al, 2007; Smith et al, 2008; Sohn et al, 2009).

8. Mechanisms for B vitamin control of one-carbon metabolism

8.1 Folate polyglutamate length modulation of one-carbon metabolism

Folylpolygammaglutamates are substrates for folate-dependent enzymes and generally have lower Km values (stronger enzyme binding) than corresponding monoglutamates. They result from reacting with folylpolygammaglutamyl synthetase (FPGS) (Cook et al,

1987; Lowe et al, 1993; Moran & Colman, 1984; Shane, 2010; Sun et al, 2001; Ward & Nixon, 1990). Polyglutamate tails increase folate cellular retention and coenzyme activity. Only folylmonoglutamates traverse cell membranes (Antony, 1992; Alemdaroglu, 2007; Perry & Chanarin, 1972; Shane, 2010). FPGS is up-regulated in cycling, dividing cells and in folate deficiency (Freemantle & Moran, 1997) Figure 15.

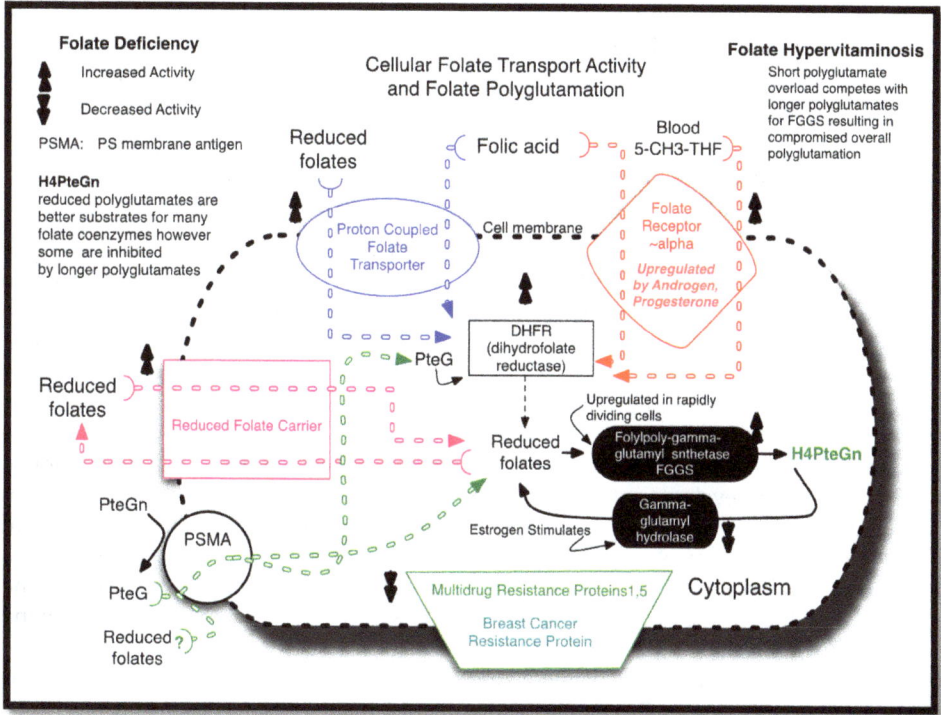

Fig. 15. Changes in folate metabolism in deficiency and sufficiency

Polyglutamation increases the affinity of folate forms (Krumdieck et al, 1992; Matthews et al, 1987) for most folate-dependent enzymes except for dihydrofolatereductase (DHFR) (Bailey & Ayling, 2009). DHFR is a crucial rate-limiting enzyme responsible for regenerating reduced tetrahydrofolates from spent dihydrofolates generated after reduced folates transfer their one-carbon moiety Figure 8. Polyglutamation of 5,10 methyleneTHF results in the potentiation of thymidylate synthase (TS) and thus the conversion of dUMP to thymidine monophosphate (TMP) by a factor 100-fold greater than for the monoglutamate (Galivan et al, 1977; Kisliuk et al, 1974; Matthews et al, 1987; Moran, 1989).

The competing enzyme within intracellular lysosomes, folylpolygammaglutamalhydrolase (FPH) shortens polyglutamate length by splitting terminal glutamate residues (Krumdieck et al, 1976; Shane, 2010). FPGS and FPH are competing enzymes. FPH activity is duplicated in the prostate specific membrane antigen (PSMA) and its splice variants (PSM') implicated in prostate cancer carcinogenesis (Yao et al, 2010) Figure 19.

Methyltetrahydrofolate (CH3–THF) is a poor substrate for FPGS (Perry et al, 1983) and irreversible trapping of CH3–THF in B12 deficiency imposes both intracellular CH3–THF polyglutamate deficiency and loss of intracellular CH3–THF (Lowe et al, 1993). B12 deficiency was found to limit intracellular transport of CH3–THF (Tisman & Herbert, 1973), an example of B vitamin interaction compounding effects of B12 deficiency. Irreversible trapping of reduced folate as CH3–THF in B12 deficiency exhausts regeneration of reduced THF (Figure 9).

9. Sex steroid hormones and modulation of folate metabolizing enzymes and polyglutamate length

Relevant to the prostate, in rodents, estrogen and progesterone modulation of FPH affects intracellular polyglutamate length (Krumdieck et al, 1975) and thus folate polyglutamate concentrations and activity while testosterone impacts folate-metabolizing enzyme activity of the prostate and seminal vesicles (Bovina et al, 1972; Rovinetti et al, 1972). In women, estrogen administration to women lowers homocysteine and induces measurable changes of the epimethylome suggesting an effect on homocysteine remethylation and SAM methylation of DNA (Friso et al, 2007).

By shortening the folylpolyglutamate tails, increased activity of FPH can induce folate insufficiency. FPH levels of uteri of castrated rats increase in response to estrogen replacement (Krumdieck et al, 1975). FPH modulation by estrogen, a hormone active in prostate cancer, could involve regulation of folate metabolism. Estramustine (Emcyt™) and diethylstilbestrol might share similar effects on FPH. Orchiectomy and testosterone replacement induce intracellular folate-dependent enzyme concentration variations (Bovina et al, 1972; Rovinetti et al, 1972) Figures 8 and 16.

The effects of castration on folate metabolizing enzymes in rat prostate, seminal vesicle and liver tissue were reported by Rovinetti and Bovina (Bovina et al, 1972; Rovinetti et al, 1972). They found that for prostate tissue, castration caused reversible changes in content and tissue distribution of folate coenzymes Figures 8 and 16. Castration caused suppression of activity of dihydrofolate reductase (DHFR), 10- formyl THF synthase, and serine hydroxymethyl transferase (SHMT). Cytoplasmic cSHMT in concert with vitamin B6 acts as a metabolic switch with at least three functions: 1) preferentially supplies one-carbon units for DNA-thymidine synthesis, Figure 17 circle-number-1, 2) lowers methylene THF used for SAM synthesis Figure 17 circle-number-3, and 3) sequesters CH3–THF by adsorption to the enzyme thus limiting SAM synthesis Figure 17 circle-c. Administration of testosterone restored castration-related enzymatic activities to near normal and higher than normal values. The changes described by Rovinetti (Rovinetti et al, 1972) within prostate tissue could produce powerful metabolic and genetic changes regulated by the testosterone and folate status of the patient.

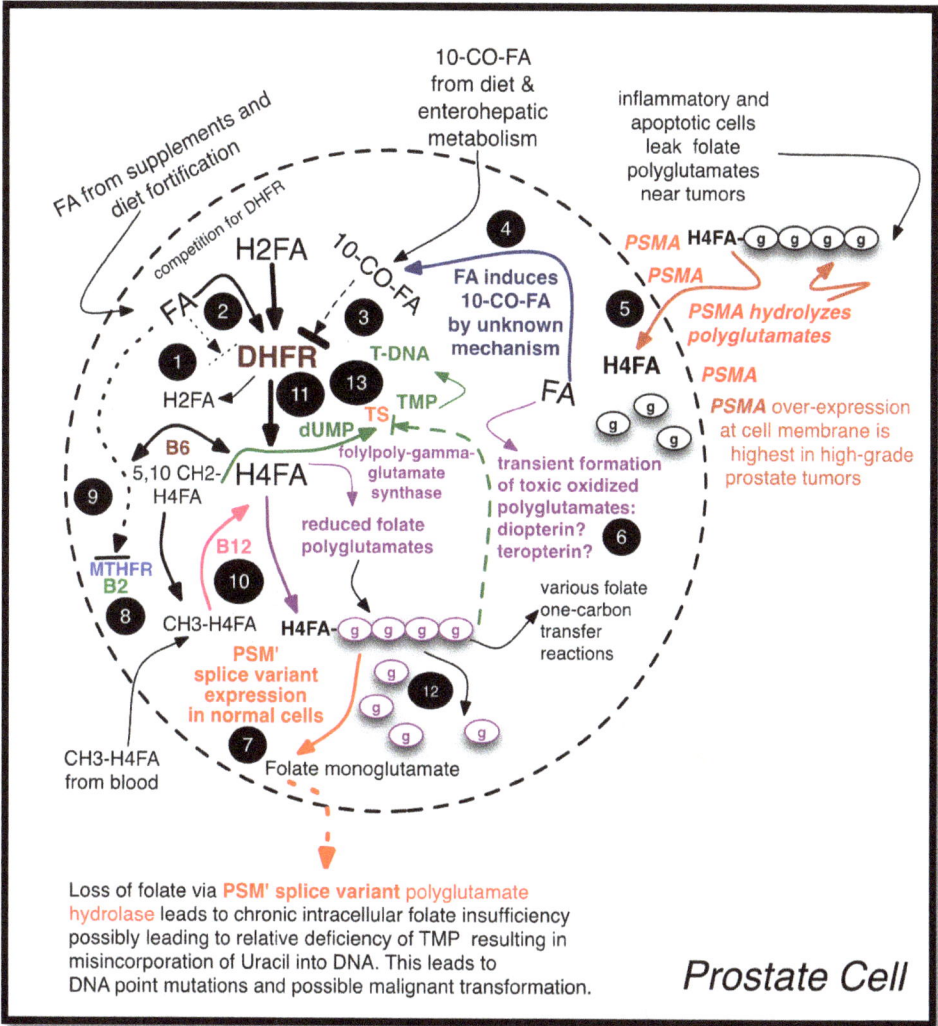

1) FA may directly inhibit DHFR (Kao et al, 2008) 2) FA competes with H2FA for reduction 3) 10-CO-FA
inhibits DHFR 4) FA induces 10-CO-FA (D'Urso-Scott et al, 1974; Pratt & Cooper, 1971)? 5) PSMA of
prostate cell membrane enhances folate monoglutamate of microenvironment 6) Possible transient
production of toxic diopterin and teropterin and other polyglutamates by action of FPGS on FA
(Hoffbrand et al, 1976; Shane, 2010) 7) PSM' splice variant FPH produces folate monoglutamates
intracellularly 8) B2 modulates MTHFR (Bates & Fuller, 1986; Matthews & Baugh, 1980; Matthews &
Haywood, 1979; McNulty et al, 2002) 9) DHFA SAM (Matthews & Daubner, 1982), and FA-(slightly)
(Matthews & Haywood, 1979) inhibit MTHFR 10) CH3 — THF trapped by B12 deficiency
11)Testosterone increases DHFR activity (Bovina et al, 1972; Rovinetti et al, 1972) 12) Estrogen increases
FPH activity.

Fig. 16. Folate pathways affected by sex steroid concentrations and FA and other B vitamins.

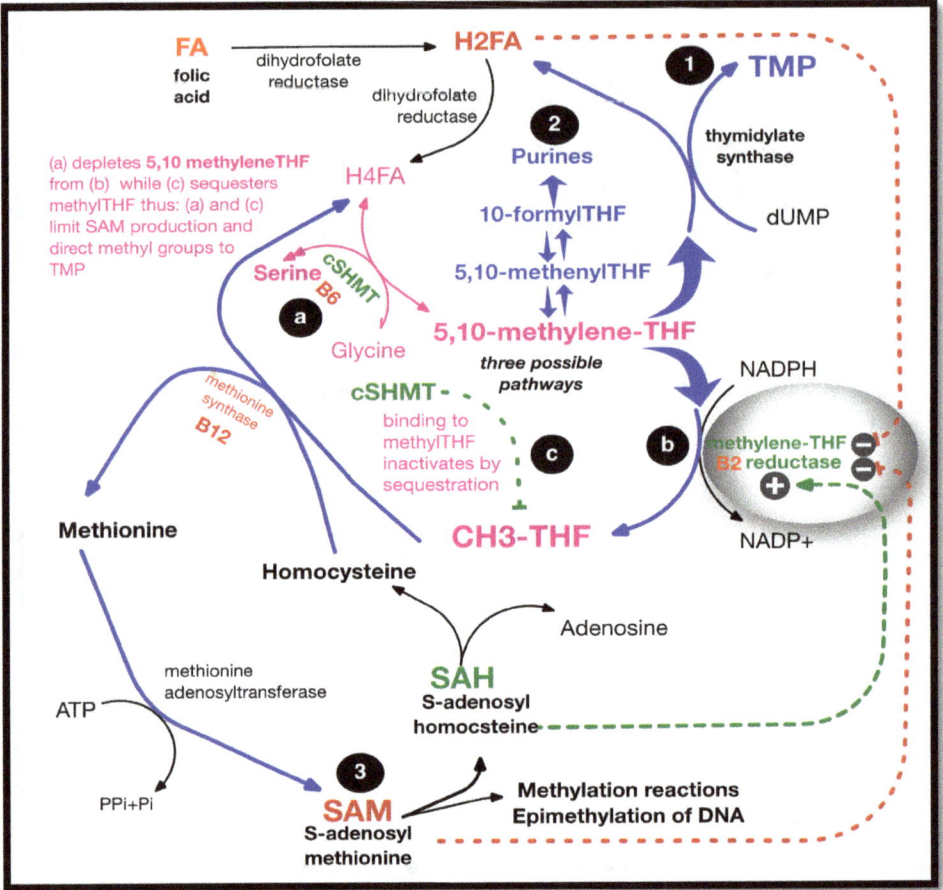

Fig. 17. DHFA, SAM, and S-adenosylhomocysteine (SAH) regulate 5, 10-methylene-THF reductase through inhibition and stimulation of the enzyme (see oval). Cytoplasmic serinehydroxymethylenetransferase (cSHMT) activity influences methylation of dUMP to DNA-thymine vs. homocysteine thru sequestration and inactivation of CH3−THF. Taken together, these compounds modulate methyl group flow to (1) dUMP for DNA-thymine (2) or purine synthesis (3) or for DNA epimethylation and other methylation reactions.

10. Modulation of folate polyglutamate tail length by folate hypersufficiency

Raising the folate concentration with FA competes for FPGS binding sites thereby lowering average polyglutamate length. This can reduce folate coenzyme substrate activity (Cook et al, 1987; Lowe et al, 1993; Shane, 2010), Figure 18.

As folate polyglutamate coenzymes increase in length, substrate-binding strength for FPGS decreases and polyglutamates are released from the enzyme limiting the maximum length to approximately 8 glutamate residues for mammalian cells. Polyglutamate tail length can change an active folate coenzyme to metabolically inert or to an anti-fol (Allegra et al, 1985; Kisliuk et al, 1974; Kisliuk & Gaumont, 1983; Kisliuk et al, 1981; Kisliuk, 1981; Matthews et al, 1987). As indicated in Figure 18, large doses of folate monoglutamates would compete for folate substrate binding, causing premature release of substrates resulting in shorter, less active folate coenzymes.

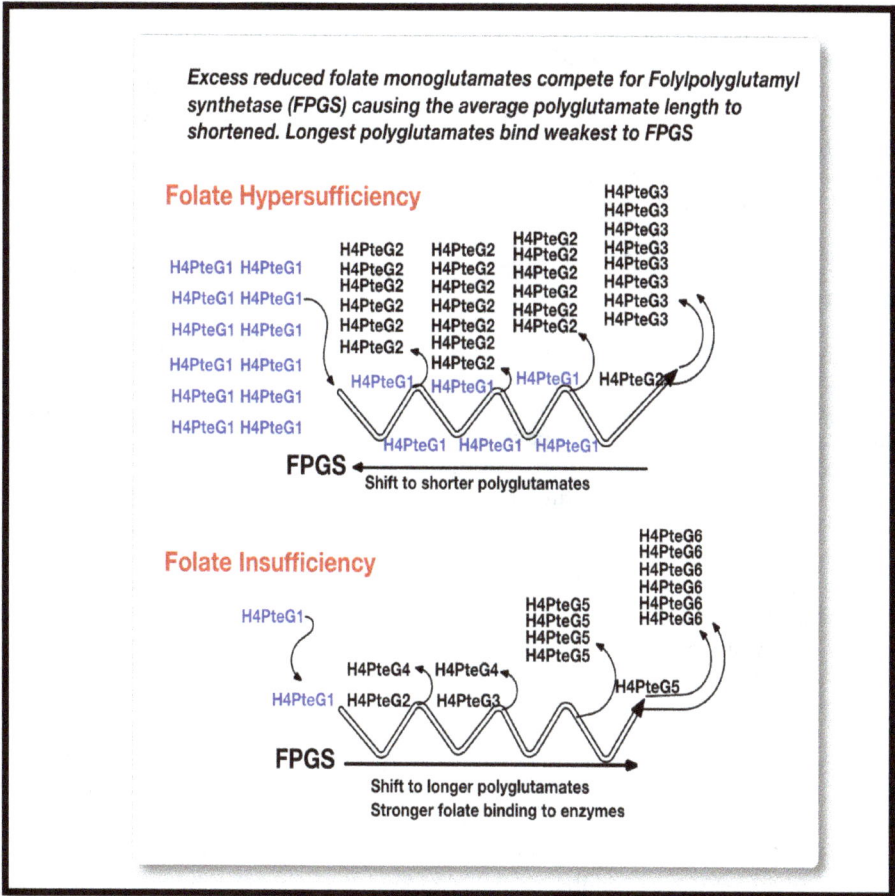

Fig. 18. Increasing reduced folatemonoglutamates competes for reduced folate substrate sites of FPGS tending to decrease overall lengths of folate polyglutamates (Lowe et al, 1993; Cook et al, 1987).

11. Modulation of folate activity by pteridine ring oxidation and DHFR polymorphisms

Matthews showed that several folate-dependent enzymes are inhibited by elevated concentrations of oxidized folate substrates. Dihydrofolate polyglutamates inhibit thymidylate synthase, AICAR transformylase and methylenetetrahydrofolate reductase (Krumdieck et al, 1992; Matthews et al, 1987; Matthews & Haywood, 1979; Ross et al, 1984). As discussed by Kisliuk, oxidation of the pteridine ring from the active tetrahydro to the dihydro state can change a stimulatory coenzyme to a powerful anti-fol (Kisliuk, 1981).

10-formylfolic acid is a potent inhibitor of dihydrofolate reductase of rat liver slices (Rauen et al, 1952; Bertino et al, 1965; D'Urso-Scott et al, 1974; Friedkin et al, 1975; Rauen et al, 1952; Silverman et al, 1954). However, the literature is inconsistent concerning the *in vivo* activity of 10-formylfolic acid in man. Whether this oxidized folate is active *in vivo*, a natural part of the diet (Butterworth & Santini, 1963; Konings et al, 2002; Konings et al, 2001) or an artifact of oxidation when purified is controversial. Pratt (Pratt & Cooper, 1971) and others (Ratanasthien et al, 1974) conjecture that this folate could be formed within the jejunum by bacteria and subject to entero-hepatic circulation and jejunal absorption. Long-term feeding of 10-formylfolic acid produces bioactive folates found to support the growth of chickens (Gregory III et al, 1984) and produces a relatively weak but measurable hematological response in humans with pernicious anemia (Spies & Garcia-Lopez, 1948). Needless to say, more work is needed here.

12. Prostate Specific Membrane Antigen (PSMA), PSMA splice variants (PSM'): Putative biology

PSMA, Figure 19, is a prostate cell membrane receptor with extracellular, transmembrane and intracellular components. The extracellular portion expresses both folylpolyglutamyl hydrolase and neurocarboxypeptidase activity. PSMA is expressed on epithelial cells of benign prostate, prostate hyperplasia, premalignant proliferative inflammatory atrophy (PIA), prostate intraepithelial neoplasia (PIN), and most intensely on high Gleason grade prostate carcinoma cells. PSMA was successfully targeted for radio-imaging vis-a-vis Prostascint scan (Taneja, 2004) and immunotherapy of prostate cancer (Bander et al, 2005; Harzstark & Small, 2009). Almost all Gleason grade 4 tumor cells express excessive amounts of surface PSMA. PSMA staining was positive for 49% of high-grade PIN and only 6% of normal prostate cells (Marchal et al, 2004). Surprisingly, PSMA, first thought to be specific for prostate cancer cells, is expressed on endothelial cells of neovessels involved in angiogenesis of most cancers and with normal wound healing (Chang et al, 1999; Gordon et al, 2008). PSMA expression on prostate epithelium is decreased by testosterone and increased in patients with prostate cancer refractory to testosterone withdrawal. As Gleason's grade and clinical stage increase, acceleration of cell proliferation requires an increased supply of nutrients and PSMA could help cells acquire folate by scavenging folatemonoglutamates from surrounding apoptotic inflammatory cells. Lighter molecular weight, so-called splice variants of PSMA, termed PSM', are present in large amounts within the cytoplasm of normal prostate cells. PSM' and its congeners are highly expressed in the normal prostate and in low-grade tumors retaining both FPH and neurocarboxypeptidase enzymatic activity (O'Keefe, Bacich, et al., 2001; Yao et al, 2008). As illustrated in Figure 18, and as suggested by Yao and O'Keefe, extensive expression of PSM' makes cells vulnerable to loss of folatemonoglutamates putatively causing intracellular folate deficiency (O'Keefe, Bacich, et al., 2001; Yao et al, 2008; Yao et al, 2010). Over time, it is conceivable that such chronic, cell-specific deficiency could transform cells to a malignant phenotype (Yao et al, 2008).

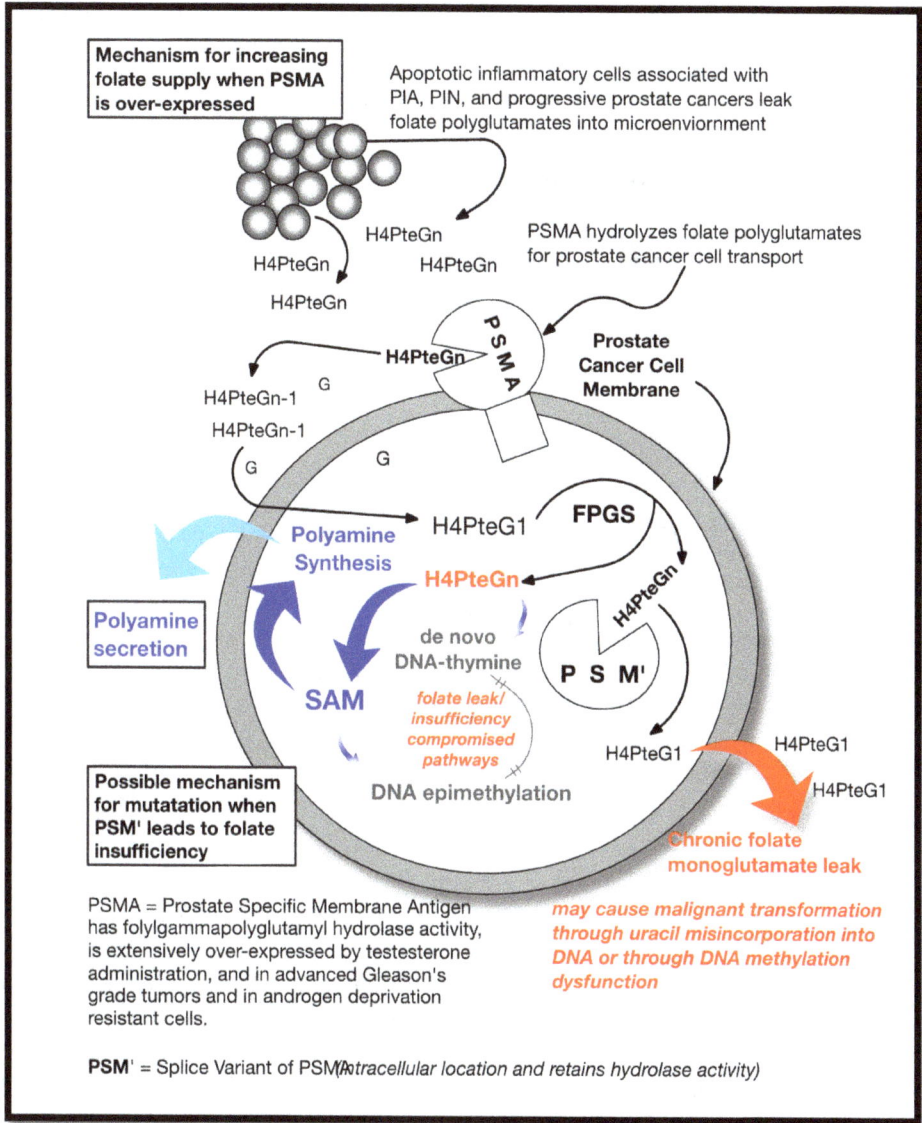

Fig. 19. Proposed balance between PSMA and PSM'. Prostate specific membrane antigen (PSMA) and its splice variant cogeners, PSM'. PSMA supplies intracellular folate monoglutamates from surrounding degenerating inflammatory cells that supply polyglutamates. PSM', present in high concentration in normal prostate cells, through its FPH activity generates folatemonoglutamates for extracellular transport leaving cells relatively deficient of folates.

13. Polyamines

These compounds contain two or more amine groups, such as spermidine and spermine and function as essential growth factors. The prostate is the major source of polyamine production and secretion. Metabolic demands for polyamine synthesis divert intracellular folate methyl groups from other metabolic processes including the synthesis of DNA-thymine and epimethylation of DNA (Bistulfi et al, 2009) Figure 14.

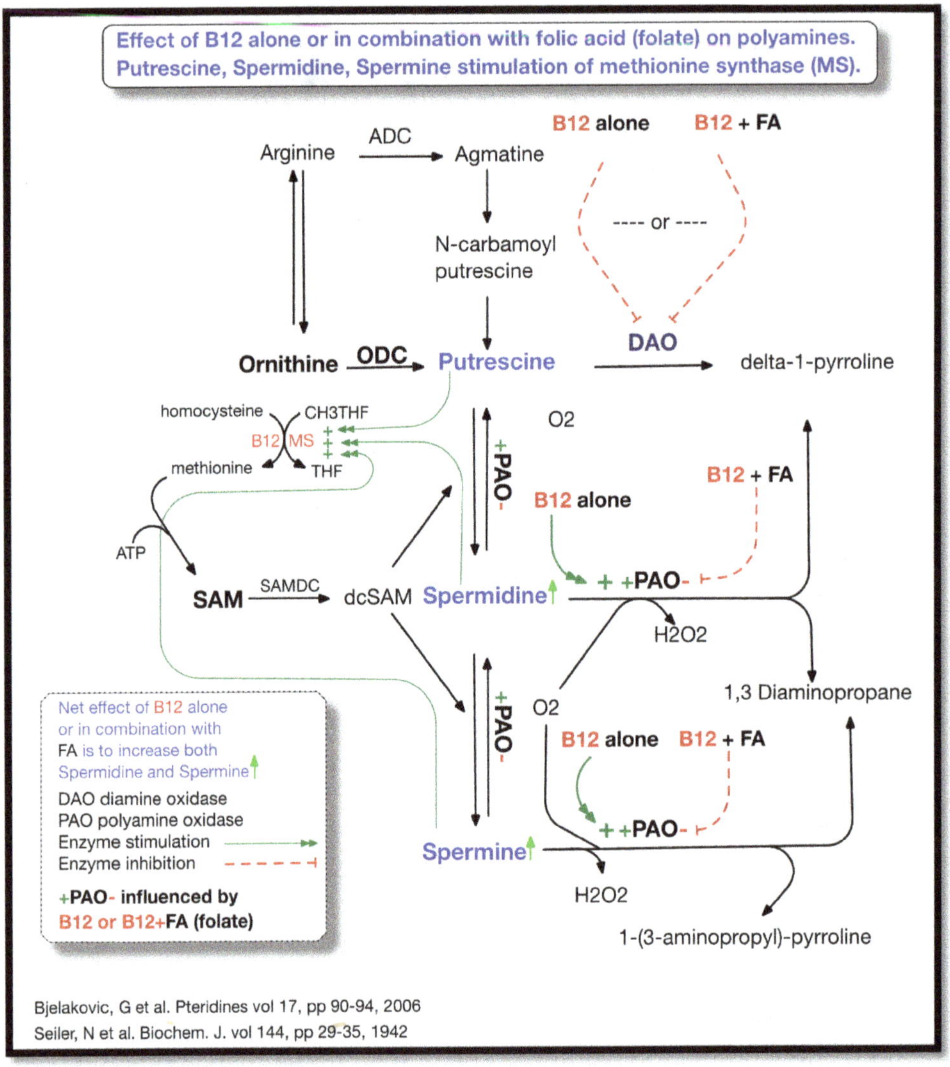

Fig. 20. Polyamine metabolism: B12 and FA influence polyamine metabolism and polyamines may modulate methionine synthase (MS)

Polyamines regulate cellular growth and participate in the evolution of prostate cancer. As
noted in Figure 20 the enzyme ornithine decarboxylase (ODC) initiates polyamine synthesis.
Testosterone increases the activity of ODC, S-adenosylmethionine decarboxylase and
spermidine synthase of prostate epithelial cells. Figure 20 shows modulation by B12 and
folate of the enzymes of polyamine oxidation, diamine oxidase (DAO) and polyamine
oxidase (PAO). Spermine and spermidine modulate the key B12-requiring enzyme,
methionine synthase, illustrating other areas of regulation between B vitamins, one-carbon
transfer and polyamine metabolism critical for prostate cells.
In 1996 Kenyon's group reported that spermine increased methionine synthase (MS) activity
by 400% and spermidine by 270% (Kenyon et al, 1996). In 2006 Bjelakovic (Bjelakovic et al,
2006) reported effects of mega doses of B12 alone and B12 plus folic acid on the activity of
the polyamine metabolizing enzymes DAO and PAO, Figure 20. Dongmei Sun placed rats
on a low folate diet inducing folate insufficiency and observed hepatic spermidine,
spermine and putrescine increase by 58%, 67% and 27% respectively compared to controls
fed a folate-replete diet (Sun et al, 2002). The polyamine concentrations of the jejunum,
ileum, colon and brain remained stable. There was a tissue-specific polyamine response to
folate deficiency. Low folate (Sun et al, 2002) as well large doses of folic acid alone, B12
alone, or B12 plus folic acid produced increased hepatic levels of spermidine and spermine
(Bjelakovic et al, 2003; Bjelakovic et al, 2006). B12 and folate are thus modulators of
polyamine metabolism and vice versa.

13.1 Other regulatory mediators of one-carbon metabolism: DHFR, SAM, GHMT and cSHMT

The pentaglutamate of CH_3-THF modulates GNMT enzyme activity by non-substrate
binding. CH_3-THF, only as the pentaglutamate-G5, strongly inhibits GNMT activity
(Wagner et al, 1985; Yeo et al, 1999). Likewise, cytoplasmic serinehydroxymethyltra-nsferase
(cSHMT), by non-enzymatic sequestration of CH_3-THF controls its metabolism to THF.
These interactions add further diversity to mechanisms for control of one-carbon
metabolism and surely wreak havoc on those trying to study them Figures 10 and 17.
When SAM levels are high, MTHFR is inhibited (Ubbink et al, 1996) and CH_3-THF
formation is reduced, resulting in active GNMT, which reduces excess SAM (Wang et al,
2011) Figures 10 and 17. SAM diversion to polyamine synthesis leads to active MTHFR
increasing CH_3-THF, which is polyglutamated to $CH_3-THFG5$ leading to inhibition of
GNMT (Williams & Schalinske, 2007; Yeo et al, 1999). GNMT catalyzes SAM mediated
methylation of glycine to sarcosine (Rowling et al, 2002) Figures 8 and 10. Testosterone up-
regulates GNMT, producing more sarcosine. Blood and urinary sarcosine has been the
subject of intense debate in the literature. Sarcosine was initially identified as a valuable
marker for aggressive prostate cancer (Sreekumar et al, 2009) but this has not yet been
confirmed by others (Jentzmik et al, 2010; Jentzmik et al, 2011; Struys et al, 2010).

13.2 General genomic and chromosomal structure

Figures 21 and 22 summarize promoter and genomic architecture. The genome includes
both the genes and the non-coding sequences of DNA. The DNA helix coiled around
histones contains the genetic code. DNA coiled around a set of 4 histone dimers is
referred to as a nucleosome (illustrated as a single bead). When the nucleosomes are

loosely packed in a relaxed state and spread apart they are collectively referred to as "euchromatin" and as such allow "epimethylation", the transfer of methyl groups delivered by S-adenosylmethionine to the cytosine bases of DNA (some arranged as CpG islands/groupings while others are more diffusely scattered about the global genome). CpG cytosine bases extend out from the DNA helix. Alternatively, tightly packed histones within chromosomes are termed "heterochromatin" and under this condition access to methylation of cytosine bases is prohibited. The packed beads of histones (loose or tight) are further folded into segments called chromosomes of which there are normally 46 in number.

14. Epigenetics, control of the epigenome, folic acid and malignant transformation

As a primer on the epigenome, methylation reactions and genetic control, we would recommend excellent comprehensive reviews (Choi & Friso, 2010; Dobosy et al, 2007; Foley et al, 2009; Jones & Takai, 2001;Perry et al, 2006). The definition of epigenetics given by Peter Jones at USC School of Medicine is "the study of heritable changes in gene expression that occur independent of changes in the primary DNA sequence or genetic code" (Jones & Laird, 1999; Sharma et al, 2010). The presence of a genetic code within DNA, though obviously necessary, is not sufficient for gene transcription. Only through gene expression do observable phenotypic changes become apparent. The prostate is under environmental controls mediated through DNA and histone methylation (Diaw et al, 2007; Esteller, 2008; Li & Dahiya, 2007; Li et al, 2005; Perry et al, 2006).

SAM, in concert with methyl transferases, mediates DNA methylation. Transfers of SAM $CH3-$ groups occur at the carbon 5' position of cytosine within CpG dinucleotide rich islands through complex reactions involving cytosine bases that "poke out" of the double helix Figures 21 and 22. DNA CpG dinucleotide clusters/islands are extensive only at promoter regions of genes Figures 21 and 22 (Esteller, 2007). Unmethylated promoter status allows downstream portions of gene exons to be transcribed to m~RNA. The presence of methylated CpG islands at promoter sites changes regional chromatin geometry by affecting the binding properties of methylation-sensitive DNA-binding proteins. This ultimately leads to interference with gene transcription and down-regulation of gene expression.

DNA from normal tissue is globally methylated/epimethylated while their CpG promoter regions lack such methyl groups. These unmethylated promoter islands turn ON m~RNA transcription of regulatory genes, some of which are tumor suppressor genes. Global methylation of normal cells stabilizes genomes, thwarting global genetic expression of oncogenes. On the other hand, tumors are globally hypomethylated allowing for oncogene expression while at the same time promoter areas of tumors are hypermethylated turning OFF transcription (Ehrlich, 2002) of regulatory and tumor suppressor genes. Promoter or CpG island hypermethylation and global hypomethylation occur during malignant transformation Figures 21 and 22.

Each tumor subtype can be assigned a DNA hypermethylome profile, a CpG island hypermethylation pattern that closely defines a specific cancer. It is estimated that each tumor contains between 100-400 tumor-specific hypermethylated CpG islands (Esteller, 2007). These hypermethylated promoters appear before overt malignancy.

(Ac) **H3 lysine 9 acetylation**

(Me) **H3 lysine 4 methylation**

(Me) **H3 lysine 9 methylation**

HISTONE CODE
Methylation of lys 4 & lys 14 & phosphorylation
of serine 10 on H3 = gene activation while methylation of lys 9 of H3 = gene silencing.

DNA helix
Histone
Nucleosome
with amino
terminal
histone
tails

The Normal Cell

5% of cytosines are as CH3-
cytosine. Regulatory CpG
Island of (promotor) area of
DNA sequence are present in
50% of all human genes.

Histone acetylation by histone acetyl transferase (HAT) and methylation
by SAM and DNMT's and absence of promotor methylation (see left)
allow open chromosomal structure and inflow of transcription factors,
thus initiating active transcription of m-RNA and its products. This Tumor
Suppressor Gene normally suppresses genes that drive tumor growth
when over expressed.

In normal cells CpG
Island promotors are
not methylated.

H3 lysine 9 acetylation

Ac Ac Ac Ac Ac Ac Ac

Gene
Expression

Normal global methylation:80%
of global CpG dinucleotides
are methylated.

m~RNA

DNA

CpG CpG CpG CpG

Me Me Me Me Me Me Me

CpG   CpG

CPG Island
5' upstream untranslated region

H3 lysine 4 methylation

Global CpG dinucleotides
3' downstream region

Transcriptionally active DNA Coding Region
of typical Tumor Suppressor Gene

Euchromatin (open chromatin available for transcription)

70-80% of all CpG sites are normally methylated. Most of these sites are diffusely spread among the genome where CpG
density is low and not arranged in concentrated CpG islands. Low density CpG methylation helps quiet transcription of
non-coding regions of DNA, endogenous retroviruses and transposons that take up 35% of the human genome. One
percent of the human genome consists of CpG islands of densley packed CpG consisting of 500 base pairs with a G-C
content of 55% with a CpG frequency of at least 65%. These motifs span the 5' end of at least 50% of all the genes in the
human DNA helix.

The Tumor Cell

Histone and promotor methylation does not allow
open chromosomal structure thus inhibiting active
transcription of m-RNA for this tumor suppressor gene

Regulatory (promotor)
area of DNA sequence

Methylation of promotor
of Tumor Suppressor
Gene in tumor cells

H3 lysine 9 methylation

Me Me Me Me Me Me

No Gene
Expression

Global hypomethylation
occurs early in
carcinogenesis

none

DNA

CpG CpG CpG CpG

CpG   CpG

5' upstream untranslated region
CpG islands

60% of Tumor Suppressor and mismatch
repair genes are methylated in cancer.
CpG sites act as "Hot Spots" for
germline point mutations by
deamination of 5'mC to T by DNMT
(DNA methyl transferases) . mC is
mutagenic itself yielding C—>T
mutations!

Transcriptional DNA Coding Region of typical
Tumor Suppressor Gene
transcription factors "locked out" by histone/
chromosome compression associated with
histone deacetylation and methylation

Heterochromatin (closed chromatin not available
for transcription)

Chromosomal instability
Increased mutation rates
LOH & rearrangements
Aneuploidy
Loss of imprinting
Activation of transposons
Gene upregulation of
protooncogenes.

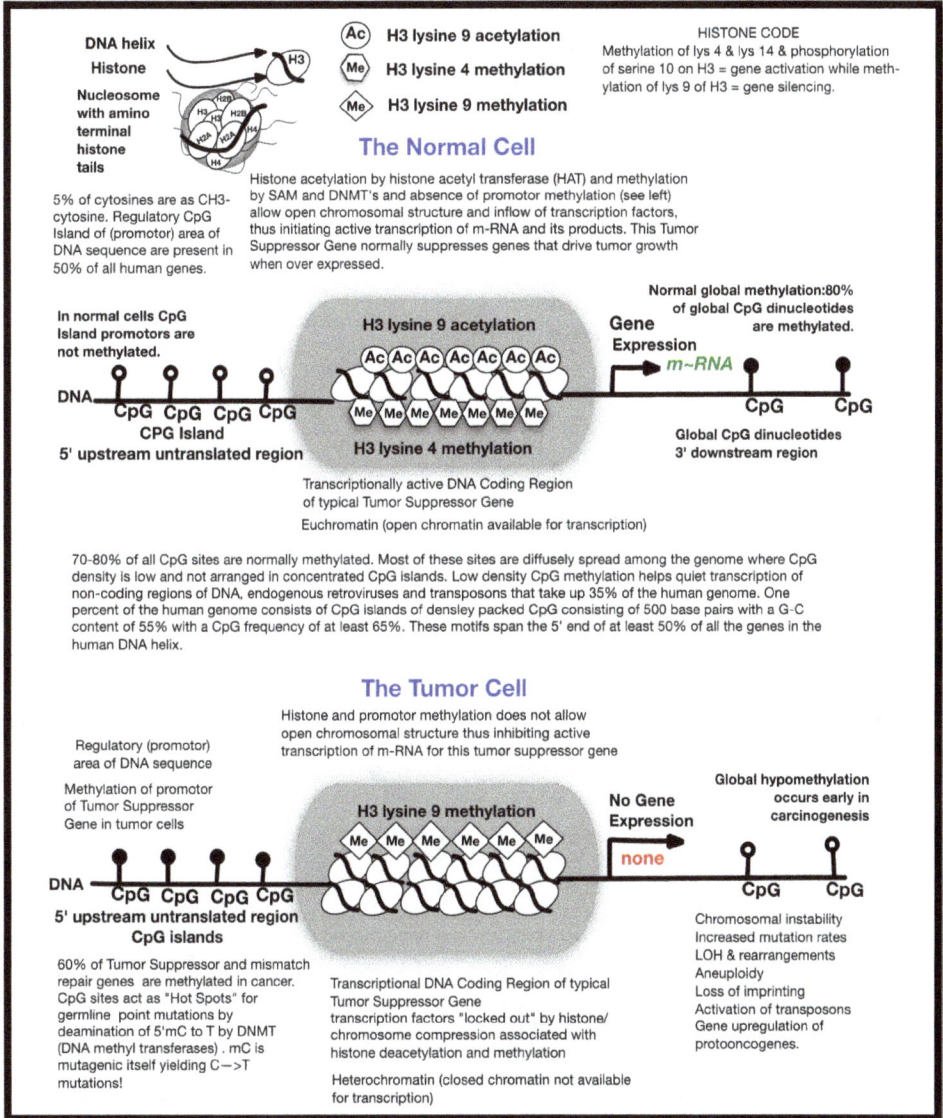

Fig. 21. Epigenetic methylations in normal and tumor cells.

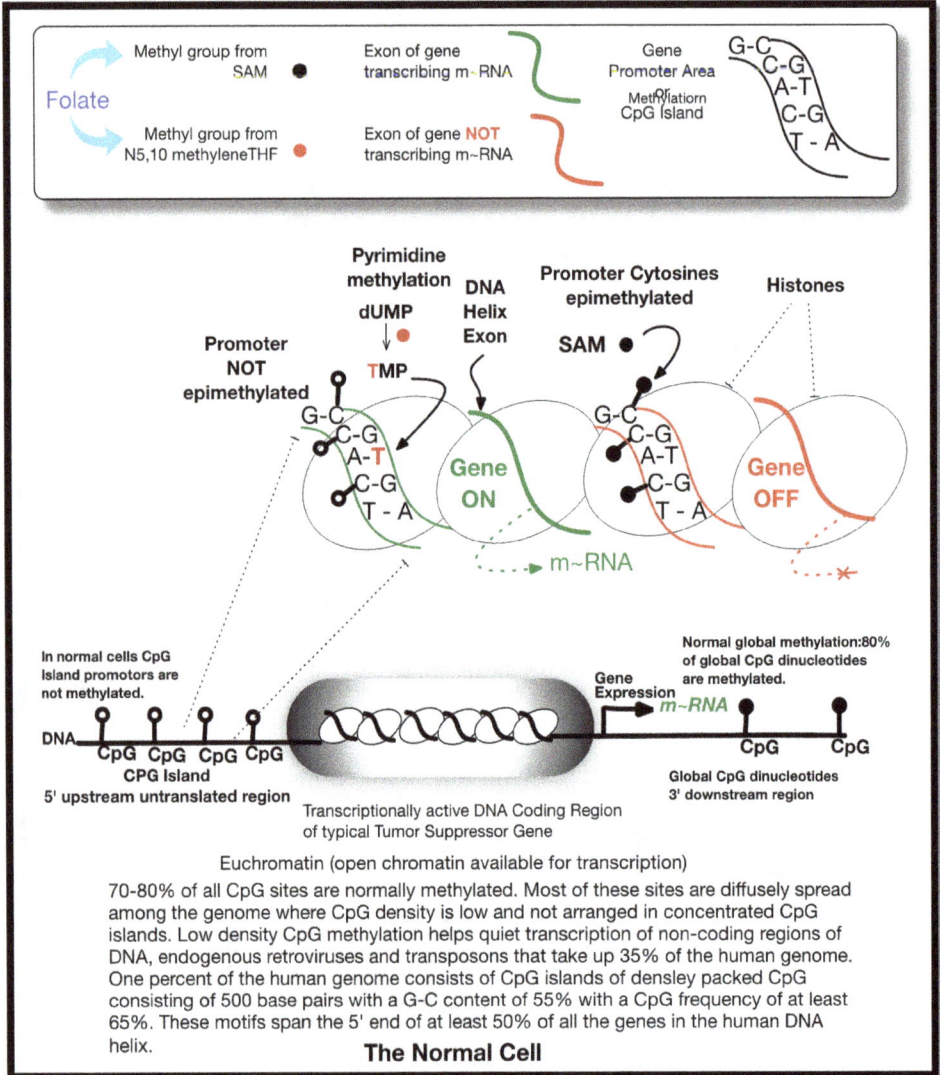

The Normal Cell

70-80% of all CpG sites are normally methylated. Most of these sites are diffusely spread among the genome where CpG density is low and not arranged in concentrated CpG islands. Low density CpG methylation helps quiet transcription of non-coding regions of DNA, endogenous retroviruses and transposons that take up 35% of the human genome. One percent of the human genome consists of CpG islands of densley packed CpG consisting of 500 base pairs with a G-C content of 55% with a CpG frequency of at least 65%. These motifs span the 5' end of at least 50% of all the genes in the human DNA helix.

Fig. 22. Gene promoter ON/OFF control, a closer look.

15. Folate modifies the epigenome

In our opinion the US population suffers from dietary "iatrogenic hyperfolatemia." Study of the effects of both high and low concentrations of FA on the epigenome are important. Linette Pellis (Pellis et al, 2008) exposed colon cancer cells to elevated concentrations of FA, 100 ng/ml, levels routinely achieved by supplement users in the USA and compared growth to cells chronically exposed to 10 ng/ml. Exposure to FA 100 ng/ml induced greater proliferation and apoptosis compared to lower doses. Gene expression analysis of the 100 ng/ml cells revealed lower expression of E-cadherin. Rennie pointed to DNA hypermethylation as an important mechanism in prostate cancer for inactivation of key regulatory genes including E-cadherin (Rennie & Nelson, 1998). Reduction of E-cadherin expression in carcinomas correlates positively to the potential for invasion and metastasis. These changes occur in many tumors including hepatoma, advanced prostate, lobular breast and others (Hirohashi, 1998).

Studies by Wainfan (Wainfan & Poirier, 1992) disclosed that within seven days of initiating a methyl-deficient diet, depletion of S-adenosylmethionine pools resulted in DNA hypomethylation leading to expression of growth regulatory genes. There were decreases in overall levels of DNA methylation yielding patterns that closely resembled those reported to occur in livers of animals exposed to hepatoma-inducing carcinogens. Studies such as these indicate the importance of dietary FA as a regulator of gene expression. The rapidity of folate-induced changes of the epimethylome is alarming.

Man is not necessarily entirely hostage to fortune. As we learned, epigenetic changes dictated by diet can turn genes ON and OFF. The epimethylome is dictated in part by ingestion of nutrients and chemicals including B vitamins, medications, sun exposure (Vitamin D3), exercise induced decreases in insulin levels (Hsing et al, 2001) and methyl groups supplied by the diet such as methionine, choline, betaine, B12, folic acid and other supplements. We are in part a product of our environment, which can be changed (Hayashi et al, 2007; Kim, 2005; Kim, 2007).

16. DNA methylation and prostate cancer

The link between nutrition, epimethylation and cancer is now well established (Choi et al, 2004; Davis & Uthus, 2004, Esteller, 2007; Friso & Choi, 2005; Mason et al, 2008). In addition to gene-specific changes, studies of methylation of colonic mucosa indicate that age-specific, as well as organ site-specific (right or left colon) changes are demonstrable (Wallace et al, 2010). Genomic DNA aberrant methylation of tumor specific genes is almost always abnormal in malignant and transforming cells. These changes progress during carcinogenesis through clinical metastases and are more frequent than chromosomal mutations (Bastian et al, 2004; Diaw et al, 2007; Li & Dahiya, 2007; Perry et al, 2006; Sasaki et al, 2002; Song et al, 2002). Epimethylation's relevance to the genesis of prostate cancer is illustrated by sequential hypermethylation and hypomethylation of genes as prostate tumors dedifferentiate and clinically progress over time (Maruyama et al, 2002). Yegnasubramanian showed that CpG promoter hypermethylation occurs early in prostate tumors, before global genomic hypomethylation. Genomic hypomethylation occurs late in metastasis and varies at different metastatic sites (Yegnasubramanian et al, 2008) and is possibly responsible for heterogeneity of the therapeutic response. As illustrated in Figure 23 the glutathione S-transferase (GSTP1) gene is methylated early in the evolution of prostate cancer. GSTP1 codes for proteins involved in processing carcinogenic metabolites and its dysfunction is understandably associated with malignant transformation.

Methylation of the GSTP1 promoter area is absent in normal prostate tissue and present in 6.4% of proliferative inflammatory atrophy, the precursor lesion of prostate cancer. GSTP1 hypermethylation is observed in 70% of high-grade PIN and in 90% of prostate cancer patients. As prostate tissue progresses from proliferative inflammatory atrophy (PIA) and PIN through hormone refractory metastatic disease a series of hypermethylated genes appear, see Figure 23 (Li & Dahiya, 2007). As tumors develop androgen independence, methylation of androgen and estrogen receptor genes becomes evident (Diaw et al, 2007; Sasaki et al, 2002).

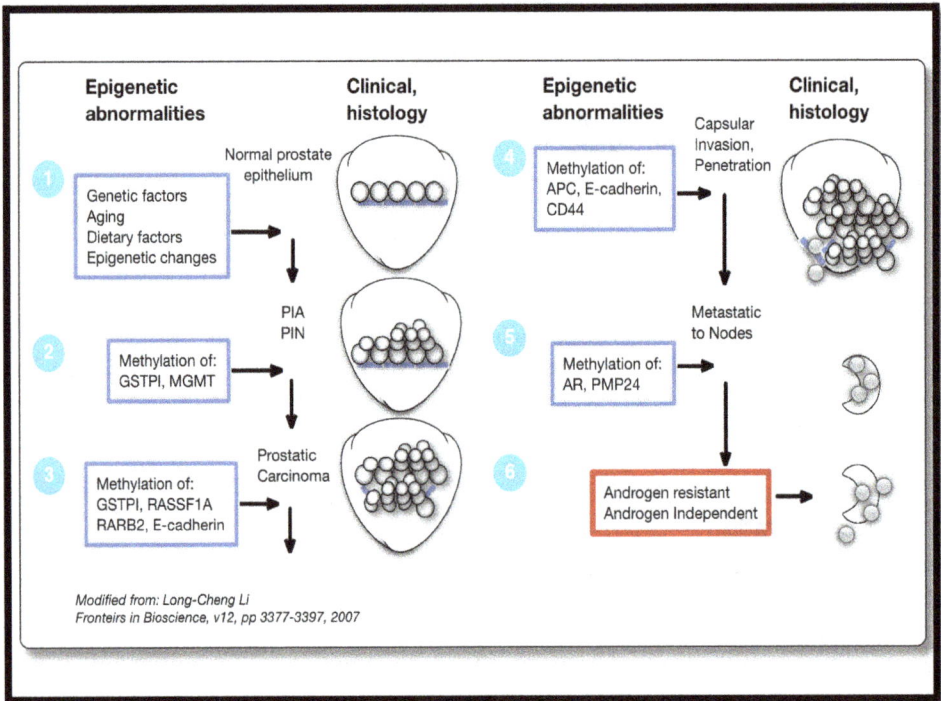

Fig. 23. Transformation of prostate tissue to malignancy involves sequential aberrant methylation of the genome.

17. Demethylating agents: Reversal of aberrant methylation in the clinic

Hypomethylation of oncogenes may activate cMYC , H-RAS (Das & Singal, 2004) and K-RAS (Feinberg & Vogelstein, 1983) contributing to oncogenesis while simultaneous promoter hypermethylation silences growth regulating tumor suppressor genes. Hypomethylation of prostate DNA is associated with BPH and metastatic prostate cancer but remarkably not with localized prostate cancer (Bedford & van Helden, 1987). Keep in mind that either high or low (Duthie, 1999) concentrations of folate and its intermediates may induce simultaneous tissue-specific (Kawakami et al, 2003) and gene-specific aberrant hyper- and hypo-methylation (Duthie, 1999; Kawakami et al, 2003). Who said life would be easy?

As is now readily demonstrable in the clinic, 5-azacitidine (Vidaza™) therapy for patients with myelodysplastic syndromes variably reverses DNA hypermethylation after several weeks to months of therapy restoring phenotypic expression towards normal vis a' vis reversal of severe anemia and life-threatening thrombocytopenia to moderate transfusion-independent anemia and mild thrombocytopenia. Based on our clinical observations, responders may have complete reversal of disease for many years, or more often, clinical symptoms are walked back to a previous, tolerable stage no longer requiring aggressive blood product support.

5-azacitidine is a demethylating agent capable of activating genes repressed by promoter hypermethylation. In preclinical studies, demethylating agents reversed acquired androgen withdrawal-resistance of prostate cancer (Gravina et al,). Each steroid receptor gene active in prostate cancer that physicians have successfully targeted in the clinic (ER, PR, AR) may become inactive by CpG methylation both in prostate cancer tissue and cultured cell lines (Li et al, 2005; Sasaki et al, 2002).

A phase II clinical trial evaluated 5-azacitidine for men with hormone refractory prostate cancer that had progressed while on androgen deprivation therapy (Sonpavde et al, 2009). Patients with PSA doubling times (PSADT) $\leq$ 3 months were treated with 5-azacitidine 75 mg/m2 subcutaneously on days 1-5 of each 28-day cycle up to 12 cycles or until clinical progression or severe toxicity. A PSADT > 3 months was attained in 19 patients or 55.8%. Overall median PSADT was significantly prolonged compared to baseline 2.8 vs. 1.5 months. Fourteen patients had some PSA decline during therapy and 1 patient had a > 30% decline compared with baseline. It appeared the 5-azacitidine favorably modulated PSA kinetics and a correlation was made with decreasing plasma DNA methylation.

Braieth (Braiteh et al, 2008), using 5-azacitidine and valproic acid (Depakote™), a histone deacetylase inhibitor in combination treated a small group of patients with advanced, pretreated malignancies and observed stable disease lasting 4 to 12 months (median, 6 months) in 14 patients (25%), one of two patients with prostate cancer experienced stable disease. We caution that demethylating drugs lack gene specificity and may be associated with unexpected results. In our own clinic we observed decreases in PSA in occasional patients with myelodysplasia treated with 5-azacitidine without obvious prostate cancer, a possible lead that should be followed.

Global DNA hypermethylation associated with epigenetic reprogramming resulting in adriamycin chemotherapy resistance was reversed by the demethylator, hydralazine (Segura-Pacheco et al, 2006). Sensitivity to taxanes, the most active drugs in hormone resistant prostate cancer, was found to be a function of aberrant methylation of the CHFR (checkpoint with forkhead-associated and ring finger) gene in endometrial cancer (Yanokura et al, 2007). Thus, not only tumor transformation but chemotherapy resistance and sensitivity may be influenced by ones DNA epimethylome. Such may in part have been responsible for Patient 2's PSA response while on docetaxel (Taxotere™) after withdrawal of folate and B12. The therapeutic potential of demethylating agents and their pharmacology is reviewed by Szyf (Szyf, 2009) and Fenaux (Fenaux, 2005).

18. Review of epidemiological studies

18.1 Vitamin B12, folic acid, potential toxicity of dietary fortification

As is apparent in Figure 24, it doesn't take much extra FA to change serum levels to values demonstrated to impact DNA methylation (Basten et al, 2006; Jacob, 2000; Mokarram et al, 2008; Pufulete et al, 2005; Rampersaud et al, 2000; Smith et al, 2008; Tisman & Garcia, 2011; Zeisel, 2009). As previously noted, post 1998 serum levels have increased 4-6-fold in select populations. In the US, a daily bowl of FA-fortified cereal (400 µg FA) plus a routine multivitamin (400-800 µg FA) plus an afternoon "pick-me-upper" 5-Hour Energy™ drink (400µg FA+500µg B12+40mg B6), available at almost every gas station, liquor and convenience store across the US, plus a probiotic supplement supplying lactic acid bacteria-generated folates LeBlanc et al, 2007 could add up to an additional 40-200ng/ml increment to the usual basal serum level, which on average in the US is ~12 ng/ml. So, serum levels in our patient population are often greater than 30 ng/ml, median 24 ng/ml Figure 1. When reviewing epidemiological studies of folate and other vitamers often there are dose-response effects that may produce contrasting results, Figure 26.

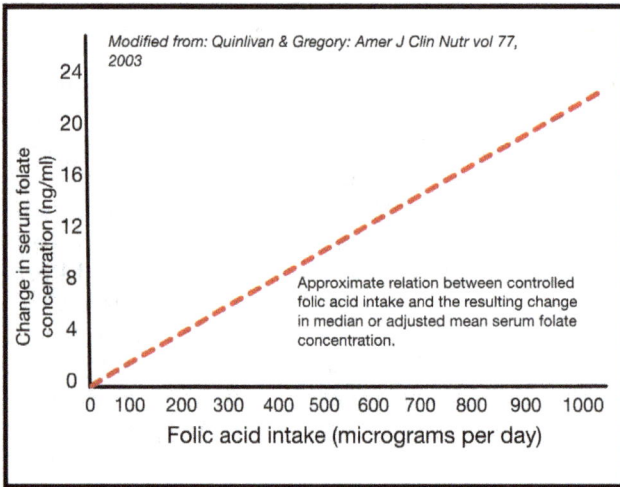

Fig. 24. Change in serum/plasma folate as a function of ingested folic acid.

There are epidemiological studies investigating prostate cancer risk based on dietary ingestion and serum folate. Most find no consistent relation (Hultdin et al, 2005; Johansson et al, 2008; Stevens et al, 2006, Weinstein et al, 2003) to prostate cancer. In one case control study by Pelucchi et al. of Italy (Pelucchi et al, 2005), folate ingestion was found to be protective against prostate cancer. The OR of prostate cancer was 0.66 for the highest versus the lowest quintile of folate intake.

A large study by Lawson (Lawson et al, 2007) of multivitamin and supplement use and risk of prostate cancer in the National Institutes of Health-AARP Diet and Health Study revealed absence of an association between multivitamin use and risk of localized prostate cancer. However, there was a statistically significant increased risk for advanced and fatal prostate cancers (RR = 1.32, and RR = 1.98, respectively) among men reporting excessive use of multivitamins (more than seven times per week) when compared with never users. The incidence rates per 100,000 person-years for advanced and fatal prostate cancers for those who took a multivitamin more than seven times per week were 143.8 and 18.9, respectively, compared with 113.4 and 11.4 in never users. Also noted was a significant increase in risk of localized prostate cancer among heavy multivitamin users who consumed a folate supplement. Use of folate, as an individual supplement independent of a multivitamin, lacked an association with prostate cancer.

An important clinical study by Figueiredo (Figueiredo et al, 2009) reviewed prostate cancer occurrence in the Aspirin/Folate Polyp Prevention Study. This was a placebo-controlled randomized trial of aspirin and folic acid supplementation for the prevention of colorectal adenomas conducted between July 1994 and December 2006. The US government mandated folic acid fortification of the food supply by the end of 1998. Participants were followed for up to 10.8 (median = 7.0) years. Aspirin alone had no effect on prostate cancer incidence, but there were unexpected and marked differences according to FA treatment. Among the 643 men who were randomly assigned to placebo or daily supplementation with 1000 µg folic acid, the estimated probability of being diagnosed with prostate cancer over a 10-year period was 9.7% in the FA group and 3.3% for the placebo group. The age-adjusted hazard ratio = 2.63 and was found statistically significant with p=0.01.

A troublesome observation by Troen (Troen et al, 2006) among women with a diet low in folate (< 233 µ/d) found that those who used folic acid-containing supplements had significantly greater natural killer (NK) cytotoxicity (p = 0.01) while those who consumed a folate-rich diet and used folic acid supplements > 400 µg/d had reduced NK cytotoxicity, p = 0.02. Ingestion of > 400µg FA is associated with measurable serum FA in addition to usual CH3−THF. Troen detected unmetabolized FA in 78% of plasma samples from fasting participants (Troen et al, 2006). There was an inverse relation between the presence of unmetabolized FA in plasma and NK cytotoxicity remembering that NK lymphocytes are important innate immune cells that target cancer cells and those infected with virus. NK cytotoxicity was 23% lower among women with detectable serum levels of FA (P = 0.04). Older women greater than 60 years were more susceptible to NK cell suppression. Complicating the picture, Young-In Kim found decreased NK-mediated cytotoxicity in rats made folate deficient (Kim et al, 2002).

Absorbed and circulating unmetabolized FA is potentially toxic (Lucock & Yates, 2005; Smith et al, 2008; Sweeney et al, 2009). Lucock studied three patients ingesting high doses of FA (5 mg/d) to lower serum homocysteine. Under these circumstances, serum folate levels may exceed 100-200 ng/ml and FA is frequently 50% of total serum folate. HPLC analysis of red cell folate coenzymes revealed an aberrant distribution from the usual. There was accumulation of methylene-, methenyl-, formyl- and unsubstituted THF at the expense of the MTHFR-downstream folate-coenzyme, CH3−THF. He conjectured that *de novo* DNA-thymine synthesis would be preferred through high intracellular FA direct inhibition of MTHFR (Lucock & Yates, 2005) Figures 9 and 25. This would limit the production of SAM and possibly DNA methylation and relative to prostate metabolism, polyamine synthesis. Importantly, he points out that administration of the recommended daily dose of ~400 µg/d, the neural tube preventing dose (Daly et al, 1997), is not associated with significant blood levels of the oxidized provitamin, FA; however, as more FA is ingested, much is circulated as potentially dangerous FA. John Scott's group has studied this pharmacology (Sweeney et al, 2009) and reported no detectable serum FA after doses of 100 or 200 µg FA were ingested for 14 weeks, however, FA was measurable at the highest level (400 µg) tested (Sweeney et al, 2007). The review by Smith discusses potential metabolic interference (Kao et al, 2008) and toxicity (Smith et al, 2008) of the provitamin FA some of which is noted in Figure 25.

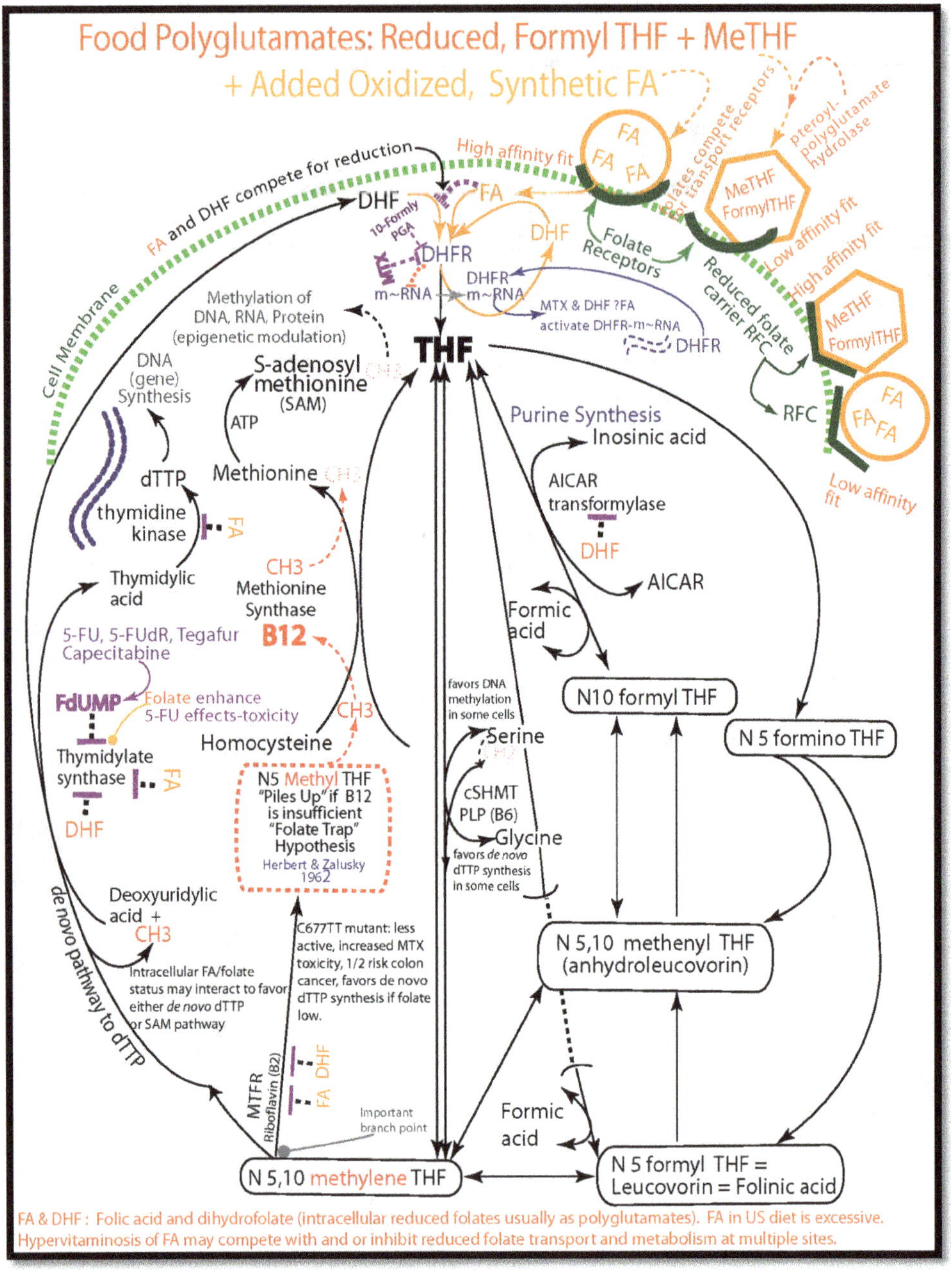

Fig. 25. Folate and one-carbon metabolism.

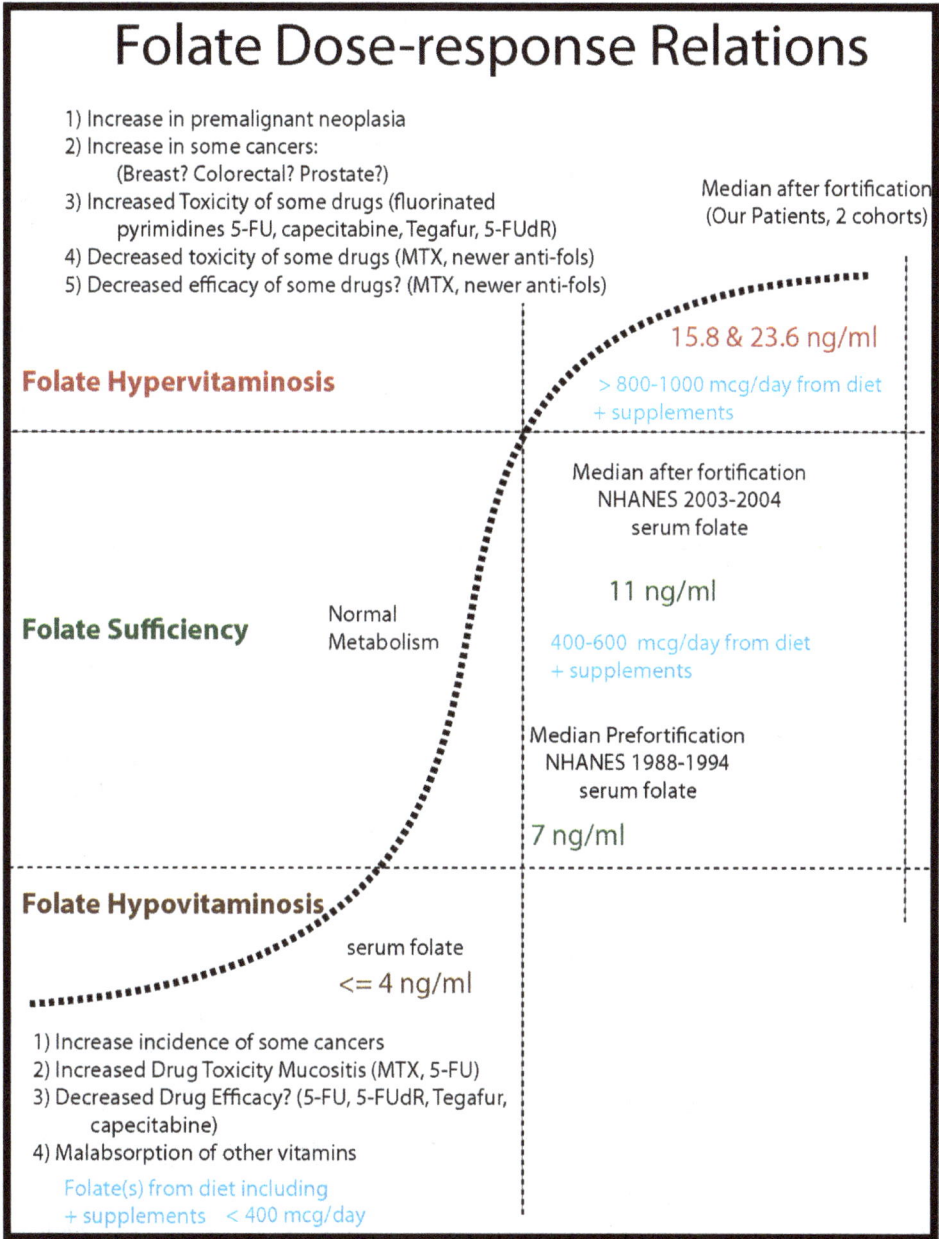

Fig. 26. Dose-response curve for folate effects. Folate dose, stage (prenatal/postnatal) and duration of exposure are critical factors in determining tissue-specific outcome

Collin (Collin et al, 2010) measured plasma concentrations of folate, B12 (cobalamin), holohaptocorrin, holotranscobalamin ("active B12") total transcobalamin, and total homocysteine in 1,461 cases and 1,507 controls. They investigated whether both B12 and folate metabolism were associated with prostate specific antigen (PSAV) as a proxy measure of prostate cancer progression in men with localized prostate cancer. Furthermore, thirteen folate pathway single nucleotide polymorphisms were genotyped for 311 participants. Post diagnosis PSAV was calculated. Median follow-up time was 2.5 years. Plasma folate was associated with an increased risk of PSAV > 2 ng/mL/yr, OR per unit increase in $\log_e$ concentration, OR = 1.57. This study provides some evidence that higher folate levels may be associated with faster prostate tumor progression. The MTRR 66A>G polymorphism was related to slower progression of localized prostate cancer. Note that the MTRR 66A>G polymorphism for methionine synthase reductase (MSR) catalyzes reductive methylation of the co-factor of [MS, B12, SAM], thus activating MS activity Figures 9 and 25. This polymorphism was associated with a reduced risk (OR, 0.33) for PSAV > 2 ng/ml/yr. The serinehydroxymethyltransferase (SHMT1) polymorphism (SHMT1 1420C>T) was associated with increased risk (per-allele OR, 1.49) for PSAV > 2 ng/ml/yr. Their work suggests that in addition to plasma levels of folate, folate-metabolizing enzyme polymorphisms are associated with the rate at which prostate tumors secrete PSA (PSAV), which relates to the rate of increase of prostate tumor volume (Berger et al, 2006). Elevated PSAV >2.0 ng/ml/yr as indicated by D'Amico increases the risk of death due to prostate cancer following radiation therapy despite having low-risk disease, Figure 2 (D'Amico et al, 2005). So it is conceivable that the combination of high plasma folate with or without associated folate enzyme polymorphisms may affect cure rates for some patients with prostate cancer.

Observations in our clinic of B12 alone and B12 plus folic acid stimulation of prostate cancer in two patients, and those of Tomaszewski's group (Tomaszewski et al, 2011) revealing direct correlation of Gleason's grade and Ki67 cellular proliferation index with both high serum and prostate tumor tissue folate, are compelling because they directly identify specific patients seen in the clinic that are adversely affected by what have largely been theoretical concepts developed from laboratory animal and large population studies.

19. Epidermal growth factor receptor (EGFR) and FA

Two colon cancer cell lines, Caco-2 and HCT-116, were maintained in medium containing 1µg/ml folic acid and supplemental folic acid was found to inhibit cell proliferation in a dose-dependent manner (Jaszewski et al, 1999). Pretreatment of the cell lines with supplemental FA (1.25 µg/ml) completely abrogated transforming growth factor-a (TGF-a)-induced proliferation in both. Tyrosine kinase activity and the relative concentration of EGFR were markedly diminished in both following a 24-h exposure to supplemental FA. FA-mediated reduced proliferation and EGFR tyrosine kinase pathway appeared to be involved.

To further establish the mechanism(s) by which FA affects EGFR, Nagothu (Nagothu et al, 2004) examined whether and to what extent supplemental FA or its metabolites modulate basal and serum-induced activation of the EGFR promoter in the HCT-116 colon cancer cell line. HCT-116 cells were pre-incubated with or without FA 10 µg/ml for 48 hours. Supplemental FA as well as its metabolites markedly inhibited EGFR promoter activity and its methylation status. Exposure of cells to 10% fetal bovine serum caused a marked stimulation of EGFR promoter activity and EGFR expression, both of which were greatly abrogated by supplemental FA or CH3 − THF. Their work suggests that FA and CH3 − THF inhibit EGFR promoter activity in colon cancer cells by enhancing promoter methylation. This could partly be responsible for FA-mediated inhibition of growth-related processes not only in colorectal but other neoplasia as well.

20. Effect of combined B vitamin insufficiency on the canonical Wnt kinase pathway

Inspection of Figures 8, 9 and 25 illustrates at least four different pathways where one-carbon vitamers of folate coenzymes depend on other B vitamins. Changes in the Wnt family of genes are prominent in prostate cancer (Yardy & Brewster, 2005; Zhu et al, 2004). In many tissues, activation of Wnt signaling is associated with neoplasia (Liu et al, 2007). Wnt-signaling was attenuated by combined B vitamin deficiency but not by singlet folate or doublet deficiencies. Increased levels of Wnt-11 found in prostate tumors contribute to tumor progression by promoting neuroendocrine dedifferentiation, tumor cell survival and cell migration/invasion (Uysal-Onganer et al, 2010). There is a positive correlation between Wnt-11 expression and PSA levels above 10 ng/ml. Beta-catenin protein, a critical molecular component of canonical Wnt signaling is capable of promoting androgen signaling through its ability to bind to the AR in a ligand-dependent (reminiscent of androgen) fashion thus allowing the beta catenin-AR complex to activate transcription of androgen-regulated genes. Based on Liu's study of colon cancer cells, one might expect that multiple deficiencies of B vitamins could modulate Wnt control of beta catenin in prostate cells. For excellent reviews of the importance of the Wnt gene and its effects in prostate metabolism, we refer Bisson and Prowse (Bisson & Prowse, 2009).

Various combinations of B vitamins and their metabolites are frequently elevated and/or low in untreated cancer patients as illustrated in Figure 11.

21. Conclusion

This review of B vitamin effects on one-carbon metabolism and neoplasia with focus on the prostate comes at a time when several countries are contemplating fortification of their nations' food supply with B12 and folic acid due to the known benefit in reducing neural tube defects in newborns. At the same time, "supplement mania" is rampant in the US and especially prominent in the prostate cancer patient population. FA-associated cancer acceleration as first reported by Lewisohn (Lewisohn et al, 1946) for mouse mammary cancer, Heinle (Heinle & Welch, 1948) for CGL, Tisman Tisman et al, 2009, Figueiredo (Figueiredo et al, 2009), Collin Collin et al, 2010 and Tomaszewski (Tomaszewski et al, 2011) for prostate cancer, is of utmost importance to those with potential or manifest occult prostate disease. Based on this review and our clinical experience we suggest a more targeted approach to vitamin supplementation, so that the benefit for one demographic does not come at the expense of another. Until more is learned, it may be best to adjust frequently abnormal serum levels of B vitamins into the normal range. It is clear that both vitamin deficiency and hypersufficiency have profound physiological effects that differentially affect select tissues. In the laboratory, the effects can be measured within days to weeks and have potential to cause life-threatening results that could have immediate effects on drug efficacy and toxicity or latent effects which may take years to manifest.

Intracellular one-carbon transfer reactions are essential for nucleotide (thymidylate from dUMP) and purine synthesis and diffuse methylation reactions that deliver methyl (CH3−) groups to DNA, RNA, proteins, and phospholipids. The one-carbon transfer reactions use intracellular polyglutamated reduced derivatives of FA. CH3-THF is the predominant form of folate in serum/plasma. The reduced folate carrier (RFC) delivers most CH3−THF into cells. RFC has a higher affinity for reduced folate and the chemotherapy folate inhibitor methotrexate than oxidized, pharmaceutical FA, and it accounts for the transport of most dietary, naturally occurring, reduced folate(s) (Brzezinska et al, 2000). Membrane-bound folate receptors, including folate receptor (FR) with very high affinity for pharmaceutical FA, are expressed in epithelial tissues and its expression is elevated in some malignant tumors. The predominant cytoplasmic folate, CH3−THF, donates its one-carbon moiety to methylate homocysteine to methionine, regenerating usable THF. THF is the much-preferred substrate to folypolygammaglutamyl synthetase (FPGS) that extends the glutamate chain enhancing intracellular retention and folate substrate binding strength to folate metabolizing enzymes. Methionine, from methylation of homocysteine and dietary ingestion, is converted to S-adenosylmethionine (SAM), a universal donor of CH3− groups to numerous methylation reactions through methyl transferase enzymes. SAM supplies CH3 − groups to cytosine bases positioned across from guanine as CpG islands of DNA and histones surrounding the DNA double helix. The methylation patterns are both heritable and subject to acute (drug) and chronic dietary effects restricting or enhancing methyl group precursors responsible for epigenetic control of both tumor suppressor and tumor promoter genes. The active coenzyme THF acquires a one-carbon moiety from the amino acid serine via serine hydroxy methyl transferase, a vitamin B6 requiring coenzyme. There are at least two forms of SHMT enzyme, one active in mitochondria, (mSHMT or SHMT2) and one active in cytoplasm (cSHMT or SHMT1). This metabolic catalysis of glycine with THF yields 5,10-methyleneTHF, a critical compound at the center of a switching point of CH3− delivery. The cSHMT form shuttles CH3−methylation reactions in the direction of the *de novo* synthesis of thymine from deoxyuridine. cSHMT activity is enhanced by the heavy chain of ferritin, a compound critical in iron metabolism. Many reactions depend on genetic coenzyme polymorphisms such as MTHFR C677TT weakening the enzyme's usual function by up to 70%. Regional B vitamin concentrations (B9, B12, B6, B2) affect delivery of CH3− from 5,10-methyleneTHF to either dUMP to form DNA thymine/thymidine (required in rapidly growing cells) or to methylation of homocysteine via B12-requiring transfer of CH3− from CH3−THF thus generating more SAM. Concentrations of SAM and DNA epimethylation enzymes control gene promoter and global gene epimethylation. This turns ON and OFF various tumor suppressor (TSG) and tumor associated (TAG) genes.

The robustness of the homocysteine methylation/SAM generation depends on the concentration and functional state of the methionine synthase-B12-enzyme complex. B12 deficiency from adsorptive, dietary, drug interference, N2O anesthesia inactivation (still common during routine surgeries) and anomalies of holotranscobalamin will eventually shut down global methylation through impaired synthesis of SAM and the ternary complex formed between thymidylate synthase, 5,10-methyleneTHF and dUMP which supplies TMP for DNA synthesis. This leads to uracil misincorporation into DNA resulting in DNA point mutations and finally to chromosomal breaks, and malignant transformation.

22. Acknowledgements

The author acknowledges the extensive assistance in development and organization of this
manuscript by MS Melanie Tisman, B.S.

23. References

Achón M, Alonso-Aperte E, Reyes L, Ubeda N, & Varela-Moreiras G. (2000). High-Dose folic
acid supplementation in rats: Effects on gestation and the methionine cycle. *Br J
Nutr*, 83, pp. 177-83

Alemdaroglu (2007) Impact of Folate Absorption and Transport for Nutrition and Drug
Targeting.

Allegra CJ, Drake JC, Jolivet J, & Chabner BA. (1985). Inhibition of phosphoribosylaminoimidazolecarboxamide transformylase by methotrexate and dihydrofolic acid
polyglutamates. *Proc Natl Acad Sci U S A*, 82, pp. 4881-5

Ames BN. (2006). Low micronutrient intake may accelerate the degenerative diseases of
aging through allocation of scarce micronutrients by triage. *Proc Natl Acad Sci U S
A*, 103, pp. 17589-94

Angier RB, Boothe JH, Hutchings BL, Mowat JH, Semb J, Stokstad EL, SubbaRow Y, Waller
CW, Cosulich DB, & Fahrenbach MJ. (1946). The structure and synthesis of the liver
L. Casei factor. *Science (New York, NY)*, 103, 667

Antony AC. (1992). The biological chemistry of folate receptors. *Blood*, 79, pp. 2807-2820

Bailey SW, & Ayling JE. (2009). The extremely slow and variable activity of dihydrofolate
reductase in human liver and its implications for high folic acid intake. *Proc Natl
Acad Sci U S A*, 106, pp. 15424-9

Bailey RL, Dodd KW, Gahche JJ, Dwyer JT, McDowell MA, Yetley EA, Sempos CA, Burt VL,
Radimer KL, & Picciano MF. (2010). Total folate and folic acid intake from foods and
dietary supplements in the united states: 2003-2006. *Am J Clin Nutr*, 91, pp. 231-7

Bander NH, Milowsky MI, Nanus DM, Kostakoglu L, Vallabhajosula S, & Goldsmith SJ.
(2005). Phase I trial of 177lutetium-labeled J591, a monoclonal antibody to prostate-
specific membrane antigen, in patients with androgen-independent prostate cancer.
J Clin Oncol, 23, pp. 4591-601

Basten GP, Duthie SJ, Pirie L, Vaughan N, Hill MH, & Powers HJ. (2006). Sensitivity of
markers of DNA stability and DNA repair activity to folate supplementation in
healthy volunteers. *Br J Cancer*, 94, pp. 1942-7

Basten GP, Hill MH, Duthie SJ, & Powers HJ. (2004). Effect of folic acid supplementation on
the folate status of buccal mucosa and lymphocytes. *Cancer Epidemiol Biomarkers
Prev*, 13, pp. 1244-9

Bastian PJ, Yegnasubramanian S, Palapattu GS, Rogers CG, Lin X, De Marzo AM, & Nelson
WG. (2004). Molecular biomarker in prostate cancer: The role of cpg island
hypermethylation. *Eur Urol*, 46, pp. 698-708

Bates CJ, & Fuller NJ. (1986). The effect of riboflavin deficiency on methylenetetrahydrofolate reductase (NADPH) (EC 1.5.1.20) and folate metabolism in the rat. *Br J
Nutr*, 55, pp. 455-64

Bedford MT, & van Helden PD. (1987). Hypomethylation of DNA in pathological conditions
of the human prostate. *Cancer Res*, 47, pp. 5274-6

Berger AP, Deibl M, Strasak A, Bektic J, Pelzer A, Steiner H, Spranger R, Fritsche G, Bartsch
G, & Horninger W. (2006). Relapse after radical prostatectomy correlates with

preoperative PSA velocity and tumor volume: Results from a screening population. *Urology*, 68, pp. 1067-71

Bertino JR, Perkins JP, & Johns DG. (1965). Purification and properties of dihydrofolatereductase from ehrlich ascites carcinoma cells. *Biochemistry*, 4, pp. 839-46

Bertrand R, MacKenzie RE, & Jolivet J. (1987). Human liver methenyltetrahydrofolate synthetase: Improved purification and increased affinity for folate polyglutamate substrates. *Biochim Biophys Acta*, 911, pp. 154-61

Bisson I, & Prowse DM. (2009). WNT signaling regulates self-renewal and differentiation of prostate cancer cells with stem cell characteristics. *Cell Res*, 19, pp. 683-97

Bistulfi G, Diegelman P, Foster BA, Kramer DL, Porter CW, & Smiraglia DJ. (2009). Polyamine biosynthesis impacts cellular folate requirements necessary to maintain s-adenosylmethionine and nucleotide pools. *FASEB J*, 23, pp. 2888-97

Bjelakovic G, Kocic G, Pavlovic D, Nikolic J, Stojanovic I, Bjelakovic BG, Jevtovic T, & Sokolovic D. (2003). Effects of folic acid on polyamine concentrations and polyamine oxidase activity in regenerating rat liver. *Pteridines*, 14, pp. 109-113

Bjelakovic G, Pavlovic D, Jevtovic T, Stojanovic I, Sokolovic D, Bjelakovic GB, Nikolic J, & Ba\vsic J. (2006). VITAMIN B 12 AND FOLIC ACID EFFECTS ON POLYAMINE METABOLISM IN RAT LIVER. *Pteridines*, 17, pp. 90-94

Blount BC, Mack MM, Wehr CM, MacGregor JT, Hiatt RA, Wang G, Wickramasinghe SN, Everson RB, & Ames BN. (1997). Folate deficiency causes uracil misincorporation into human DNA and chromosome breakage: Implications for cancer and neuronal damage. *Proc Natl Acad Sci U S A*, 94, pp. 3290-5

Bovina C, Tolomelli B, Rovinetti C, & Marchetti M. (1972). Acute effects of testosterone propionate on folate coenzyme synthesis in the rat. *J Endocrinol*, 54, pp. 457-64

Braiteh F, Soriano AO, Garcia-Manero G, Hong D, Johnson MM, Silva Lde P, Yang H, Alexander S, Wolff J, & Kurzrock R. (2008). Phase I study of epigenetic modulation with 5-azacytidine and valproic acid in patients with advanced cancers. *Clin Cancer Res*, 14, pp. 6296-301

Brzezinska A, Winska P, & Balinska M. (2000). Cellular aspects of folate and antifolate membrane transport. *Acta Biochimica Polonica*, 47, pp. 735-749

Butterworth CE, & Santini R. (1963). The pteroylglutamate components of american diets as determined by chromatographic separation. *Journal of Clinical Investigation*, 42,

De Cabo SF, Santos J, & Fernández-Piqueras J. (1995). Molecular and cytological evidence of s-adenosyl-l-homocysteine as an innocuous undermethylating agent in vivo. *Cytogenet Cell Genet*, 71, pp. 187-92

Cai D, Ning L, Pan C, Liu X, Bu R, Chen X, Wang K, Cheng Y, & Wu B. (2010). Association of polymorphisms in folate metabolic genes and prostate cancer risk: A case-control study in a chinese population. *J Genet*, 89, pp. 263-7

Chanarin (1969) *The Megaloblastic Anemias*, Blackwell Scientific Publications.

Chang SS, O'Keefe DS, Bacich DJ, Reuter VE, Heston WD, & Gaudin PB. (1999). Prostate-Specific membrane antigen is produced in tumor-associated neovasculature. *Clin Cancer Res*, 5, pp. 2674-81

Chango A, Abdel Nour AM, Niquet C, & Tessier FJ. (2009). Simultaneous determination of genomic DNA methylation and uracil misincorporation. *Med Princ Pract*, 18, pp. 81-4

Chen J, Gammon MD, Chan W, Palomeque C, Wetmur JG, Kabat GC, Teitelbaum SL, Britton JA, Terry MB, Neugut AI, & Santella RM. (2005). One-Carbon metabolism, MTHFR polymorphisms, and risk of breast cancer. *Cancer Res,* 65, pp. 1606-14

Chen, J (J), Xu, X (X), et al. (2010)" Folate and Vascular Disease: Epidemiological Perrspective" in Folate in Health and Disease: Edited by Lynn B. Bailey. Boca Raton, FL, CRC Press & Taylor and Francis Group, 263-323.

Choi SW, & Friso S. (2010). Epigenetics: A new bridge between nutrition and health. *Advances in Nutrition: An International Review Journal,* 1, 8

Choi SW, Friso S, Ghandour H, Bagley PJ, Selhub J, & Mason JB. (2004). Vitamin B-12 deficiency induces anomalies of base substitution and methylation in the DNA of rat colonic epithelium. *J Nutr,* 134, pp. 750-5

Collin SM, Metcalfe C, Refsum H, Lewis SJ, Davey Smith G, Cox A, Davis M, Marsden G, Johnston C, Lane JA, Donovan JL, Neal DE, Hamdy FC, Smith AD, & Martin RM. (2010). Associations of folate, vitamin B12, homocysteine, and folate-pathway polymorphisms with prostate-specific antigen velocity in men with localized prostate cancer. *Cancer Epidemiol Biomarkers Prev,* 19, pp. 2833-8

Collin SM, Metcalfe C, Refsum H, Lewis SJ, Zuccolo L, Smith GD, Chen L, Harris R, Davis M, Marsden G, Johnston C, Lane JA, Ebbing M, Bønaa KH, Nygård O, Ueland PM, Grau MV, Baron JA, Donovan JL, Neal DE, Martin RM. (2010). Circulating folate, vitamin B12, homocysteine, vitamin B12 transport proteins, and risk of prostate cancer: A case-control study, systematic review, and meta-analysis. *Cancer Epidemiol Biomarkers Prev,* 19, pp. 1632-42

Cook JD, Cichowicz DJ, George S, Lawler A, & Shane B. (1987). Mammalian folylpoly-gamma-glutamate synthetase. 4. In vitro and in vivo metabolism of folates and analogues and regulation of folate homeostasis. *Biochemistry,* 26, pp. 530-9

Cooper CS, & Foster CS. (2009). Concepts of epigenetics in prostate cancer development. *Br J Cancer,* 100, pp. 240-5

Corcino JJ, Zalusky R, Greenberg M, & Herbert V. (1971). Coexistence of pernicious anaemia and chronic myeloid leukaemia: An experiment of nature involving vitamin B12 metabolism. *Br J Haematol,* 20, pp. 511-20

Daly S, Mills JL, Molloy AM, Conley M, Lee YJ, Kirke PN, Weir DG, & Scott JM. (1997). Minimum effective dose of folic acid for food fortification to prevent neural-tube defects. *Lancet,* 350, pp. 1666-9

D'Amico AV, Renshaw AA, Sussman B, & Chen MH. (2005). Pretreatment PSA velocity and risk of death from prostate cancer following external beam radiation therapy. *JAMA,* 294, pp. 440-7

Das KC, Das M, Mohanty D, Jadaon MM, Gupta A, Marouf R, & Easow SK. (2005). Megaloblastosis: From morphos to molecules. *Med Princ Pract,* 14 Suppl 1, pp. 2-14

Das KC, Manusselis C, & Herbert V. (1980). Simplifying lymphocyte culture and the deoxyuridine suppression test by using whole blood (0.1 ml) instead of separated lymphocytes. *Clin Chem,* 26, pp. 72-7

Das PM, & Singal R. (2004). DNA methylation and cancer. *J Clin Oncol,* 22, pp. 4632-42

Davis CD, & Uthus EO. (2004). DNA methylation, cancer susceptibility, and nutrient interactions. *Exp Biol Med (Maywood),* 229, pp. 988-95

Diaw L, Woodson K, & Gillespie JW. (2007). Prostate cancer epigenetics: A review on gene regulation. *Gene Regulation and Systems Biology,* 1, pp. 313-325

Dietrich M, Brown CJ, & Block G. (2005). The effect of folate fortification of cereal-grain products on blood folate status, dietary folate intake, and dietary folate sources among adult non-supplement users in the united states. *J Am Coll Nutr*, 24, pp. 266-74

Dobosy JR, Roberts JL, Fu VX, & Jarrard DF. (2007). The expanding role of epigenetics in the development, diagnosis and treatment of prostate cancer and benign prostatic hyperplasia. *J Urol*, 177, pp. 822-31

Dormandy KM, Waters AH, & Mollin DL. (1963). Folic-Acid deficiency in coeliac disease. *The Lancet*, 281, pp. 632-635

D'Urso-Scott M, Uhoch J, & Bertino JR. (1974). Formation of 10-formylfolic acid, a potent inhibitor of dihydrofolate reductase, in rat liver slices incubated with folic acid. *Proc Natl Acad Sci U S A*, 71, pp. 2736-9

Duthie SJ. (1999). Folic acid deficiency and cancer: Mechanisms of DNA instability. *British medical bulletin*, 55, 578

Duthie SJ. (2010). Folate and cancer: How DNA damage, repair and methylation impact on colon carcinogenesis. *J Inherit Metab Dis*,

Duthie SJ, Narayanan S, Brand GM, Pirie L, & Grant G. (2002). Impact of folate deficiency on DNA stability. *J Nutr*, 132, pp. 2444S-2449S

Ehrlich M. (2002). DNA methylation in cancer: Too much, but also too little. *Oncogene*, 21, pp. 5400-13

Ericson UC, Ivarsson MI, Sonestedt E, Gullberg B, Carlson J, Olsson H, & Wirfält E. (2009). Increased breast cancer risk at high plasma folate concentrations among women with the MTHFR 677T allele. *Am J Clin Nutr*, 90, pp. 1380-9

Ernst T, Hergenhahn M, Kenzelmann M, Cohen CD, Bonrouhi M, Weninger A, Klären R, Gröne EF, Wiesel M, Güdemann C, Küster J, Schott W, Staehler G, Kretzler M, Hollstein M, & Gröne HJ. (2002). Decrease and gain of gene expression are equally discriminatory markers for prostate carcinoma: A gene expression analysis on total and microdissected prostate tissue. *Am J Pathol*, 160, pp. 2169-80

Esteller M. (2003). Relevance of DNA methylation in the management of cancer. *The lancet oncology*, 4, pp. 351-358

Esteller M. (2007). Cancer epigenomics: DNA methylomes and histone-modification maps. *Nat Rev Genet*, 8, pp. 286-98

Esteller M. (2008). Molecular origins of cancer: Epigenetics in cancer. *New England Journal of Medicine*, 358, 1148

Esteller M, Gaidano G, Goodman SN, Zagonel V, Capello D, Botto B, Rossi D, Gloghini A, Vitolo U, Carbone A, & others. (2002). Hypermethylation of the DNA repair gene o6-methylguanine DNA methyltransferase and survival of patients with diffuse large b-cell lymphoma. *JNCI Journal of the National Cancer Institute*, 94, 26

Farber S, Cutler EC, Hawkins JW, Harrison JH, Peirce EC, & Lenz GG. (1947). The action of pteroylglutamic conjugates on man. *Science*, 106, pp. 619-21

Farber S, Diamond LK, Mercer RD, Sylvester Jr RF, & Wolff JA. (1948). Temporary remissions in acute leukemia in children produced by folic acid antagonist, 4-aminopteroyl-glutamic acid (aminopterin). *New England Journal of Medicine*, 238, pp. 787-793

Feinberg AP, & Vogelstein B. (1983). Hypomethylation of ras oncogenes in primary human cancers. *Biochem Biophys Res Commun*, 111, pp. 47-54

Fenaux P. (2005). Inhibitors of DNA methylation: Beyond myelodysplastic syndromes. *Nat Clin Pract Oncol*, 2 Suppl 1, pp. S36-44

Figueiredo JC, Grau MV, Haile RW, Sandler RS, Summers RW, Bresalier RS, Burke CA, McKeown-Eyssen GE, & Baron JA. (2009). Folic acid and risk of prostate cancer: Results from a randomized clinical trial. *J Natl Cancer Inst*, 101, pp. 432-5

Finch CA, Hegsted M, Kinney TD, Thomas ED, Rath CE, Haskins D, Finch S, & Fluharty Rexg. (1950). Iron metabolism: The pathophysiology of iron storage. *Blood*, 5, 983

Foley DL, Craig JM, Morley R, Olsson CA, Olsson CJ, Dwyer T, Smith K, & Saffery R. (2009). Prospects for epigenetic epidemiology. *Am J Epidemiol*, 169, pp. 389-400

Freemantle SJ, & Moran RG. (1997). Transcription of the human folylpoly-gamma-glutamate synthetase gene. *J Biol Chem*, 272, pp. 25373-25379

Friedkin M, Plante LT, Crawford EJ, & Crumm M. (1975). Inhibition of thymidylate synthetase and dihydrofolate reductase by naturally occurring oligoglutamate derivatives of folic acid. *J Biol Chem*, 250, pp. 5614-21

Friso S, & Choi SW. (2005). Gene-Nutrient interactions in one-carbon metabolism. *Curr Drug Metab*, 6, pp. 37-46

Friso S, Lamon-Fava S, Jang H, Schaefer EJ, Corrocher R, & Choi SW. (2007). Oestrogen replacement therapy reduces total plasma homocysteine and enhances genomic DNA methylation in postmenopausal women. *Br J Nutr*, 97, pp. 617-21

Galivan J, Maley F, & Baugh CM. (1977). Protective effect of the pteroylpolyglutamates and phosphate on the proteolytic inactivation of thymidylate synthetase. *Arch Biochem Biophys*, 184, pp. 346-54

Gordon IO, Tretiakova MS, Noffsinger AE, Hart J, Reuter VE, & Al-Ahmadie HA. (2008). Prostate-Specific membrane antigen expression in regeneration and repair. *Mod Pathol*, 21, pp. 1421-7

Gravina GL, Marampon F, Di Staso M, Bonfili P, Vitturini A, Jannini EA, Pestell RG, Tombolini V, & Festuccia C. (5-Azacitidine restores and amplifies the bicalutamide response on preclinical models of androgen receptor expressing or deficient prostate tumors. *The Prostate*,

Green R. (1994). Typical and atypical manifestations of pernicious anemia. *Advances in Thomas Addison's Diseases*, 1, pp. 377-90

Gregory III JF, Ristow KA, Sartain DB, & Damron BL. (1984). Biological activity of the folacin oxidation products 10-formylfolic acid and 5-methyl-5, 6-dihyrofolic acid. *Journal of agricultural and food chemistry*, 32, pp. 1337-1342

Harzstark AL, & Small EJ. (2009). Immunotherapeutics in development for prostate cancer. *Oncologist*, 14, pp. 391-8

Hayashi I, Sohn KJ, Stempak JM, Croxford R, & Kim YI. (2007). Folate deficiency induces cell-specific changes in the steady-state transcript levels of genes involved in folate metabolism and 1-carbon transfer reactions in human colonic epithelial cells. *J Nutr*, 137, pp. 607-13

Heaney RP. (2003). Long-Latency deficiency disease: Insights from calcium and vitamin D. *Am J Clin Nutr*, 78, pp. 912-9

Heinle RW, & Welch AD. (1948). Experiments with pteroylglutamic acid and pteroylglutamic acid deficiency in human leukemia. *J Clin Invest*, 27, 539

Hennessy BT, Gauthier AM, Michaud LB, Hortobagyi G, & Valero V. (2005). Lower dose capecitabine has a more favorable therapeutic index in metastatic breast cancer: Retrospective analysis of patients treated at M. D. Anderson cancer center and a review of capecitabine toxicity in the literature. *Ann Oncol*, 16, pp. 1289-96

Herbert (1959) *The Megaloblastic Anemias*, New York, New York, Grune and Stratton.

Herbert V. (1987). The 1986 herman award lecture. Nutrition science as a continually unfolding story: The folate and vitamin B-12 paradigm. *Am J Clin Nutr,* 46, pp. 387-402

Hirohashi S. (1998). Inactivation of the e-cadherin-mediated cell adhesion system in human cancers. *Am J Pathol,* 153, pp. 333-9

Hirsch S, Sanchez H, Albala C, de la Maza MP, Barrera G, Leiva L, & Bunout D. (2009). Colon cancer in chile before and after the start of the flour fortification program with folic acid. *Eur J Gastroenterol Hepatol,* 21, pp. 436-9

Hoffbrand AV, Tripp E, & Lavoie A. (1976). Synthesis of folate polyglutamates in human cells. *Clinical science and molecular medicine,* 50, 61

Holmes RS, Zheng Y, Baron JA, Li L, McKeown-Eyssen G, Newcomb PA, Stern MC, Haile RW, Grady WM, Potter JD, Le Marchand L, Campbell PT, Figueiredo JC, Limburg PJ, Jenkins MA, Hopper JL, Ulrich CM, & Colon Cancer Family Registry. (2010). Use of folic acid-containing supplements after a diagnosis of colorectal cancer in the colon cancer family registry. *Cancer Epidemiol Biomarkers Prev,* 19, pp. 2023-34

Honein MA, Paulozzi LJ, Mathews TJ, Erickson JD, & Wong LY. (2001). Impact of folic acid fortification of the US food supply on the occurrence of neural tube defects. *JAMA,* 285, pp. 2981-6

Hron G, Lombardi R, Eichinger S, Lecchi A, Kyrle PA, & Cattaneo M. (2007). Low vitamin B6 levels and the risk of recurrent venous thromboembolism. *Haematologica,* 92, pp. 1250-3

Hsing AW, Chua S, Gao YT, Gentzschein E, Chang L, Deng J, & Stanczyk FZ. (2001). Prostate cancer risk and serum levels of insulin and leptin: A population-based study. *J Natl Cancer Inst,* 93, pp. 783-9

Hultdin J, Van Guelpen B, Bergh A, Hallmans G, & Stattin P. (2005). Plasma folate, vitamin B12, and homocysteine and prostate cancer risk: A prospective study. *Int J Cancer,* 113, pp. 819-24

Jacob RA. (2000). Folate, DNA methylation, and gene expression: Factors of nature and nurture. *American Journal of Clinical Nutrition,* 72, 903

James SJ, Pogribny IP, Pogribna M, Miller BJ, Jernigan S, & Melnyk S. (2003). Mechanisms of DNA damage, DNA hypomethylation, and tumor progression in the folate/methyl-deficient rat model of hepatocarcinogenesis. *J Nutr,* 133, pp. 3740S-3747S

Jang H, Mason JB, & Choi SW. (2005). Genetic and epigenetic interactions between folate and aging in carcinogenesis. *J Nutr,* 135, pp. 2967S-2971S

Jaszewski R, Khan A, Sarkar FH, Kucuk O, Tobi M, Zagnoon A, Dhar R, Kinzie J, & Majumdar AP. (1999). Folic acid inhibition of egfr-mediated proliferation in human colon cancer cell lines. *Am J Physiol,* 277, pp. C1142-8

Jentzmik F, Stephan C, Lein M, Miller K, Kamlage B, Bethan B, Kristiansen G, & Jung K. (2011). Sarcosine in prostate cancer tissue is not a differential metabolite for prostate cancer aggressiveness and biochemical progression. *Journal Urology,* 185, pp. 385-6

Jentzmik F, Stephan C, Miller K, Schrader M, Erbersdobler A, Kristiansen G, Lein M, & Jung K. (2010). Sarcosine in urine after digital rectal examination fails as a marker in prostate cancer detection and identification of aggressive tumours. *Eur Urol,* 58, pp. 12-8; discussion 20-1

Johansson M, Appleby PN, Allen NE, Travis RC, Roddam AW, Egevad L, Jenab M, Rinaldi S, Kiemeney LA, Bueno-de-Mesquita HB, Vollset SE, Ueland PM, Sánchez MJ, Quirós JR, González CA, Larrañaga N, Chirlaque MD, Ardanaz E, Sieri S, Palli D, Key TJ. (2008). Circulating concentrations of folate and vitamin B12 in relation to

prostate cancer risk: Results from the european prospective investigation into
cancer and nutrition study. *Cancer Epidemiol Biomarkers Prev*, 17, pp. 279-85

Johansson M, Van Guelpen B, Vollset SE, Hultdin J, Bergh A, Key T, Midttun O, Hallmans
G, Ueland PM, & Stattin P. (2009). One-Carbon metabolism and prostate cancer
risk: Prospective investigation of seven circulating B vitamins and metabolites.
Cancer Epidemiol Biomarkers Prev, 18, pp. 1538-43

Jones PA, & Baylin SB. (2002). The fundamental role of epigenetic events in cancer. *Nat Rev
Genet*, 3, pp. 415-28

Jones PA, & Laird PW. (1999). Cancer epigenetics comes of age. *Nat Genet*, 21, pp. 163-7

Jones PA, & Takai D. (2001). The role of DNA methylation in mammalian epigenetics.
Science, 293, pp. 1068-70

Kao TT, Wang KC, Chang WN, Lin CY, Chen BH, Wu HL, Shi GY, Tsai JN, & Fu TF. (2008).
Characterization and comparative studies of zebrafish and human recombinant
dihydrofolate reductases--inhibition by folic acid and polyphenols. *Drug Metab
Dispos*, 36, pp. 508-16

Kasperzyk JL, Fall K, Mucci LA, Håkansson N, Wolk A, Johansson JE, Andersson SO, &
Andrén O. (2009). One-Carbon metabolism-related nutrients and prostate cancer
survival. *Am J Clin Nutr*, 90, pp. 561-9

Kawakami K, Ruszkiewicz A, Bennett G, Moore J, Watanabe G, & Iacopetta B. (2003). The
folate pool in colorectal cancers is associated with DNA hypermethylation and with
a polymorphism in methylenetetrahydrofolate reductase. *Clin Cancer Res*, 9, pp.
5860-5

Kenyon SH, Nicolaou A, Ast T, & Gibbons WA. (1996). Stimulation in vitro of vitamin b12-
dependent methionine synthase by polyamines. *Biochem J*, 316 (Pt 2), pp. 661-5

Key TJ, Silcocks PB, Davey GK, Appleby PN, & Bishop DT. (1997). A case-control study of
diet and prostate cancer. *British journal of cancer*, 76, 678

Kim YI. (2004). Folate and DNA methylation: A mechanistic link between folate deficiency
and colorectal cancer?. *Cancer Epidemiol Biomarkers Prev*, 13, pp. 511-9

Kim YI. (2005). Does a high folate intake increase the risk of breast cancer?. *Nutrition
Reviews*, 63,

Kim YI. (2005). Nutritional epigenetics: Impact of folate deficiency on DNA methylation and
colon cancer susceptibility. *J Nutr*, 135, pp. 2703-9

Kim YI. (2007). Folate and colorectal cancer: An evidence-based critical review. *Mol Nutr
Food Res*, 51, pp. 267-92

Kim YI. (2007). Folic acid fortification and supplementation – good for some but not so good
for others. *Nutrition Reviews*, 65, pp. 504-511

Kim YI. (2008). Folic acid supplementation and cancer risk: Point. *Cancer Epidemiol
Biomarkers Prev*, 17, pp. 2220-5

Kim YI. (2009). Role of the MTHFR polymorphisms in cancer risk modification and
treatment. *Future Oncol*, 5, pp. 523-42

Kim YI, Hayek M, Mason JB, & Meydani SN. (2002). Severe folate deficiency impairs natural
killer cell-mediated cytotoxicity in rats. *J Nutr*, 132, pp. 1361-7

Kisliuk RL. (1981). Pteroylpolyglutamates. *Molecular and Cellular Biochemistry*, 39, pp. 331-345

Kisliuk L, & Gaumont Y. (1983). An hypothesis on the role of pteroylpolyglutamate
derivatives as coenzymes. *Adv Exp Med Biol*, 163, pp. 71-4

Kisliuk RL, Gaumont Y, & Baugh CM. (1974). Polyglutamyl derivatives of folate as
substrates and inhibitors of thymidylate synthetase. *J Biol Chem*, 249, pp. 4100-3

Kisliuk RL, Gaumont Y, Lafer E, Baugh CM, & Montgomery JA. (1981). Polyglutamyl derivatives of tetrahydrofolate as substrates for lactobacillus casei thymidylate synthase. *Biochemistry*, 20, pp. 929-34

Konings EJ, Goldbohm RA, Brants HA, Saris WH, & van den Brandt PA. (2002). Intake of dietary folate vitamers and risk of colorectal carcinoma: Results from the netherlands cohort study. *Cancer*, 95, pp. 1421-33

Konings EJ, Roomans HH, Dorant E, Goldbohm RA, Saris WH, & van den Brandt PA. (2001). Folate intake of the dutch population according to newly established liquid chromatography data for foods. *Am J Clin Nutr*, 73, pp. 765-76

Krumdieck CL, Boots LR, Cornwell PE, & Butterworth CE. (1975). Estrogen stimulation of conjugase activity in the uterus of ovariectomized rats. *Am J Clin Nutr*, 28, pp. 530-4

Krumdieck CL, Boots LR, Cornwell PE, & Butterworth CE. (1976). Cyclic variations in folate composition and pteroylpolyglutamyl hydrolase (conjugase) activity of the rat uterus. *Am J Clin Nutr*, 29, pp. 288-94

Krumdieck CL, Eto I, & Baggott JE. (1992). Regulatory role of oxidized and reduced pteroylpolyglutamates. *Ann N Y Acad Sci*, 669, pp. 44-57; discussion 57-8

Kuster GG, ReMine WH, & Dockerty MB. (1972). Gastric cancer in pernicious anemia and in patients with and without achlorhydria. *Annals of Surgery*, 175, 783

Lawson KA, Wright ME, Subar A, Mouw T, Hollenbeck A, Schatzkin A, & Leitzmann MF. (2007). Multivitamin use and risk of prostate cancer in the national institutes of health-aarp diet and health study. *J Natl Cancer Inst*, 99, pp. 754-64

LeBlanc JG, de Giori GS, Smid EJ, Hugenholtz J, & Sesma F. (2007). Folate production by lactic acid bacteria and other food-grade microorganisms. *Commun Curr Res Educ Topics Trends Appl Microbiol*, 1,

Leuchtenberger R, Leuchtenberger C, Laszlo D, & Lewisohn R. (1945). The influence of "folic acid" on spontaneous breast cancers in mice. *Science*, 101, 406

Lewisohn R, Leuchtenberger C, Leucetenberger R, & Keresztesy JC. (1946). The influence of liver L. Casei factor on spontaneous breast cancer in mice. *Science*, 104, pp. 436-7

Li LC, Carroll PR, & Dahiya R. (2005). Epigenetic changes in prostate cancer: Implication for diagnosis and treatment. *J Natl Cancer Inst*, 97, pp. 103-15

Li LC, & Dahiya R. (2007). Epigenetics of prostate cancer. *Frontiers in Bioscience*, 12, pp. 3377-3397

Lindzon GM, Medline A, Sohn KJ, Depeint F, Croxford R, & Kim YI. (2009). Effect of folic acid supplementation on the progression of colorectal aberrant crypt foci. *Carcinogenesis*, 30, pp. 1536-43

Liu Z, Choi SW, Crott JW, Keyes MK, Jang H, & Mason JB. (2006). Mild depletion of vitamin B2, B6 and B12 superimposed on mild folate depletion: Effects on DNA methylation, uracil incorporation and gene expression in the mouse colon. *Proceedings of the American Association for Cancer Research*, 2006, 916

Liu Z, Choi SW, Crott JW, Keyes MK, Jang H, Smith DE, Kim M, Laird PW, Bronson R, & Mason JB. (2007). Mild depletion of dietary folate combined with other B vitamins alters multiple components of the wnt pathway in mouse colon. *J Nutr*, 137, pp. 2701-8

Lowe KE, Osborne CB, Lin BF, Kim JS, Hsu JC, & Shane B. (1993). Regulation of folate and one-carbon metabolism in mammalian cells. II. Effect of folylpoly-gamma-glutamate synthetase substrate specificity and level on folate metabolism and folylpoly-gamma-glutamate specificity of metabolic cycles of one-carbon metabolism. *Journal of Biological Chemistry*, 268, 21665

Lucock M, & Yates Z. (2005). Folic acid - vitamin and panacea or genetic time bomb?. *Nat Rev Genet*, 6, pp. 235-40

Luka Z, Mudd SH, & Wagner C. (2009). Glycine n-methyltransferase and regulation of s-adenosylmethionine levels. *J Biol Chem*, 284, pp. 22507-11

Ly A, Lee H, Chen J, Sie KK, Renlund R, Medline A, Sohn KJ, Croxford R, Thompson LU, & Kim YI. (2011). Effect of maternal and postweaning folic acid supplementation on mammary tumor risk in the offspring. *Cancer Res*, 71, pp. 988-97

Marchal C, Redondo M, Padilla M, Caballero J, Rodrigo I, García J, Quian J, & Boswick DG. (2004). Expression of prostate specific membrane antigen (PSMA) in prostatic adenocarcinoma and prostatic intraepithelial neoplasia. *Histol Histopathol*, 19, pp. 715-8

Maring JG, Groen HJ, Wachters FM, Uges DR, & de Vries EG. (2005). Genetic factors influencing pyrimidine-antagonist chemotherapy. *Pharmacogenomics J*, 5, pp. 226-43

Marsillach J, Ferré N, Camps J, Riu F, Rull A, & Joven J. (2008). Moderately high folic acid supplementation exacerbates experimentally induced liver fibrosis in rats. *Exp Biol Med (Maywood)*, 233, pp. 38-47

Maruyama R, Toyooka S, Toyooka KO, Virmani AK, Zöchbauer-Müller S, Farinas AJ, Minna JD, McConnell J, Frenkel EP, & Gazdar AF. (2002). Aberrant promoter methylation profile of prostate cancers and its relationship to clinicopathological features. *Clin Cancer Res*, 8, pp. 514-9

Mason JB, Choi SW, & Liu Z. (2008). Other one-carbon micronutrients and age modulate the effects of folate on colorectal carcinogenesis. *Nutr Rev*, 66 Suppl 1, pp. S15-7

Mason JB, Dickstein A, Jacques PF, Haggarty P, Selhub J, Dallal G, & Rosenberg IH. (2007). A temporal association between folic acid fortification and an increase in colorectal cancer rates may be illuminating important biological principles: A hypothesis. *Cancer Epidemiol Biomarkers Prev*, 16, pp. 1325-9

Matthews RG, & Baugh CM. (1980). Interactions of pig liver methylenetetrahydrofolate reductase with methylenetetrahydropteroylpolyglutamate substrates and with dihydropteroylpolyglutamate inhibitors. *Biochemistry*, 19, pp. 2040-5

Matthews RG, & Daubner SC. (1982). Modulation of methylenetetrahydrofolate reductase activity by s-adenosylmethionine and by dihydrofolate and its polyglutamate analogues. *Advances in Enzyme Regulation*, 20, pp. 123-131

Matthews RG, Ghose C, Green JM, Matthews KD, & Dunlap RB. (1987). Folylpolyglutamates as substrates and inhibitors of folate-dependent enzymes. *Adv Enzyme Regul*, 26, pp. 157-71

Matthews RG, & Haywood BJ. (1979). Inhibition of pig liver methylenetetrahydrofolate reductase by dihydrofolate: Some mechanistic and regulatory implications. *Biochemistry*, 18, pp. 4845-51

McDowell MA, Lacher DA, Pfeiffer CM, Mulinare J, Picciano MF, Rader JI, Yetley EA, Kennedy-Stephenson J, & Johnson CL. (2008). Blood folate levels: The latest NHANES results. *NCHS Data Brief*, pp. 1-8

McNulty H, McKinley MC, Wilson B, McPartlin J, Strain JJ, Weir DG, & Scott JM. (2002). Impaired functioning of thermolabile methylenetetrahydrofolate reductase is dependent on riboflavin status: Implications for riboflavin requirements. *Am J Clin Nutr*, 76, pp. 436-41

Midgley R, & Kerr DJ. (2009). Capecitabine: Have we got the dose right?. *Nat Clin Pract Oncol*, 6, pp. 17-24

Milic M, Rozgaj R, Kasuba V, Orescanin V, Balija M, & Jukic I. (2010). Correlation between folate and vitamin B_{12} and markers of DNA stability in healthy men: Preliminary results. *Acta Biochim Pol*, 57, pp. 339-45

Mokarram P, Naghibalhossaini F, Firoozi MS, Hosseini SV, Izadpanah A, Salahi H, Malek-Hosseini SA, Talei A, & Mojallal M. (2008). Methylenetetrahydrofolate reductase C677T genotype affects promoter methylation of tumor-specific genes in sporadic colorectal cancer through an interaction with folate/vitamin B12 status.

Moran RG. (1989). Leucovorin enhancement of the effects of the fluoropyrimidines on thymidylate synthase. *Cancer*, 63, pp. 1008-1012

Moran RG, & Colman PD. (1984). Mammalian folyl polyglutamate synthetase: Partial purification and properties of the mouse liver enzyme. *Biochemistry*, 23, pp. 4580-9

Nagothu KK, Rishi AK, Jaszewski R, Kucuk O, & Majumdar AP. (2004). Folic acid-mediated inhibition of serum-induced activation of EGFR promoter in colon cancer cells. *Am J Physiol Gastrointest Liver Physiol*, 287, pp. G541-6

O'Keefe, Bacich, et al. (2001)" Prostate Specific Membrane Antigen" in Chung, Leland, Isaacs, William, Simons, Jonathan, (ed.) Prostate Cancer Biology, Genetics, and the New Therapeutics. Totowa, New Jersey, Humana Press, 307-326.

Pellis L, Dommels Y, Venema D, Polanen A, Lips E, Baykus H, Kok F, Kampman E, & Keijer J. (2008). High folic acid increases cell turnover and lowers differentiation and iron content in human HT29 colon cancer cells. *Br J Nutr*, 99, pp. 703-8

Pelucchi C, Galeone C, Talamini R, Negri E, Parpinel M, Franceschi S, Montella M, & La Vecchia C. (2005). Dietary folate and risk of prostate cancer in italy. *Cancer Epidemiol Biomarkers Prev*, 14, pp. 944-8

Perry J, & Chanarin I. (1972). Observations on folate absorption with particular reference to folate polyglutamate and possible inhibitors to its absorption. *Gut*, 13, pp. 544-50

Perry J, Chanarin I, Deacon R, & Lumb M. (1983). Chronic cobalamin inactivation impairs folate polyglutamate synthesis in the rat. *J Clin Invest*, 71, pp. 1183-90

Perry AS, Foley R, Woodson K, & Lawler M. (2006). The emerging roles of DNA methylation in the clinical management of prostate cancer. *Endocr Relat Cancer*, 13, pp. 357-77

Pratt RF, & Cooper BA. (1971). Folates in plasma and bile of man after feeding folic acid--3h and 5-formyltetrahydrofolate (folinic acid). *J Clin Invest*, 50, pp. 455-62

Pufulete M, Al-Ghnaniem R, Rennie JA, Appleby P, Harris N, Gout S, Emery PW, & Sanders TA. (2005). Influence of folate status on genomic DNA methylation in colonic mucosa of subjects without colorectal adenoma or cancer. *Br J Cancer*, 92, pp. 838-42

Rampersaud GC, Kauwell GP, Hutson AD, Cerda JJ, & Bailey LB. (2000). Genomic DNA methylation decreases in response to moderate folate depletion in elderly women. *Am J Clin Nutr*, 72, pp. 998-1003

Ratanasthien K, Blair JA, Leeming RJ, Cooke WT, & Melikian V. (1974). Folates in human serum. *Journal of Clinical Pathology*, 27, 875

Rauen HM, Stamm W, & Kimbel KH. (1952). [N(12)-formyl-folic acid, a fermentative metabolic product of folic acid]. *Hoppe Seylers Z Physiol Chem*, 289, pp. 80-4

Remacha AF, Souto JC, Rámila E, Perea G, Sarda MP, & Fontcuberta J. (2002). Enhanced risk of thrombotic disease in patients with acquired vitamin B12 and/or folate deficiency: Role of hyperhomocysteinemia. *Ann Hematol*, 81, pp. 616-21

Rennie PS, & Nelson CC. (1998). Epigenetic mechanisms for progression of prostate cancer. *Cancer Metastasis Rev,* 17, pp. 401-9

Robinson K, Arheart K, Refsum H, Brattström L, Boers G, Ueland P, Rubba P, Palma-Reis R, Meleady R, Daly L, Witteman J, & Graham I. (1998). Low circulating folate and vitamin B6 concentrations: Risk factors for stroke, peripheral vascular disease, and coronary artery disease. European COMAC group. *Circulation,* 97, pp. 437-43

Ross J, Green J, Baugh CM, MacKenzie RE, & Matthews RG. (1984). Studies on the polyglutamate specificity of methylenetetrahydrofolate dehydrogenase from pig liver. *Biochemistry,* 23, pp. 1796-801

Rovinetti C, Bovina C, Tolomelli B, & Marchetti M. (1972). Effects of testosterone on the metabolism of folate coenzymes in the rat. *Biochem J,* 126, pp. 291-4

Rowling MJ, McMullen MH, & Schalinske KL. (2002). Vitamin A and its derivatives induce hepatic glycine n-methyltransferase and hypomethylation of DNA in rats. *J Nutr,* 132, pp. 365-9

Sanderson P, Stone E, Kim YI, Mathers JC, Kampman E, Downes CS, Muir KR, & Baron JA. (2007). Folate and colo-rectal cancer risk. *Br J Nutr,* 98, pp. 1299-304

Santini R, Brewster C, & Butterworth CE. (1964). The distribution of folic acid active compounds in individual foods. *Am J Clin Nutr,* 14, pp. 205-10

Sasaki M, Tanaka Y, Perinchery G, Dharia A, Kotcherguina I, Fujimoto S, & Dahiya R. (2002). Methylation and inactivation of estrogen, progesterone, and androgen receptors in prostate cancer. *J Natl Cancer Inst,* 94, pp. 384-90

Segura-Pacheco B, Perez-Cardenas E, Taja-Chayeb L, Chavez-Blanco A, Revilla-Vazquez A, Benitez-Bribiesca L, & Duenas-González A. (2006). Global DNA hypermethylation-associated cancer chemotherapy resistance and its reversion with the demethylating agent hydralazine. *J Transl Med,* 4, 32

Shane (2010)" Folate Chemistry and Metabolism" in Folate in Health and Disease: Edited by Lynn B. Bailey. Boca Raton, FL, CRC Press & Taylor and Francis Group, 1-24.

Sharma R, Hoskins JM, Rivory LP, Zucknick M, London R, Liddle C, & Clarke SJ. (2008). Thymidylate synthase and methylenetetrahydrofolate reductase gene polymorphisms and toxicity to capecitabine in advanced colorectal cancer patients. *Clin Cancer Res,* 14, pp. 817-25

Sharma S, Kelly TK, & Jones PA. (2010). Epigenetics in cancer. *Carcinogenesis,* 31, 27

Shukeir N, Pakneshan P, Chen G, Szyf M, & Rabbani SA. (2006). Alteration of the methylation status of tumor-promoting genes decreases prostate cancer cell invasiveness and tumorigenesis in vitro and in vivo. *Cancer Res,* 66, pp. 9202-10

Sie KK, Medline A, van Weel J, Sohn KJ, Choi SW, Croxford R, & Kim YI. (2011). Effect of maternal and postweaning folic acid supplementation on colorectal cancer risk in the offspring. *Gut,*

Silverman M, Keresztesy JC, & Koval GJ. (1954). Isolation of n-10-formylfolic acid. *Journal of Biological Chemistry,* 211, 53

Skipper HE, Chapman JB, & Bell M. (1950). Studies on the role of folic acid in the leukemic process. *Cancer,* 3, pp. 871-3

Smith AD, Kim YI, & Refsum H. (2008). Is folic acid good for everyone?. *Am J Clin Nutr,* 87, pp. 517-33

Sohn KJ, Jang H, Campan M, Weisenberger DJ, Dickhout J, Wang YC, Cho RC, Yates Z, Lucock M, Chiang EP, Austin RC, Choi SW, Laird PW, & Kim YI. (2009). The methylenetetrahydrofolate reductase C677T mutation induces cell-specific changes in genomic DNA methylation and uracil misincorporation: A possible molecular basis for the site-specific cancer risk modification. *Int J Cancer*, 124, pp. 1999-2005

Song JZ, Stirzaker C, Harrison J, Melki JR, & Clark SJ. (2002). Hypermethylation trigger of the glutathione-s-transferase gene (GSTP1) in prostate cancer cells. *Oncogene*, 21, pp. 1048-61

Sonpavde G, Aparicio AM, Zhan F, North B, Delaune R, Garbo LE, Rousey SR, Weinstein RE, Xiao L, Boehm KA, Asmar L, Fleming MT, Galsky MD, Berry WR, & Von Hoff DD. (2009). Azacitidine favorably modulates PSA kinetics correlating with plasma DNA LINE-1 hypomethylation in men with chemonaïve castration-resistant prostate cancer. *Urol Oncol*,

Spies TD, & Garcia-Lopez G. (1948). Further observations on the specificity of the folic acid molecule. *Blood*, 3, pp. 121-6

Sreekumar A, Poisson LM, Rajendiran TM, Khan AP, Cao Q, Yu J, Laxman B, Mehra R, Lonigro RJ, Li Y, Nyati MK, Ahsan A, Kalyana-Sundaram S, Han B, Cao X, Byun J, Omenn GS, Ghosh D, Pennathur S, Alexander DC, Chinnaiyan AM. (2009). Metabolomic profiles delineate potential role for sarcosine in prostate cancer progression. *Nature*, 457, pp. 910-4

Stevens VL, McCullough ML, Sun J, & Gapstur SM. (2010). Folate and other one-carbon metabolism-related nutrients and risk of postmenopausal breast cancer in the cancer prevention study II nutrition cohort. *Am J Clin Nutr*,

Stevens VL, Rodriguez C, Pavluck AL, McCullough ML, Thun MJ, & Calle EE. (2006). Folate nutrition and prostate cancer incidence in a large cohort of US men. *Am J Epidemiol*, 163, pp. 989-96

Struys EA, Heijboer AC, van Moorselaar J, Jakobs C, & Blankenstein MA. (2010). Serum sarcosine is not a marker for prostate cancer. *Annals of Clinical Biochemistry*, 47, 282

Sun X, Cross JA, Bognar AL, Baker EN, & Smith CA. (2001). Folate-Binding triggers the activation of folylpolyglutamate synthetase. *J Mol Biol*, 310, pp. 1067-78

Sun D, Wollin A, & Stephen AM. (2002). Moderate folate deficiency influences polyamine synthesis in rats. *J Nutr*, 132, pp. 2632-7

Sweeney MR, McPartlin J, & Scott J. (2007). Folic acid fortification and public health: Report on threshold doses above which unmetabolised folic acid appear in serum. *BMC Public Health*, 7, 41

Sweeney MR, Staines A, Daly L, Traynor A, Daly S, Bailey SW, Alverson PB, Ayling JE, & Scott JM. (2009). Persistent circulating unmetabolised folic acid in a setting of liberal voluntary folic acid fortification. Implications for further mandatory fortification?. *BMC Public Health*, 9, 295

Szyf M. (2009). Epigenetics, DNA methylation, and chromatin modifying drugs. *Annu Rev Pharmacol Toxicol*, 49, pp. 243-63

Taneja SS. (2004). Prostascint(R) scan: Contemporary use in clinical practice. *Rev Urol*, 6 Suppl 10, pp. S19-28

Tisman (2005)" Pernicious anemia and other megaloblastic anemias: method of Glenn Tisman" in Conn's Current Therapy. Philadelphia, Elsevier Saunders, 443-448.

Tisman & Garcia (2011) B Vitamins in Cancer Patients are Frequently Abnormal, Stimulate and Inhibit Prostate Cancer and Modulate Chemotherapy Toxicity. . Advances and Controversies in Clinical Nutrition , 17.

Tisman G, & Herbert V. (1973). B12 dependence of cell uptake of serum folate: An explanation for high serum folate and cell folate depletion in B12 deficiency. *Blood*, 41,

Tisman G, Herbert V, & Edlis H. (1973). Determination of therapeutic index of drugs by in vitro sensitivity tests using human host and tumor cell suspensions. *Cancer Chemother Rep*, 57, pp. 11-9

Tisman G, Kutik S, & Rainville C. (2009). Coexistence of pernicious anemia and prostate cancer - 'an experiment of nature' involving vitamin B(12)modulation of prostate cancer growth and metabolism: A case report. *J Med Case Reports*, 3, 9295

Tomaszewski JJ, Cummings JL, Parwani AV, Dhir R, Mason JB, Nelson JB, Bacich DJ, & O'Keefe DS. (2011). Increased cancer cell proliferation in prostate cancer patients with high levels of serum folate. *Prostate*,

Troen AM, Mitchell B, Sorensen B, Wener MH, Johnston A, Wood B, Selhub J, McTiernan A, Yasui Y, Oral E, Potter JD, & Ulrich CM. (2006). Unmetabolized folic acid in plasma is associated with reduced natural killer cell cytotoxicity among postmenopausal women. *J Nutr*, 136, pp. 189-94

Ubbink JB, van der Merwe A, Delport R, Allen RH, Stabler SP, Riezler R, & Vermaak WJ. (1996). The effect of a subnormal vitamin B-6 status on homocysteine metabolism. *J Clin Invest*, 98, pp. 177-84

Ulrey CL, Liu L, Andrews LG, & Tollefsbol TO. (2005). The impact of metabolism on DNA methylation. *Hum Mol Genet*, 14 Spec No 1, pp. R139-47

Uysal-Onganer P, Kawano Y, Caro M, Walker MM, Diez S, Darrington RS, Waxman J, & Kypta RM. (2010). Wnt-11 promotes neuroendocrine-like differentiation, survival and migration of prostate cancer cells. *Mol Cancer*, 9, 55

van Engeland M, Weijenberg MP, Roemen GM, Brink M, de Bruïne AP, Goldbohm RA, van den Brandt PA, Baylin SB, de Goeij AF, & Herman JG. (2003). Effects of dietary folate and alcohol intake on promoter methylation in sporadic colorectal cancer: The netherlands cohort study on diet and cancer. *Cancer Res*, 63, pp. 3133-7

Velicer CM, & Ulrich CM. (2008). Vitamin and mineral supplement use among US adults after cancer diagnosis: A systematic review. *J Clin Oncol*, 26, pp. 665-73

Vlajinac HD, Marinkovi JM, Ili MD, & Kocev NI. (1997). Diet and prostate cancer: A case-control study. *European Journal of Cancer*, 33, pp. 101-107

Wagner C, Briggs WT, & Cook RJ. (1985). Inhibition of glycine n-methyltransferase activity by folate derivatives: Implications for regulation of methyl group metabolism. *Biochem Biophys Res Commun*, 127, pp. 746-52

Wainfan E, Dizik M, Stender M, & Christman JK. (1989). Rapid appearance of hypomethylated DNA in livers of rats fed cancer-promoting, methyl-deficient diets. *Cancer Res*, 49, pp. 4094-7

Wainfan E, & Poirier LA. (1992). Methyl groups in carcinogenesis: Effects on DNA methylation and gene expression. *Cancer Res*, 52, pp. 2071s-2077s

Wallace K, Grau MV, Levine AJ, Shen L, Hamdan R, Chen X, Gui J, Haile RW, Barry EL, Ahnen D, McKeown-Eyssen G, Baron JA, & Issa JP. (2010). Association between folate levels and cpg island hypermethylation in normal colorectal mucosa. *Cancer Prev Res (Phila)*, 3, pp. 1552-64

Wang X, Qin X, Demirtas H, Li J, Mao G, Huo Y, Sun N, Liu L, & Xu X. (2007). Efficacy of folic acid supplementation in stroke prevention: A meta-analysis. *Lancet*, 369, pp. 1876-82

Wang YC, Tang FY, Chen SY, Chen YM, & Chiang EP. (2011). Glycine-N methyltransferase expression in hepg2 cells is involved in methyl group homeostasis by regulating transmethylation kinetics and DNA methylation. *J Nutr*,

Ward GJ, & Nixon PF. (1990). Modulation of pteroylpolyglutamate concentration and length in response to altered folate nutrition in a comprehensive range of rat tissues. *J Nutr*, 120, pp. 476-84

Weinstein SJ, Hartman TJ, Stolzenberg-Solomon R, Pietinen P, Barrett MJ, Taylor PR, Virtamo J, & Albanes D. (2003). Null association between prostate cancer and serum folate, vitamin B(6), vitamin B(12), and homocysteine. *Cancer Epidemiol Biomarkers Prev*, 12, pp. 1271-2

Weinstein SJ, Stolzenberg-Solomon R, Pietinen P, Taylor PR, Virtamo J, & Albanes D. (2006). Dietary factors of one-carbon metabolism and prostate cancer risk. *Am J Clin Nutr*, 84, pp. 929-35

Williams KT, & Schalinske KL. (2007). New insights into the regulation of methyl group and homocysteine metabolism. *J Nutr*, 137, pp. 311-4

Yang Q, Cogswell ME, Hamner HC, Carriquiry A, Bailey LB, Pfeiffer CM, & Berry RJ. (2010). Folic acid source, usual intake, and folate and vitamin B-12 status in US adults: National health and nutrition examination survey (NHANES) 2003-2006. *Am J Clin Nutr*, 91, pp. 64-72

Yanokura M, Banno K, Kawaguchi M, Hirao N, Hirasawa A, Susumu N, Tsukazaki K, & Aoki D. (2007). Relationship of aberrant DNA hypermethylation of CHFR with sensitivity to taxanes in endometrial cancer. *Oncol Rep*, 17, pp. 41-8

Yao V, Berkman CE, Choi JK, O'Keefe DS, & Bacich DJ. (2010). Expression of prostate-specific membrane antigen (PSMA), increases cell folate uptake and proliferation and suggests a novel role for PSMA in the uptake of the non-polyglutamated folate, folic acid. *Prostate*, 70, pp. 305-16

Yao V, Parwani A, Maier C, Heston WD, & Bacich DJ. (2008). Moderate expression of prostate-specific membrane antigen, a tissue differentiation antigen and folate hydrolase, facilitates prostate carcinogenesis. *Cancer Res*, 68, pp. 9070-7

Yardy GW, & Brewster SF. (2005). Wnt signalling and prostate cancer. *Prostate Cancer Prostatic Dis*, 8, pp. 119-26

Yegnasubramanian S, Haffner MC, Zhang Y, Gurel B, Cornish TC, Wu Z, Irizarry RA, Morgan J, Hicks J, DeWeese TL, Isaacs WB, Bova GS, De Marzo AM, & Nelson WG. (2008). DNA hypomethylation arises later in prostate cancer progression than cpg island hypermethylation and contributes to metastatic tumor heterogeneity. *Cancer Res*, 68, pp. 8954-67

Yeo EJ, Briggs WT, & Wagner C. (1999). Inhibition of glycine n-methyltransferase by 5-methyltetrahydrofolate pentaglutamate. *J Biol Chem*, 274, pp. 37559-64

Yunis JJ, & Soreng AL. (1984). Constitutive fragile sites and cancer. *Science*, 226, 1199

Zeisel SH. (2009). Epigenetic mechanisms for nutrition determinants of later health outcomes. *Am J Clin Nutr*, 89, pp. 1488S-1493S

Zhu H, Mazor M, Kawano Y, Walker MM, Leung HY, Armstrong K, Waxman J, & Kypta RM. (2004). Analysis of wnt gene expression in prostate cancer: Mutual inhibition by WNT11 and the androgen receptor. *Cancer Res*, 64, pp. 7918-26

13

MAP Kinases and Prostate Cancer

Gonzalo Rodríguez-Berriguete, Benito Fraile, Laura Galvis,
Ricardo Paniagua and Mar Royuela
Department of Cell Biology and Genetics. University of Alcalá, Madrid
Spain

1. Introduction

One of the most relevant aspects in cell death regulation is the signaling of apoptosis by serine/threonine kinases, a broad category of kinases that includes, among others, the mitogen-activated protein kinases (MAPKs) (Cross et al., 2000; Khlodenko & Birtwistle, 2009). The three main members that integrate the MAPK family in mammalian cells are: the stress-activated protein kinase c-Jun NH_2-terminal kinases (JNK), the stress-activated protein kinase 2 (SAPK2, p38), and the extracellular signal-regulated protein kinases (ERK1/2, p44/p42) (Fig. 1). In addition, other less well-characterized MAPK pathways exist, such as the extracellular regulated kinase 5 (ERK5) pathway (Hayashi &Lee, 2004; Junttila & Li, 2008) (Fig. 1). Albeit with multiple exceptions, JNK and ERK5 are generally associated with apoptosis induction; while ERK1/2 are generally associated to mitogenesis, and therefore inversely related to apoptosis (Hayashi &Lee, 2004; Junttila & Li, 2008); and contradictory effects on cell death have been described to p38 (Chang et al., 2008; Joo & Yoo, 2009; Khwaja et al., 2008; Ricote et al., 2006a; Shimada et al., 2006; Vayalil et al., 2004; Zhang &Kong, 2008).

ERK is a threonine-glutamic acid-tyrosine (Thr-Glu-Tyr) motif (Hunter, 2000; Liu et al., 2010) that play a central role in stimulation of cell proliferation (Marais & Marshall, 1990; Peng et al., 2010). Two isoforms of ERK, referred as ERK1 (or p44) and ERK2 (or p42), are ubiquitously expressed and represent a convergence point for mitogenic signaling from a diverse array of pathways (Cullen &Lockyer, 2002; Eisinger &Ammer, 2008; Gao et al., 2010). Both are ubiquitously expressed, although their relative abundance in tissues is variable. For example, in many immune cells ERK2 is the predominant species, while in several cells of neuroendocrine origin they may be equally expressed (Zebisch et al., 2007). ERK 1/2 is activated by MEK1/2 specifically by phosphorylating a tyrosine and a threonine residue, separated by a glutamate residue (TEY) (Zebisch et al., 2007). Activated ERK1 and ERK2 can translocate to the nucleus, where it activates several transcription factors such as ATF-2, Elk-1, c-Fos, c-myc or Ets-1 (Junttila & Li, 2008). At the same time, it can also phosphorylate cytoplasmic and nuclear kinases, such as MNK1, MNK2, MPKAP-2, RSK or MSK1 (Zebisch et al., 2007). The ERK1/2 cascade is triggered by growth factors and cytokines acting through receptor tyrosine kinases, G-protein-coupled receptors, and non-nuclear activated steroid hormone receptors. The biological consequences of ERK1/2 substrate phosphorylation include pro-proliferative (Pearson et al., 2001), pro-differentiation (Pearson et al., 2001), pro-survival (Pearson et al., 2001), pro-angiogenic (Pàges et al., 2000), pro-motility (Joslin et al., 2007) and pro-invasive effects (Price et al., 2002).

P38 plays roles in cell differentiation, growth inhibition and apoptosis, proliferation and cell survival (Hui et al., 2007; Raingeaud et al., 1995; Thornton & Rincon, 2009). p38 is activated in cells in response to stress signals, growth factors, inflammatory cytokines, UV, heat and osmotic shock (Raingeaud et al., 1995; Whyte et al., 2009). Four isoforms of p38 exist (p38α, β, γ and δ), although p38α is the most widely expressed. MKK3/6 (MAPKKK) and SEK (MAPKK) activate p38. A great number MAPKKs and MAPKKKs (e.g. Mlk1-3, MEKK1-4, TAK, ASK1/2) upstream of p38 have been identified. Both MAPKKs and MAPKKKs are generally activated by G small proteins as Rac1, Cdc42, RhoA and RhoB (Fenf et al., 2009). Activated p38 phosphorylates and regulates many transcription factors (including activating transcription factor-2, NF-kB, Elk-1, Max, myocyte enhancer factor-2, Mac, p53 or Stat1) (Royuela et al., 2008; Whyte et al., 2009; Zhao et al., 1999), and other cell cycle and apoptosis mediators (e.g. Cdc25A, Bcl-2) (Thornton & Rincon, 2009). p38 has been defined as tumor suppressor and generally exert a pro-apoptotic role. However, it has been also shown to enhance cell survival in response to stress stimuli, for instance, in response to DNA damage (Thornton& Rincon., 2009; Whyte et al., 2009; Jiang et al., 1997; Wang XS et al., 1997; Feng et al., 2009; Zhao et al., 1999; Royuela et al., 2008; Wood et al., 2009). Triggering of pro- or anti-apoptotic p38-mediated response seems to depend on the stimuli, the cell system and the involved p38 isoform (Feng et al., 2009).

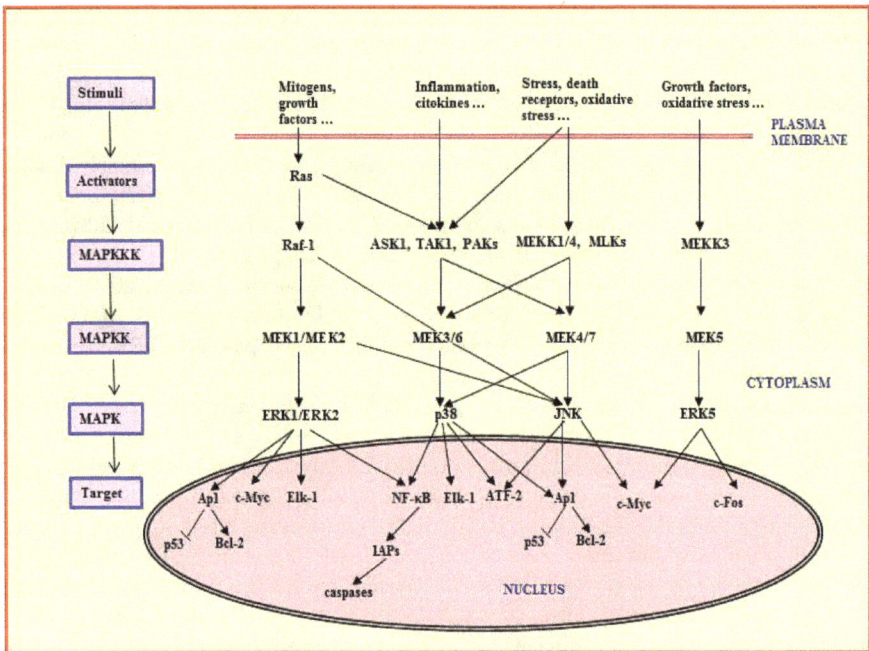

Fig. 1. Mitogen activated protein kinase (MAPK) signaling. MAP kinases are activated by upstream kinases such as MAP kinase kinase (MAPKK), that include MEKs 1, 2, 3, 4, 5, 6 and 7. In turn, MAPKKs are activated by several different MAP kinase kinase kinases (MAPKKKs). Numerous stimulatory factors such as cytokines, mitogens or death receptors, can activate MAPKKKs. Each MAPK, depending on the stimulus and cell type, can phosphorylate different transcription factors.

JNK proteins, also called stress activated protein kinases (SAPKs), are activated in response to a variety of extracellular stimuli, including UV irradiation, mitogens and cytokines (De Graeve et al., 1999). Notably, the earliest discoveries included the identification of the three mammalian JNK genes called JNK1, JNK2, and JNK3 (also termed stress-activated protein kinase (SAPK)-γ, SAPK-α and SAPK-β, respectively) which can be subdivided into 10 isoforms by alternative splicing (Bogoyevitch et al., 2010; Dérijard et al., 1994). Alternative splicing further increases the diversity of JNK proteins, however apart from early biochemical studies on these splice forms (Gupta et al., 1996) their functional significance *in vivo* has remained largely unexplored (Bogoyevitch et al., 2010). The products of JNK1 and JNK2 are ubiquitously expressed in every cells and tissues, whereas JNK3 is localized primarily in brain, heart and testis. Due to the specificity of tissue, JNK3 presents different functions than JNK1 and JNK2. In addition, several authors believe that JNK1 and JNK2 present redundant functions. Several studies suggest that JNK are involved in regulation of the cell cycle (Bode & Dong, 2007.). JNK signaling contributes to the ability of p53 to mediate apoptosis through stabilization and activation of p53 (Bode & Dong, 2007; Fuchs et al., 1998). The fourth MAPK of interest in this review is ERK5. ERK5 is a large molecular size kinase (Lee et al., 1995) identified independently by two groups. One used a two hybrid screen with an upstream activator MEK5 as the bait; the other used a degenerate PCR strategy to clone novel MAPK (Lee et al., 1995; Zhou et al., 2005). ERK5 is activated by growth factors (Kato et al., 1998), integrin engagement (Sawhney et al., 2009) and cell stress (Pi et al., 2004), and its important molecular targets would seem to include the induction of transcription of components of the transcription factor Ap1 (cJun (Kayahama et al., 2005) and Fos (Kamakura et al., 1999) and activation of transcription factors of the myocyte enhancer family group (for example, MEF2C, a well characterized target (Kato et al., 1997)), and cMyc (English et al., 1998).

In an *in vitro* study directed using androgen-dependent PC3 cells, McCracken et al. (2008) described ERK5-overexpresion related with proliferative, migrative and invasive capabilities, establishing the potential importance of ERK5 in aggressive prostate cancer. In similar studies Sawhney et al. (Sawhney et al., 2009) hypothesized that ERK5 activation could promote cancer metastasis.

In mammalian cells, ERK, p38 and JNK activities are respectively regulated by three different MAPK cascades, which provide a link between transmembrane signaling and changes in transcription and are activated in response to different environmental or developmental signals (Junttila & Li, 2008) (Fig. 1). Depending on the cell type, a particular MAPK cascade may be involved in different cellular responses. The JNK and p38 signaling pathways are activated by pro-inflammatory (TNFα, IL-6 or IL-1) or anti-inflammatory (EGF, TGF-β) cytokines, but also in response to cellular stresses such as genotoxic, osmotic, hypoxic, or oxidative stress. The JNK pathway consists of JNK, a MAPKK such as SEK1 (also known as MEK4) or MEK7, and a MAPKKK such as ASK1, MEKK1, mixed-lineage kinase (MLK), or transforming growth factor-β-activated kinase 1 (TAK1) (Davis, 2000; Kim & Choi, 2010). In the p38 signaling pathway, distinct MAPKKs such as MEK3 and MEK6 activate p38 and these are activated by the same MAPKKKs (such as ASK1 and TAK1) that function in the JNK pathway. In the ERK signaling pathway, ERK1 or ERK2 (ERK1/2) is activated by MEK1/2, which in turn is activated by a Raf isoform such as A-Raf, B-Raf, or Raf-1 (also known as C-Raf) but also by TRAF-2 and TRAF-6. The kinase Raf-1 is activated by the small Ras-like GTPase, whose activation is mediated by the receptor tyrosine kinase

(RTK)-Grb2-SOS signaling axis (Dhillon et al., 2007). Members of the Ras family of proteins, including K-Ras, H-Ras, and N-Ras, play a key role in transmission of extracellular signals into cells (Ancrile et al., 2008) (Fig. 1).

The aim of this review was to focus on the possible involvement of MAPKs in several transduction pathways related with prostate cancer development as well as the possible functional role of MAPKs in cell death/ survival/ proliferation decisions depending on the cell type, stage and cell stimulus. We also discuss the possible use of some members of this pathway as a potential therapeutic target.

2. IL-6/TNF/JNK pathway

Depending on the stimulus and cell type, JNKs can phosphorylate different substrates such as Ap1, ATF-2, Elk-1, c-Myc, p53, MLK2 and several members of the Bcl-2 family. JNKs are implicated in development, morphogenesis and cell differentiation (Heasley & Han, 2006). Several studies suggest that in apoptosis JNKs have opposite functions depending on the cellular stimulus. In this way, JNKs can induce apoptosis, but also can enhance cell survival and proliferation. JNKs are also involved in regulation of the cell cycle (Bode & Dong, 2007). JNK signaling contributes to the ability of p53 to mediate apoptosis through stabilization and activation of p53 (Bode & Dong, 2007; Fuchs et al., 1998). Several authors suggest that JNK activity is chronically altered in various cancer types such as prostate (Meshki et al., 2010; Royuela et al., 2002), breast (Wang HY et al., 2003; Wang J et al., 2010), pancreatic or lung (Lee et al., 2010; Su et al., 1998) carcinomas.

Investigations of JNKs have focused on their activation in response to diverse stresses including ultraviolet and gamma radiation, inflammatory cytokines and cytotoxic drugs. In this way, pro inflammatory cytokines such as IL-6 or TNF activate different transduction pathway (Khalaf et al., 2010).

IL-6 exerts its effects through a membrane receptor complex composed by IL-6 receptor a (IL-6Ra) and glycoprotein 130 (gp130). Silver and Hunter (Silver & Hunter, 2010) described the role of gp130 in promoting or preventing the development of autoimmunity and cancer, two processes that are associated with aberrant inflammatory responses. In addition to an immunological role, IL-6 is involved in cell proliferation in other tissues such as bone (Kurihara et al., 1990), testis (spermatogenesis) (Huleihel & Lunenfeld, 2004), skin (Krueguer et al., 1990) or nervous system (Hama et al., 1989). It has been shown that IL-6 also stimulates the development of many tumors, including melanoma, renal cell carcinoma, Kaposi's sarcoma, ovarian carcinoma, lymphoma and leukemia, multiple myeloma, prostate carcinoma and breast carcinoma (García-Tuñon et al., 2005; Hong et al., 2007; Rabinovich et al., 2007; Royuela et al., 2004).

First, IL-6 binds to IL-6Ra, which is unable to initiate signal transduction, and this complex attracts gp130 molecules, which dimerize leading to the intracellular signal by the activation of constituvely-associated gp130 Jak proteins (Heinrich et al., 1998; Hong et al., 2007; Silver & Hunter, 2010). In PC (prostate cancer) immunoreaction to IL-6 and gp-130 were increased. IL-6 signalling could be enhanced not only due to increased autocrine production but also increasing levels of this receptor (Rodriguez-Berriguete et al., 2010a; Royuela et al., 2004). Jak proteins can simultaneously trigger functionally distinct and even contradictory signaling pathways. One of them leads to the recruitment at the complex receptor of SHP2, Sos and Grb2, which in turn activates Ras by stimulating the exchange of GDP bound to Ras for GTP. Then, Ras initiates a MAPK cascade by phosphorylation of Raf-1 (Ancrile &

O'Hayer, 2008). Raf-1 activation might stimulate two different pathways. One pathway is initiated by MEK1/2 and the other with the activation of JNK. In prostate cancer expression of to Raf-1, MEK-1 and p-MEK were increased with Gleason grade (Rodruguez et al., 2010a). TNF-α is a 17 kDa polypeptide that has been implicated in skin carcinogenesis and in metastatic tumor spread of a variety of carcinomas and sarcomas. The action of TNF- α is mediated by two distinct receptors named TNF-receptor I (55 kDa, TNFRI) and receptor II (75 kDa, TNFRII) with similar affinity for TNF- α in human tissues (Loetscher et al., 1990; Smith et al., 1990). The domains of these receptors are different (Tartaglia et al., 1991). TNFRI is the major mediator of most TNF-α activity (Wiegmann et al., 1992). The expression and action of TNF- α and its receptors has been reported in several tumors such as esophageal (Hubel et al., 2000), prostate (De Miguel et al., 2000; Meshki et al., 2010), follicular thyroid (Zubelewicz et al., 2002), skin (Arnott et al., 2004), ovarian (Qiu et al., 2010; Rzymski et al., 2005) and breast (García-Tuñon et al., 2006) cancers.

In human prostate cancer, TNFα cascade seems to be over-stimulated since TNFα receptors (TNFRI and TNFRII) present high immunoexpression (Ricote et al., 2003). Binding of TNF-α/TNFRI complex to TNF receptor associated death domain proteins (TRADD) activates TRAF-2 (1 of the 6 members of the TNF receptor associated factor), which represents an integration point for pro-apoptotic and antiapoptotic signals (Wajant & Scheurich, 2001). TRAF-2 activation might stimulate two different pathways. One pathway is initiated by the interaction of TRAF-2 with the activation of NF-kB inducing kinase termed NIK, which is a MAP3K-related kinase that activates the IKK complex composed of IKK-α and IKK-β (Wu & Kral, 2005). In prostate cancer, NIK seems to be triggered by TNF/TRAF-2 or IL-1/IRAK/TRAF-6, since the presence of TNF, TNFRI and TRAF-2 has been described (De Miguel et al., 2000; Ricote et al., 2003), but also the presence of IL-1 family members (Nuñez et al., 2008; Ricote et al., 2004). NIK stimulate IKK-β, which induces IKK-α degradation. IKK complex phosphorylates IkB, following its ubiquitination and rapid degradation causing the nuclear translocation of NF-kB, which in turn, activates target genes involved in carcinogenesis: tumor initiation, malignant transformation and metastasis (Wu & Kral., 2005; Chengedza & Benbrook, 2010). In PC, TRAF-2 might be involved in the NIK activation pathway, although immunoexpression to TRAF-2 was detected in a low number of cases (decrease with Gleason grade), at the same time that the most of these patients were positives to NF-kB/p50 and NF-kB/p65 (Nuñez et al., 2008). These data, in addition with the elevated immunoexpressions to IL-1, IRAK, TRAF-6 and NIK observed in the same samples, suggest that NIK is stimulated by IL-1. Using the prostate carcinoma cell lines LNCaP, DU45 and PC3, Gasparian et al. (2009) found that increased IKK activation leads to the activation of NF-kB. A potential role of NF-kB in the development of different tumors as breast (Miller et al., 2000; Wu & Kral, 2005), colon (Dejardin et al., 1999; Wang S et al., 2009), pancreas (Wang W et al 1999; Eldor et al., 2009), thyroid (Visconti et al., 1997) or prostate (Nuñez et al., 2008; Domingo-Domenech et al., 2005) have been reported.

The other pathway activates the cascade ASK-1 (signal regulating kinase), MEK-4 (mitogen activated protein kinase-kinase 4) and Jun N-terminal kinase (JNK) (Royuela et al., 2008). When JNK is translocated to the nucleus is phosphorylated and activates transcription factors such as AP-1 or ATF-2. In all normal human prostates, positive immunoreactions to TRAF-2 and ASK1 (cytoplasm localization) MEK-4 (cytoplasm and nucleus localization) and JNK were found. Although in prostate cancer the transduction pathway from TRAF-2 to AP-1 seems to be inanctive, since immunoreaction to TRAF-2, ASK-1 And MEK-4 decreased and no immunoreaction to AP-1 was even found (Ricote et al., 2003; Royuela et al., 2008). The mechanism that accounts for the nuclear location MEK-4 is unclear, since this protein is activated by a cytoplasmic protein and phosphorylates JNK in the cytoplasm. However, MEK-4 function may not be restricted to the JNK signal transduction pathway because MEK-4 also phosphorylate and activates p38, and this latter is prelocalized in the nucleus and is rapidly exported to the cytoplasm upon activation (Taylor et al., 2008).

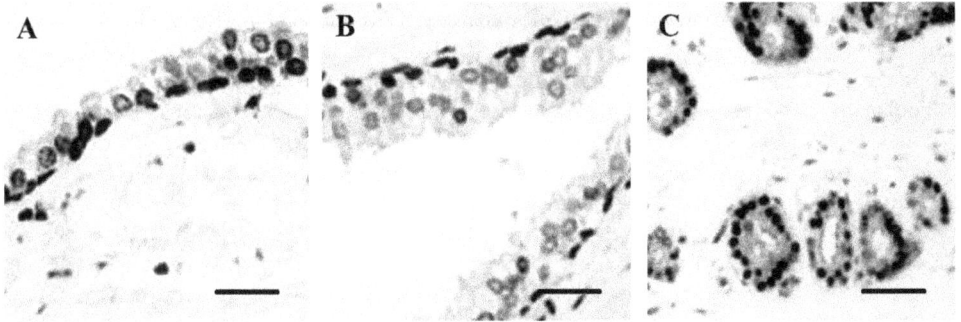

Fig. 2. JNK immunostaining appeared in normal (A), BPH (B) and PC (B) samples. Scale bars: 20 μm (A-B) and 30 μm (C).

JNK immunoreactiveness is increased in the glandular epithelium of PC specimens (Royuela et al., 2002; Shimada et al., 2006). With these data, Ricote et al. (2003) suggest that MEK-4 is not involved in JNK/AP-1 pathway, although it might be involved in p38 activation pathway. This hypothesis agrees with the high p38 levels found in normal prostate in our laboratory (Royuela et al., 2002). In this pathology there must be several extracellular or intracellular factors that are blocking the activation of this transduction pathway in different steps. ASK1 might be a critical blockage point of this transduction pathway. P21 has been reported as an ASK1 inhibitor and has been found significantly associated with a high Gleason score (Aaltomaa et al., 1999; Royuela et al., 2001). Bcl-2 has been postulated as a potential modulator of JNK activation in fibroblasts. Since an increase of bcl-2 has been reported in prostate cancer specimens, bcl-2 might be another potential inhibitor of JNK in prostate cancer (Haeusgen et al., 2010; Royuela et al., 2000). Ricote et al. (2006) reported in an *in vitro* study that JNK phosphorylation was found to be increased by TNF-α dose-dependent manner in LNCaP cells (but not in PC3 cells), and the rate of apoptosis was reduced by the administration of a specific JNK inhibitor, suggesting that JNK positively regulates apoptosis induction by TNF-α in this cell model.

Two opposite roles in the cell cycle control have been reported for JNK: cell proliferation and apoptosis. In contrast, JNK activation by some cytokines, such as TNF-α and IL-6, stimulates apoptosis. Since these two cytokines have been found increased in the prostatic epithelium of PC patients (Rodriguez-Berriguete et al., 2010a; Royuela et al., 2008), it might be that the increased apoptotic indexes in PC are related to the elevated levels of TNF-α, IL-6 and JNK. Nevertheless, the apoptotic mechanism stimulated by JNK is via p53 (Fuchs et al., 1998), but the p53 present in PC patients (Lee y cols., 2008), as occurs in most cancers is a mutant form with deletions or mutations which obstruct its association to JNK (Fuchs et al., 1998). Therefore, the elevated apoptotic rates in PC does not seem to be related to the high levels of cytokines and JNK in these patients but to other factors including the increased p38 levels mentioned above. Therefore, the most probable action of JNK in PC would be cell proliferation stimulation rather than apoptosis.

3. IL-1/ TNF/ p38

Several studies suggested that p38 play an important role in leukemia (Feng et al., 2009); lymphomas (Zheng et al., 2003) or tumor such as breast (Ancrile et al., 2008), prostate (Ricote et al., 2006a), gastrical (Guo et al., 2008) or lung (Zhang et al., 2010).

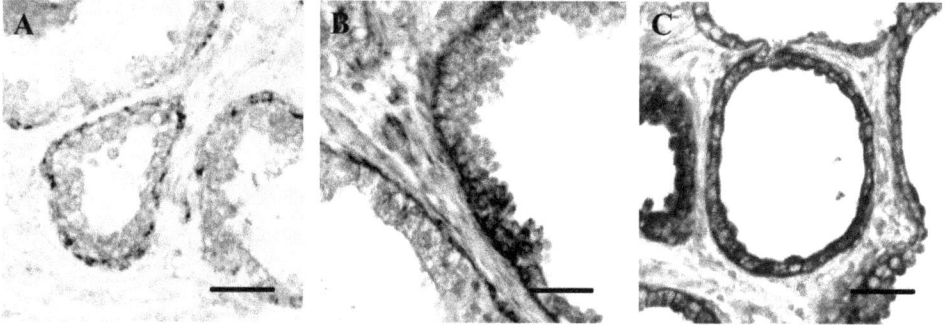

Fig. 3. p38 immunostaining appeared in normal (A), BPH (B) and PC (B) samples. Scale bars: 25 μm (B) 30 μm (A, C).

In addition to TNFα/AP1 pathway (by ASK-1 or MEK-4), Interleukin-1 (IL-1) is another physiological regulator of p38. IL-1 activates PAK-1 through its binding to two GTPases, called Cdc42 and Rac. These ones activate PAK-1, which induces MEK-6 activation that in turns activates p38 (Raingeaud et al., 1995).

Several reports about IL-1 family in cancer have been reported. IL-1α, IL-1β and IL-1Ra have been detected in human breast cancer, and have been related to protumorigenic activity (Miller et al., 2010). The number of men showing IL-1β immunoexpression is lower in prostate cancer group than in normal prostate group but most cancer patients studied presented immunoreaction to IL-1α, IL-1RI, IL-1RII and IL-1Ra [60]. The interaction between IL-1α and IL-RI would be involved in the high proliferation degree of these tumors. No association between IL-1 and IL-1Ra has also been reported in premalignant gastric conditions (Kupcinskas et al., 2010).

In human prostate cancer, intense immnoreaction to PAK-1, MEK-6 and p38 were found but also to p-Elk-1 and p-ATF-2 whose location change from the nucleus to the cytoplasm (Ricote et al., 2006a; Rodriguez-Berriguete et al., 2010b). This fact may be related with its biological function. In mammalian cells, endogenous p38 is present in the nucleus but it can be exported to the cytoplasm upon activation (Ricote et al., 2006). Recently, Wood et al. (2009) described nuclear localization of p38 in response to DNA damage. In the nucleus, p38 phosphorylates Elk-1, ATF-2 and also NF-kB (Junttila et al., 2008; Raingeaud et al., 1995; Royuela et al., 2008). ATF-2 (Li & Wicks, 2001) and Elk-1 (Amorino & Parsons, 2004) are not only a target of p38 but also a target for JNK. Since immunoreaction to JNK was found in normal human prostate, but not in prostate cancer, is reasonable to suggest that the activation of ATF-2 and Elk-1 are the consequence of p38 pathway activation (Ricote et al.,

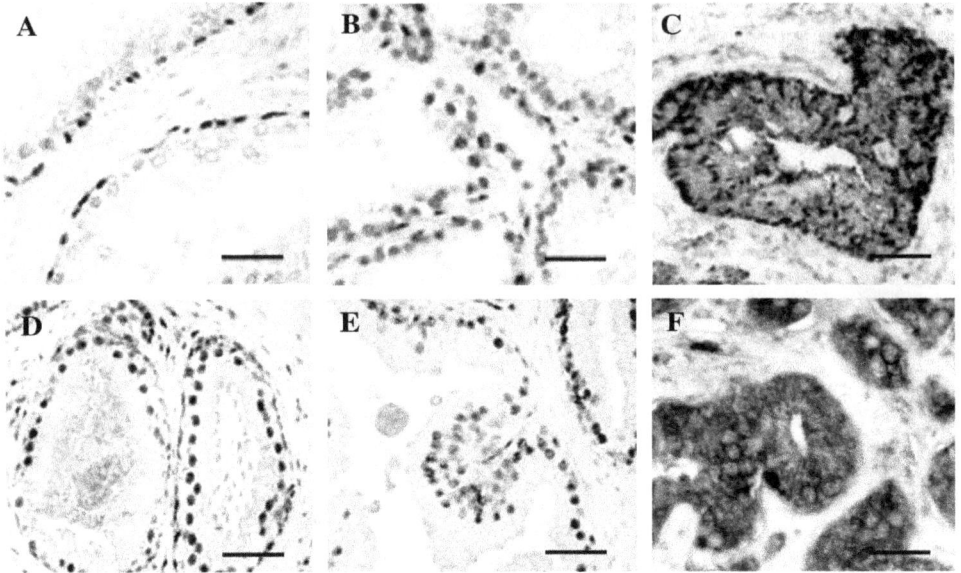

Fig. 4. Nuclear immunoreaction to p-Elk-1 appeared in the epithelial basal cells of normal prostate (A) or all epithelial cells in BPH (B). In PC samples p-Elk-1 (C) was observed in the cytoplasm. p-ATF-2 immunostaining was localised in the nuclei of epithelial cells in normal prostate (D) but more intense in BPH (E) and PC (F). Scale bar: 20 μm (B, E) and 25 μm (A, C-D, F).

2006a). However, the TNF-α signal may be diverted from the Ap-1 pathway towards the p38 pathway, because MEK-4 may also phosphorylate and activate p38 and ASK-1 may activate MEK-6, which, in turn, phosphorylates p38 (Stein et al., 1996). Proapoptotic effects of TNFα/AP-1 pathway decrease, because this pathway is inhibited by p21 at ASK1 step (Ricote et al., 2003). Cell proliferation stimulation triggered by TNFα via p38 occurs, since intense immunoreaction to PAK-1 and MEK-6 was found (Ricote et al., 2006a), but previous studies have shown elevated levels of IL-1 (Ricote et al., 2004) and p38 (Royuela et al., 2002). Ricote et al. (2006)b using LNCaP cells suggest that p38 plays an important role in prostatic tumor promotion by TNFα stimulation, and hence may represent a target for the treatment of prostatic cancer. Treatment with the p38 inhibitor SB203580 caused a notable increase in the frequency of apoptosis in LNCaP cell cultures, indicating that p38 exerts an anti-apoptotic action in this cell line (Ricote et al., 2006). Noted that LNCaP cells represent a good model of well-differentiated tumor and as such its behavior is more comparable to the in vivo tumor condition. In this way, Thornton and Rincon (2009) considered the potential use of pharmacological inhibitors of p38 in therapeutic treatment for several diseases.

4. TNF/IL-1/IL-6/ERK

When IL-6 and IL-6Rα induces dimerization of gp130, and subsequently the activation of constituvely-associated gp130 Jak proteins, simultaneously trigger functionally distinct and even contradictory signaling pathways. One of them leads to the recruitment at the complex receptor of SHP2, Sos and Grb2, which in turn activates Ras by stimulating the exchange of

GDP bound to Ras for GTP (Silver & Hunter, 2010). Then, Ras phosphorylate of Raf-1. In this way is iniciate a MAPK cascade when Raf-1 (via IL-6 pathway), TRAF-2 (via TNF pathway) or TRAF-6 (via Il-6 pathway) phosphorylate sequentially MEK1/2 and ERK1/2, in a process that culminates in modulation of gene transcription through the activation of several transcription factors such as c-Myc, Elk-1 (Werlen et al., 2003) or NF-kB (Turjanski et al., 2007).

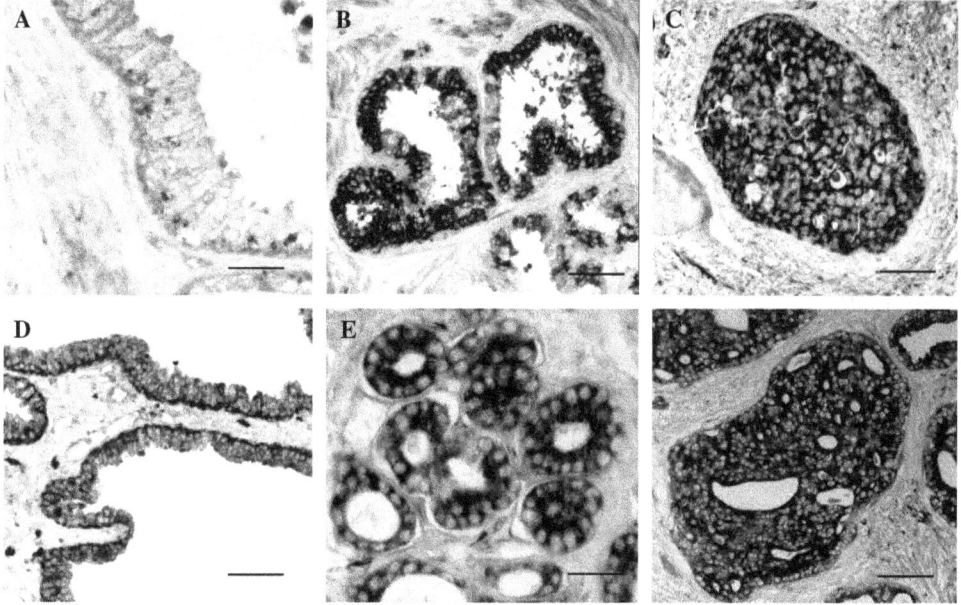

Fig. 5. P50 was scantly in the cytoplasm epithelial cells of normal (A) but in PC immunostaining also was nuclear, increasing the expression in medium (B) and after, in high (C) Gleason. No immunoreaction was found to p65 in normal prostate but was localized in the cytoplasm of epithelial cells in BPH (D) and PC (E-F) samples; but in PC was also localized in the nuclei of epithelial increasing nuclear localization with Gleason grade. Scale bars: 20 μm (A), 25 μm (B-C, E-F) and 30 μm (D).

Some components of the Raf-MEK-ERK pathway are activated in solid tumors and hematological malignaces (Grant, 2008; McCubrey et al., 2007).
In approximately 30% of human breast cancers, mutations are found in the ERK1/2 MAPK pathway (Whyte et al., 2009). ERK1/2 and downstream ERK1/2 targets are hyper-phosphorylated in a large subset of mammary tumors (Mueller et al., 2000). Increased expressions of Raf pathway has been associated with advance prostate cancer, hormonal independence, metastasis and a poor prognosis (Keller et al., 2004). Moreover, prostate cancer cell lines isolated from advanced cancer patients (LNCaP, PC3, DU145) expressed low levels of active Raf kinase inhibitors (McCubrey et al., 2007). TNFα acts as an ERK activator in some cases related to inflammation and cell proliferation. In this way, Ricote et al. (2006b) showed that ERK phosphorylation was notably increased by TNFα dose dependent manner in LNCaP cells. In prostate cancer, presence of Raf-1 and MEK-1 in

conjunction with elevated ERK-1 and ERK-2 suggest that stimulation of cell proliferation could be triggered by IL-6 via the ERK pathway (Rodriguez-Berriguete et al., 2010a). In this way, Ricote et al. (2006b) in *in vitro* studies with LNCaP cells, showed that the use of specific ERK inhibitor minimally affected apoptosis, suggesting that ERK activation does not play a significant role in apoptosis regulation.

Moreover, ERK may also induce the phosphorilation of apoptotic regulatory molecules including bcl-2 family members (e.g. Bad, Bim and controversially Bcl-2) and caspase 9 (McCubrey et al., 2007). There are evidences suggesting a protective effect in cells by NF-kB activation via ERK (Chu et al., 2008; Zhu et al., 2004). This transcription factor in a basal state is retained in the cytoplasm by binding to specific inhibitors, the inhibitors of NF-kB (IkBs). Upon cell stimulation IkBs are degradated and consequently NF-kB is translocated into the nucleus (Karin, 2006), where it promotes the expression of several anti-apoptotic genes such as inhibitors of apoptosis proteins (IAPs) (Rodriguez-Berriguete et al., 2010) and bcl-2 family members (Aggarwal, 2000).

5. New perspectives

In summary, it is reasonable to speculate that MAPK could be involved in prostate cancer development, maintenance and/or progression, since are involucrate in several transduction pathway related with prostate cancer development. These transduction pathways were interrelated and activated by pro-inflammatory (IL-6, IL-1 and TNF). At the end are activated several transcription factor such as NF-kB, Elk-1, ATF-2, p53, or mcl-1. Translocation of NF-kB to the nucleus in PC might be due to the overactivation of several transduction pathways triggered by pro-inflammatory cytokines (IL-1, IL-6 and TNF-α). NF-kB has been considered a marker of predicting PC since nuclear localization was only observed in PC, but another transcription factor activate by these pro-inflammatory cytokines relate with cell proliferation such as Elk-1, ATF-2 or c-myc were also increased in PC. For this, might be that overexpression of MAPKs might be secondary to overexpression of these cytokines and, subsequently, MAPKs also might be involved in the development of prostatic hyperplasia and neoplasia. Therefore, since PC is a heterogeneous disease in which multiple transduction pathways may contribute to uncontrolled apoptosis/cell proliferation balance, we concluded that significant attention would be focused to the rational combination of novel agents directed toward the inactivation of pro-inflammatory cytokines, because could be disrupt complementary tumor cell proliferation pathways.

6. Acknowledgements

Supported by grants from the "Ministerio de Educación y Ciencia", Spain (SAF2007-61928) and the "Fundación Mutua Madrileña, 2010" (Spain). Gonzalo Rodríguez-Berriguete had a predoctoral fellowship from the Alcalá University (Madrid, Spain) during the course of this work.

7. References

Aaltomaa, S.; Lipponen, P.; Eskelinen, M.; Ala-Opas, M.; Kosma, V.M. (1999). Prognostic value and expression of p21 (waf1/cip1) protein in prostate cancer. *The Prostate*, Vol. 39, No. 1 (Apr 1), pp. 8-15, ISSN: 0270-4137.

Aggarwal, B.B. (2000). Tumour necrosis factors receptor associated signalling molecules and their role in activation of apoptosis, JNK and NF-kappaB. *Annals of the Rheumatic Diseases*, Vol. 59, Supp l (Nov), pp.i6-16., ISSN: 1468-2060.

Amorino, G.P. & Parsons, S.J. (2004). Neuroendocrine cells in prostate cancer. *Critical Reviews in Eukaryotic Gene Expression*, Vol. 14, No. 4, pp. 287-300. ISSN: 1045-4403.

Ancrile, B.B.; O'Hayer, K.M.; Counter, C.M. (2008). Oncogenic ras-induced expression of cytokines: a new target of anti-cancer therapeutics. *Molecular Interventions*, Vol. 8, No. 1 (Feb), pp: 22-27, ISSN: 1534-0384.

Arnott, C.H.; Scott, K.A.; Moore, R.J.; Robinson, S.C.; Thompson, R.G.; Balkwill, F.R. (2004). Expression of both TNF-alpha receptor subtypes is essential for optimal skin tumour development. *Oncogene*, Vol. 23, No. 10 (Mar 11), pp. 1902-1910, ISSN: 0950-9232.

Bode, A.M. & Dong, Z. (2007). The functional contrariety of JNK. *Molecular Carcinogenesis*, Vol. 46, No. 8 (Aug), pp. 591-598, ISSN: 0899-1987.

Bogoyevitch, M.A.; Ngoei, K.R.; Zhao, T.T.; Yeap, Y.Y.; Ng, D.C. (2010). c-Jun N-terminal kinase (JNK) signaling: recent advances and challenges. *Biochimica et Biophysica Acta*, Vol. 1804, No.3 (Mar), pp. 463-475, ISSN: 0006-3002.

Chang, H.L.; Wu, Y.C.; Su, J.H.; Yeh, Y.T.; Yuan, S.S. (2008). Protoapigenone, a novel flavonoid, induces apoptosis in human prostate cancer cells through activation of p38 mitogen-activated protein kinase and c-Jun NH2-terminal kinase 1/2. *Journal of Pharmacology and Experimental Therapeutics*, Vol. 325, No. 3 (Jun), pp. 841-849, ISSN: 0022-3565.

Chengedza, S. & Benbrook, D.M. (2010). NF-kappaB is involved in SHetA2 circumvention of TNF-alpha resistance, but not induction of intrinsic apoptosis. *Anticancer Drugs*, Vol. 21, No. 3 (Mar), pp. 297-305, ISSN: 0959-4973.

Chu, L.F.; Wang, W.T.; Ghanta, V.K.; Lin, C.H.; Chiang, Y.Y.; Hsueh, C,M. (2008). Ischemic brain cell-derived conditioned medium protects astrocytes against ischemia through GDNF/ERK/NF-kB signaling pathway. *Brain Research*, Vol. 1239 (Nov 6), pp. 24-35, ISSN: 0006-8993.

Cross, T.G.; Scheel-Toellner, D.; Henriquez, N.V.; Deacon, E.; Salmon, M.; Lord, J.M. (2000). Serine/threonine protein kinases and apoptosis. *Experimental Cell Research*, Vol. 256, No. 1 (Apr 10), 34-41, ISSN: 0014-4827.

Cullen, P.J. & Lockyer, P.J. (2002). Intergration of calcium and Ras signaling. *Nature Reviews Molecular Cell Biology*, Vol. 3, No. 5 (May), pp. 339-348. ISSN: 1471-0072.

Dejardin, E.; Deregowski, V.; Chapelier, M.; Jacobs, N.; Gielen, J.; Merville, M.; Bours, V. (1999). Regulation of NF-iB activity by IiBrelated proteins in adenocarcinoma cells. *Oncogene*, Vol. 18, No. 16 (Apr 22), pp. 2567-2577, ISSN: 0950-9232.

De Graeve, F.; Bahr, A.; Sabapathy, K.T.; Hauss, C.; Wagner, E.F.; Kedinger, C.; Chatton, B. (1999). Role of the ATFa/JNK2 complex in Jun activation. *Oncogene*, Vol. 18, No. 23 (Jun 10), pp. 3491-3500, ISSN: 0950-9232.

De Miguel, M.P.; Royuela, M.; Bethencourt, F.R.; Santamaria, L.; Fraile, B.; Paniagua, R. (2000). Immuno-expression of tumor necrosis factor-a and its receptors 1 and 2 correlates with proliferation/apoptosis equilibrium in normal, hyperplasic and carcinomatous human prostate. *Cytokine*, Vol. 12, No. 5, (May), pp. 535-538, ISSN: 1043-4666.

Dérijard, B.; Hibi, M.; Wu, I-H.; Barrett, T.; Su, B.; Deng, T.; Karin, M.; Davis, R.J. (1994). JNK1: a protein kinase stimulated by UV light and Ha-Ras that binds and phosphorylates the c-Jun activation domain. *Cell*, Vol. 76, No. 6 (Mar 25), pp. 1025-1037, ISSN: 0092-8674.

Dhillon, A.S.; Hagan, S.; Rath, O.; Kolch, W. (2007). MAP kinase signalling pathways in cancer. *Oncogene*, Vol. 26, No. 22 (May 14) pp. 3279-3290, ISSN: 0950-9232.

Domingo-Domenech, J.; Mellado, B.; Ferrer, B.; Truan, D.; Codony-Servat, J.; Sauleda, S.; Alcover, J.; Campo, E.; Gascon, P.; Rovira, A.; Ross, J.S.; Fernandez, P.L.; Albanell, J. (2005). Activation of nuclear factor-kappaB in human prostate carcinogenesis and association to biochemical relapse. British Journal of Cancer, Vol. 93, No. 11 (Nov 28), pp. 1285-1294, ISSN: 0007-0920.

English, J.M.; Pearson, G.; Baer, R.; Cobb, M.H. (1998). Identification of substrates and regulators of the mitogen-activated protein kinase ERK5 using chimeric protein kinases. *The Journal of Biological Chemistry*, Vol. 273, No. 7 (Feb 13), pp. 3854-3860, ISSN: 0021-9258.

Eisinger, D.A. & Ammer, H. (2008). Delta-opioid receptors activate ERK/MAP kinase via integrinstimulated receptor tyrosine kinases. *Cellular Signalling*; Vol. 20, No. 12(Dec), pp. 2324-2331, ISSN: 0898-6568.

Davis, R.J. (2000). Signal transduction by the JNK group of MAP kinases. *Cell*, Vol. 103, No. 2 (Oct 13), pp. 239-252, ISSN: 0092-8674.

Eldor, R.; Baum. K.; Abel, R.; Sever, D.; Melloul, D. (2009). The ToI-beta transgenic mouse: a model to study the specific role of NF-kappaB in beta-cells. *Diabetes Research and Clinical Practice*, Vol. 86, Suppl 1 (Dec), pp. S7-14, ISSN: 0168-8227.

Feng, Y.; Wen, J.; Chang, C.C. (2009). p38 Mitogen-activated protein kinase and hematologic malignancies. *Archives of Pathology & Laboratory Medicine*, Vol. 133, No. 11 (Nov), pp. 1850-1856, ISSN: 0003-9985.

Fuchs, S.Y.; Adler, V.; Pincus, M.R.; Ronai, Z. (1998). MEKK1/JNK signaling stabilizes and activates p53. *Proceedings of the National Academy of Sciences of the United States of America*, Vol. 95, No. 18 (Sep 1), pp. 10541-10546, ISSN: 0027-8424.

Gao, L.; Chao, L.; Chao, J. (2010). A novel signaling pathway of tissue kallikrein in promoting keratinocyte migration: Activation of proteinase-activated receptor 1 and epidermal growth factor receptor. *Experimental Cell Research*, Vol. 316, No. 3 (Feb 1), pp. 376-389, ISSN: 0014-4827.

Garcia-Tuñon, I.; Ricote, M.; Ruiz, A.; Fraile, B.; Paniagua, R.; Royuela, M. (2005). IL-6, its receptors and its relationship with bcl-2 and bax proteins in infiltrating and in situ human breast carcinoma. *Histopathology*, Vol. 47, No. 1 (Jul), pp.82-89, ISSN: 1365-2559.

Garcia-Tuñon, I.; Ricote, M.; Ruiz, A.; Fraile, B.; Paniagua, R.; Royuela, M. (2006). Role of tumor necrosis factor-alpha and its receptors in human benign breast lesions and tumors (in situ and infiltrative). *Cancer Science*, Vol. 97, No. 10 (Oct), pp. 1044-1049, ISSN: 1349-7006.

Gasparian, A.V.; Guryanova, O.A.; Chebotaev, D.V.; Shishkin, A.A.; Yemelyanov, A.Y.; Budunova, I.V. (2009). Targeting transcription factor NFkappaB: comparative analysis of proteasome and IKK inhibitors. *Cell Cycle*, Vol. 8, No. 10 (May 15), pp. 1559-1566, ISSN: 1538-4101.

Grant, S. (2008). Cotargeting survival signaling pathways in cancer. *The Journal Of Clinical Investigation*, Vol. 118, No. 9 (Sep), pp. 3003-3006, ISSN:0021-9738.

Guo, X.; Ma, N.; Wang, J.; Song, J.; Bu, X.; Cheng, Y.; Sun, K.; Xiong, H.; Jiang, G.; Zhang, B.; Wu, M.; Wei, L. (2008). Increased p38-MAPK is responsible for chemotherapy resistance in human gastric cancer cells. *BMC Cancer*, Vol. 8 (Dec 18), pp. 375, ISSN 1471-2407.

Gupta, S.; Barrett, T.; Whitmarsh, A.J.; Cavanagh, J.; Sluss, H.K.; Dérijard, B.; Davis, R.J. (1996). Selective interaction of JNK protein kinase isoforms with transcription factors. *The EMBO Journal*, Vol. 15, No. 11 (Jun 3), pp. 2760-2770, ISSN 0261-4189.

Haeusgen, W.; Herdegen, T.; Waetzig, V. (2010). Specific regulation of JNK signalling by the novel rat MKK7gamma1 isoform. *Cellular Signalling* Vol. 22, No. 11 (Nov), pp. 1761-1772, ISSN: 0898-6568.

Hama, T.; Miyamoto, M.; Tsuki, H.; Nishio, C.; Hatanaka, M. (1989). Interleukin-6 is a neurotrophic factor for promoting the survival of cultured basal forebrain cholinergic neurons fron postnatal rats. *Neuroscience Letters*, Vol. 104, No. 3 (Oct 9), 340-344, ISSN: 0304-3940.

Hayashi, M.; Lee, J.D. (2004). Role of the BMK1/ERK5 signaling pathway: lessons from knockout mice. Journal of Molecular Medicine, Vol. 82, No. 12 (Dec), pp. 800-808, ISSN: 0946-2716.

Heasley, L.E. & Han, S.Y. (2006). JNK regulation of oncogenesis. *Molecular Cell*, Vol. 21, No. 2 (Apr 30), pp. 167-173, ISSN 1097-2765.

Heinrich, P.C.; Behrmann, I.; Mueller-Newen, G.; Shaper, F.; Graeve, L. (1998). Interleukin 6-type cytokine signaling throught the gp130/jak/stat pathways. *Biochemical Journal*, Vol. 334, Pt. 2 (Sep 1), pp. 297-314, ISSN: 0264-6021.

Hong, D.S.; Angelo, L.S.; Kurzrock, R. (2007). Interleukin-6 and its receptor in cancer: implications for Translational Therapeutics. *Cancer*, Vol. 110 No. 9 (Nov 1), pp. 1911-1928, ISSN: 1097-0142.

Hubel, K.; Mansmann, G.; Schafer, H.; Oberhauser, F.; Diehl, V.; Engert, A. (2000). Increase of anti-inflammatory cytokines in patients with esophageal cancer after perioperative treatment with G-CSF. *Cytokine*, Vol. 12, No. 12 (Dec), pp. 1797-1800, ISSN: 1043-4666.

Hui, L.; Bakiri, L.; Stepniak, E.; Wagner, E.F. (2007). p38alpha: a suppressor of cell proliferation and tumorigenesis. *Cell Cycle*, Vol. 6, No. 20 (Oct 15), pp. 2429-2433, ISSN: 1551-4005.

Huleihel, M.; Lunenfeld, E. (2004). Regulation of spermatogenesis by paracrine/autocrine testicular factors. *Asian Journal of Andrology*, Vol. 6, No. 3 (Sep), pp. 259-268, ISSN: 1008-682X.

Hunter, T. (2000). Signaling -2000 and beyond. *Cell*, Vol. 100, No. 1 (Jan 7), pp. 113-127, ISSN: 0092-8674.

Jiang, Y.; Li, Z.; Schwarz, E.M.; Lin, A.; Guan, K.; Ulevitch, R.J.; Han, J. (1997). Structure-function studies of p38 mitogen-activated protein kinase. Loop 12 influences substrate specificity and autophosphorylation, but not upstream kinase selection. *The Journal of Biological Chemistry*, Vol. 272, No. 17 (Apr 25), pp. 11096-11102, ISSN: 0021-9258.

Joo, S.S.; Yoo, Y.M. (2009). Melatonin induces apoptotic death in LNCaP cells via p38 and JNK pathways: therapeutic implications for prostate cancer. *Journal of Pineal Research*, Vol. 47, No. 1 (Aug), pp. 8-14, ISSN: 1600-079X.

Joslin, E.J.; Opresko, L.K.; Wells, A.; Wiley, H.S.; Lauffenburger, D.A. (2007). EGF-receptor-mediated mammary epithelial cell migration is driven by sustained ERK signaling from autocrine stimulation. *Journal of Cell Science*, Vol. 120, Pt. 20 (Oct 15), pp. 3688-3699, ISSN: 0370-2952.

Junttila, M.R.; Li, S.P.; Westermarck, J. (2008). Phosphatase-mediated crosstalk between MAPK signaling pathways in the regulation of cell survival. *The FASEB Journal*, Vol. 22, No. 4 (Apr), pp. 954-965, ISSN: 0892-6638.

Karin, M. (2006). Nuclear factor-kappaB in cancer development and progression. *Nature*, Vol. 441, No. 7092 (May 25), pp. 431-436, ISSN : 0028-0836.

Keller, E.T.; Fu, Z.; Yeung, K.; Brennan, M. (2004). Raf kinase inhibitor protein: a prostate cancer metastasis suppressor gene. *Cancer Letters*, Vol. 207, No. 2 (Apr 30), pp. 131-137, ISSN: 0304-3835.

Kato, Y.; Kravchenko, V.V.; Tapping, R.I.; Han, J.; Ulevitch, R.J.; Lee, J.D. (1997). BMK1/ERK5 regulates serum-induced early gene expression through transcription factor MEF2C. *The EMBO Journal*, Vol. 16, No. 23 (Dec 1), pp. 7054-7066, ISSN 0261-4189.

Kato, Y.; Tapping, R.I.; Huang, S.; Watson, M.H.; Ulevitch, R.J.; Lee, J.D. (1998). Bmk1/Erk5 is required for cell proliferation induced by epidermal growth factor. *Nature*, Vol. 395, No. 6703 (Oct 15), pp. 713-716, ISSN : 0028-0836.

Kamakura, S.; Moriguchi, T.; Nishida, E. (1999). Activation of the protein kinase ERK5/BMK1 by receptor tyrosine kinases. Identification and characterization of a signalling pathway to the nucleus. *The Journal of Biological Chemistry*, Vol. 274, No. 37 (Sep 10), pp. 26563-26571, ISSN: 0021-9258

Kayahara, M.; Wang, X.; Tournier, C. (2005). Selective regulation of c-jun gene expression by mitogen-activated protein kinases via the 12-o-tetradecanoylphorbol-13-acetate-responsive element and myocyte enhancer factor 2 binding sites. *Molecular and Cellular Biology*, Vol. 25, No. 9 (May), pp. 3784-3792, ISSN: 0270-7306.

Khalaf, H.; Jass, J.; Olsson, P.E. (2010). Differential cytokine regulation by NF-kappaB and AP-1 in Jurkat T-cells. *BMC Immunology*, Vol. 11 (May 27), pp. 26, ISSN: 1471-2172.

Kholodenko, B.N. & Birtwistle, M.R. (2009). Four-dimensional dynamics of MAPK information processing systems. *Wiley interdisciplinary reviews. Systems biology and medicine*, Vol. 1, No. 1 (Jul-Aug), pp. 28-44, ISSN:1939-5094.

Khwaja, F.S.; Quann, E.J.; Pattabiraman, N.; Wynne, S.; Djakiew, D. (2008). Carprofen induction of p75NTR-dependent apoptosis via the p38 mitogen-activated protein kinase pathway in prostate cancer cells. *Molecular Cancer Therapeutics*, Vol. 7, No. 11 (Nov), pp. 3539-3545, ISSN: 1535-7163.

Kim, E.K. & Choi, E.J. (2010)Pathological roles of MAPK signaling pathways in human diseases. *Biochimica et Biophysica Acta (BBA)*, Vol. 1802, No. 4 (Apr), 396-405, ISSN 0005-2736.

Kupcinskas, L.; Wex, T.; Kupcinskas, J.; Leja, M.; Ivanauskas, A.; Jonaitis, L.V.; Janciauskas, D.; Kiudelis, G.; Funka, K.; Sudraba, A.; Chiu, H.M.; Lin, J.T.; Malfertheiner, P. (2010). Interleukin-1B and interleukin-1 receptor antagonist gene polymorphisms are not associated with premalignant gastric conditions: a combined haplotype analysis. *European Journal of Gastroenterology and Hepatology*, Vol. 22, No. 10 (Oct), pp. 1189-1195, ISSN: 0954-691X.

Kurihara, N.; Bertolini, D.; Suda, T.; Akiyama, Y.; Roodman, G.D. (1990). IL-6 stimulates osteoclast-like multinucleated cell formation in long term human marrow cultures by inducing IL-1 release. *The Journal of Immunology*, Vol. 144, No. 11 (Jun 1), pp. 4226-30, ISSN: 0022-1767.

Krueguer, J.; Krane, J.; Carter, D.; Gottlieb, A. (1990). Role of growth factors, cytokines, and their receptors in the pathogenesis of psoriasis. *Journal of Investigative Dermatology*, Vol. 94, No. 6 Suppl (Jun), pp. 135S-140S, ISSN: 0022-202X.

Lee, J.D.; Ulevitch, R.J.; Han, J. (1995). Primary structure of BMK1: a new mammalian map kinase. *Biochemical and Biophysical Research Communications*, Vol. 213, No. 2 (Aug 15), pp. 715-724, ISSN: 0006-291X.

Lee, J.J.; Lee, J.H.; Ko, Y.G.; Hong, S.I.; Lee, J.S. (2010). Prevention of premature senescence requires JNK regulation of Bcl-2 and reactive oxygen species. *Oncogene*, Vol. 29, No. 4 (Jan 28), pp. 561-575, ISSN: 0950-9232.

Lee, J.T.; Lehmann, B.D.; Terrian, D.M.; Chappell, W.H.; Stivala, F.; Libra, M.; Martelli, A.M.; Steelman, L.S.; McCubrey, J.A. (2008). Targeting prostate cancer based on signal transduction and cell cycle pathways. *Cell Cycle*, Vol. 7, No. 12 (Jun 15), pp. 1745-1762, ISSN: 1551-4005.

Li, H. & Wicks, W.D. (2001). Retinoblastoma protein interacts with ATF2 and JNK/p38 in stimulating the transforming growth factor-beta2 promoter. *Archives of Biochemistry and Biophysics*, Vol. 394, No. 1 (Oct 1), pp. 1-12, ISSN: 0003-9861.

Liu, Y.; Formisano, L.; Savtchouk, I.; Takayasu, Y.; Szabó, G.; Zukin, R.S.; Liu, S.J. (2010). A single fear-inducing stimulus induces a transcription-dependent switch in synaptic AMPAR phenotype. *Nature Neuroscience*, Vol. 13, No. 2 (Feb), pp. 223-231, ISSN: 1097-6256.

Loetscher, H.; Pan, Y.C.; Lahm, H.W.; Gentz, R.; Brockhaus, M.; Tabuchi, H.; Lesslauer, W. (1990). Molecular cloning and expression of the human 55 kd tumor necrosis factor receptor. *Cell*, Vol. 61, No. 2 (Apr 20), pp. 351-359, ISSN: 0092-8674.

Marais, R. & Marshall, C.J. (1996). Control of the ERK MAP kinase cascade by ras and raf. Cancer Surveys, Vol. 27, pp. 101-25, ISSN: 0261-2429.

McCracken, S.R.; Ramsay, A.; Heer, R.; Mathers, M.E.; Jenkins, B.L.; Edwards, J.; Robson, C.N.; Marquez, R.; Cohen, P.; Leung, H.Y. (2008). Aberrant expression of extracellular signal-regulated kinase 5 in human prostate cancer. *Oncogene*, Vol. 27, No. 21 (May 8), pp. 2978-2988, ISSN: 0950-9232.

McCubrey, J.A.; Steelman, L.S.; Chappell, W.H.; Abrams, S.L.; Wong, E.W.; Chang, F.; Lehmann, B.; Terrian, D.M.; Milella, M.; Tafuri, A.; Stivala, F.; Libra, M.; Basecke, J.; Evangelisti, C.; Martelli, A.M.; Franklin, R.A. (2007). Roles of the Raf/MEK/ERK pathway in cell growth, malignant transformation and drug resistance. *Biochimica et Biophysica Acta (BBA)*, Vol. 1773, No. 8 (Aug), pp. 1263-1284, ISSN: 0005-2736.

Mechergui, Y.B., Ben Jemaa, A.; Mezigh, C.; Fraile, B.; Ben Rais, N.; Paniagua, R.; Royuela, M.; Oueslati, R. (2009). The profile of prostate epithelial cytokines and its impact on sera prostate specific antigen levels. *Inflammation*, Vol. 32, No. 3 (Jun), pp. 202-210, ISSN: 0360-3997.

Meshki, J.; Caino, M.C.; von Burstin, V.A.; Griner, E.M.; Kazanietz, M.G. (2010). Regulation of prostate cancer cell survival by protein kinase C {epsilon} involves Bad phosphorylation and modulation of the TNF{alpha}/JNK pathway. *The Journal of Biological Chemistry*, Vol. 285, No. 34 (Aug 20), pp. 26033-26040, ISSN: 0021-9258

Miller, L.J.; Kurtzman, S.H.; Anderson, K.; Wang, Y.; Stankus, M.; Renna, M.; Lindquist, R.; Barrows, G.; Kreutzer, D.L. (2000). Interleukin-1 family expre-ssion in human breast cancer: interleukin-1 receptor antagonist. *Cancer Investigation*, Vol. 18, No. 4, pp. 293-302, ISSN: 0735-7907.

Miller, S.C.; Huang, R.; Sakamuru, S.; Shukla, S.J.; Attene-Ramos, M.S.; Shinn, P.; Van Leer, D.; Leister, W.; Austin, C.P.; Xia, M. (2010). Identification of known drugs that act as inhibitors of NF-kappaB signaling and their mechanism of action. *Biochemical Pharmacology*, Vol. 79, No. 9 (May 1), pp. 1272-1280, ISSN: 0006-2952.

Mueller, H.; Flury, N.; Eppenberger-Castori, S.; Kueng, W.; David, F.; Eppenberger, U. (2000). Potential prognostic value of mitogen-activated protein kinase activity for disease-free survival of primary breast cancer patients. *International Journal of Cancer*, Vol. 89, No. 4 (Jul 20), pp. 384-388, ISSN: 0020-7136.

Nuñez, C.; Cansino, J.R.; Bethencourt, F.; Pérez-Utrilla, M.; Fraile, B.; Martínez-Onsurbe, P.; Olmedilla, G.; Paniagua, R.; Royuela, M. (2008). TNF/IL-1/NIK/NF-kappa B transduction pathway: a comparative study in normal and pathological human prostate (benign hyperplasia and carcinoma). *Histopathology*, Vol. 53, No. 2 (Aug), pp. 166-176, ISSN: 0213-3911.

Pagès, G.; Milanini, J.; Richard, D.E.; Berra, E.; Gothié, E.; Viñals, F.; Pouysségur, J. (2000). Signaling angiogenesis via p42/p44 MAP kinase cascade. *Annals of the New York Academy of Sciences*, Vol. 902 (May), pp. 187-200, ISSN: 0077-8923.

Pearson, G.; Robinson, F.; Beers Gibson, T.; Xu, B.E.; Karandikar, M.; Berman, K.; Cobb, M.H. (2001). Mitogen-activated protein (MAP) kinase pathways: regulation and physiological functions. *Endocrine Reviews*, Vol. 22, No. 2 (Apr), pp. 153-183, ISSN: 0163-769X.

Peng, S.; Zhang, Y.; Zhang, J.; Wang, H.; Ren B. (2010). ERK in learning and memory: A review of recent research. *International Journal of Molecular Sciences*, Vol. 11, No. 1 (Jan 13), pp. 222-232, ISSN: 1422-0067.

Pi, X.; Yan, C.; Berk, B.C. (2004). Big mitogen-activated protein kinase (BMK1)/ERK5 protects endothelial cells from apoptosis. *Circulation Research*, Vol. 94, No. 3 (Feb 20), pp. 362-369, ISSN: 0009-7330.

Price, D.J.; Avraham, S.; Feuerstein, J.; Fu, Y.; Avraham, H.K. (2002). The invasive phenotype in HMT-3522 cells requires increased EGF receptor signaling through both PI 3-kinase and ERK 1,2 pathways. *Cell Communication and Adhesion*, Vol. 9, No. 2 (Mar-Apr), pp. 87-102, ISSN: 1543-5180.

Qiu, J.; Xiao, J.; Han, C.; Li, N.; Shen, X.; Jiang, H.; Cao, X. (2010). Potentiation of tumor necrosis factor-alpha-induced tumor cell apoptosis by a small molecule inhibitor for anti-apoptotic protein hPEBP4. *The Journal of Biological Chemistry*, Vol. 285, No. 16 (Apr 16), pp. 12241-12247, ISSN: 0021-9258.

Rabinovich, A.; Medina, L.; Piura, B.; Segal, S.; Huleihel, M. (2007). Regulation of ovarian carcinoma SKOV-3 cell proliferation and secretion of MMPs by autocrine IL-6. *Anticancer Research*, Vol. 27, No. 1A (Jan-Feb;), pp. 267-272, ISSN: 0250-7005.

Raingeaud, J.; Gupta, S.; Rogers, J.S.; Dickens, M.; Han, J.; Ulevitch, R.J.; Davis, R.J. (1995). Pro-inflammatory cytokines and environmental stress cause p38 mitogen-activated protein kinase activation by dual phosphorylation on tyrosine and threonine. *The*

Journal of Biological Chemistry, Vol. 270, No. 13 (Mar 31), pp. 7420-7426, ISSN: 0021-9258.

Ricote, M.; Royuela, M.; Garcia-Tuñon, I.; Bethencourt, F.R.; Paniagua, R.; and Fraile, B. (2003). Pro-apoptotic tumor necrosis factor-alpha transduction pathway in normal prostate, benign prostatic hyperplasia and prostatic carcinoma. *Journal of Urology*, Vol. 170, No. 3 (Sep), pp. 787-790, ISSN: 0022-5347.

Ricote, M.; Garcia-Tuñon, I.; Bethencourt, F.R.; Fraile, B.; Paniagua, R.; Royuela, M. (2004). Interleukin-1 (IL-1alpha and IL-1beta) and its receptors (IL-1RI, IL-1RII, and IL-1Ra) in prostate carcinoma. *Cancer*, Vol. 100, No. 7 (Apr 1), pp. 1388-1396, ISSN: 1097-0142.

Ricote, M.; García-Tuñón, I.; Bethencourt, F.; Fraile, B.; Onsurbe, P.; Paniagua, R.; Royuela, M. (2006a). The p38 transduction pathway in prostatic neoplasia. *The Journal of Pathology*, Vol. 208, No. 3 (Feb), pp. 401-407, ISSN: 1096-9896.

Ricote, M.; García-Tuñón, I.; Fraile, B.; Fernández, C.; Aller, P.; Paniagua, R.; Royuela, M. (2006b). P38 MAPK protects against TNF-alpha-provoked apoptosis in LNCaP prostatic cancer cells. *Apoptosis*, Vol. 11, No. 11 (Nov), pp. 1969-1975, ISSN: 1360-8185.

Rodriguez-Berriguete, G.; Prieto, A.; Fraile, B.; Bouraoui, Y.; Bethencourt, F.; Martínez-Onsurbe, P.; Olmedilla, G.; Paniagua, R.; Royuela, M. (2010a). IL-6/ERK/NF-kB transduction pathway: a study in normal and pathological human prostate (benign hyperplasia, intraepithelial neoplasia and cancer). *European Cytokine Network*, Vol. 21, No. 4 (Dec 1), pp. 241-250, ISSN: 1148-5493.

Rodriguez-Berriguete, G.; Fraile, B.; de Bethencourt, F.R.; Prieto-Folgado, A.; Bartolome, N.; Nunez, C.; Prati, B.; Martinez-Onsurbe, P.; Olmedilla, G.; Paniagua, R.; Royuela, M. (2010b). Role of IAPs in prostate cancer progression: immunohistochemical study in normal and pathological (benign hyperplastic, prostatic intraepithelial neoplasia and cancer) human prostate. *BMC Cancer*,Vol. 10 (Jan 15), pp. 18, ISSN: 1471-1407.

Royuela, M.; De Miguel, M.P.; Bethencourt, F.; Fraile, B.; Arenas, M.I.; Paniagua, R. (2000). IL-2, Its receptors, and bcl-2 and bax genes in Normal, Hyperplastic and Carcinomatous human prostates: Immunohistochemical Comparative Analysis. Growth Factors; Vol. 18, No. 2, pp. 135-146, ISSN: 0897-7194.

Royuela, M.; Arenas, M.I.; Bethencourt, F.R.; Sanchez-Chapado, M.; Fraile, B.; Paniagua, R. (2001). Immuno expressions of p21, Rb, mcl-1 and bad gene products in normal, hyperplastic and carcinomatous human prostates. *European Cytokine Network*, Vol. 12, No. 4 (Oct-Dec), pp. 654-663, ISSN: 1148-5493.

Royuela, M.; Arenas, M.I.; Bethencourt, F.R.; Sánchez-Chapado, M.; Fraile, B.; Paniagua, R. (2002). Regulation of proliferation/apoptosis equilibrium by mitogen-activated protein kinases in normal, hyperplastic, and carcinomatous human prostate. *Human Pathology*, Vol. 33, No. 3 (Mar), pp. 299-306, ISSN: 0046-8177.

Royuela, M.; Ricote, M.; Parsons, M.S.; Garcia-Tuñon, I.; Paniagua, R.; De Miguel, M.P. (2004). Immunohistochemical analysis of IL-6 family of cytokines and their receptors in benign, hyperplastic and malignant human prostate. *The Journal of Pathology*, Vol. 202, No. 1 (Jan), pp. 41-49, ISSN: 1096-9896.

Royuela, M.; Rodríguez-Berriguete, G.; Fraile, B.; Paniagua, R. (2008). TNF-alpha/IL-1/NF-kappaB transduction pathway in human cancer prostate. *Histology and Histopathology*, Vol. 23, No. 10 (Oct), pp. 1279-1290, ISSN: 0213-3911.

Rzymski, P.; Opala, T.; Wilczak, M.; Wozniak, J.; Sajdak, S. (2005). Serum tumor necrosis factor alpha receptors p55/p75 ratio and ovarian cancer detection. *International Journal of Gynecology & Obstetrics*, Vol. 88, No. 3, (Mar), pp. 292-298, ISSN: 1097-6868.

Sawhney, R.S.; Liu, W.; Brattain, M.G. (2009). A novel role of ERK5 in integrin-mediated cell adhesion and motility in cancer cells via Fak signaling. *Journal of Cellular Physiology*, Vol. 219, No. 1 (Apr), pp. 152-161, ISSN: 0021-9541.

Shimada, K.; Nakamura, M.; Ishida, E.; Konishi, N. (2006). Molecular roles of MAP kinases and FADD phosphorylation in prostate cancer. *Histology and Histopathology*, Vol. 21, No. 4, (Apr), pp. 415-422, ISSN: 0213-3911.

Silver, J.S. & Hunter, C.A. (2010). gp130 at the nexus of inflammation, autoimmunity, and cancer. *Journal of Leukocyte Biology*, Vol. 88, No. 6, (Dec), pp. 1145-1156, ISSN: 0741-5400.

Smith, C.A.; Davis, T.; Anderson, D.; Solam, L.; Beckmann, M.P.; Jerzy, R.; Dower, S.K.; Cosman, D.; Goodwin, R.G. (1990). A receptor for tumor necrosis factor defines an unusual family of cellular and viral proteins. *Science*, Vol. 248, No. 4958 (May 25), pp. 1019-1023, ISSN: 1095-9203.

Stein, B.; Brady, H.; Yang, M.X.; Young, D.B.; Barbosa, M.S. (1996). Cloning and characterization of MEK-6, a novel member of the mitogen-activated protein kinase kinase cascade. *The Journal of Biological Chemistry*, Vol. 271, No. 19 (May 10), pp. 11427-11433, ISSN: 0021-9258.

Su, G.H.; Hilgers, W.; Shekher, M.C.; Tang, D.J.; Yeo, C.J.; Hruban, R.H.; Kern, S.E. (1998). Alterations in pancreatic, biliary, and breast carcinomas support MKK4 as a genetically targeted tumor suppressor gene. *Cancer Research*, Vol. 58, No. 11 (Jun 1), pp. 2339-2342, ISSN: 0008-5472.

Tartaglia, L.A.; Weber, R.F.; Figari, I.S.; Reynolds, C.; Palladino Jr, M.A.; Goeddel, D.V. (1991). The two different receptors for tumor necrosis factor mediate distinct cellular responses. *Proceedings of the National Academy of Sciences of the United States of America*, Vol. 88, No. 20(Oct 15), pp. 9292-9296, ISSN: 0027-8424.

Taylor, J.L.; Szmulewitz, R.Z.; Lotan, T.; Hickson, J.; Griend, D.V.; Yamada, S.D.; Macleod, K.; Rinker-Schaeffer, C.W. (2008). New paradigms for the function of JNKK1/MKK4 in controlling growth of disseminated cancer cells. *Cancer Letters*, Vol. 272, No. 1 (Dec 8), pp. 12-22, ISSN: 0304-3835.

Thornton, T.M. & Rincon, M. (2009). Non-classical p38 map kinase functions: cell cycle checkpoints and survival. *International Journal of Biological Sciences*, Vol. 5, No. 1 (), pp. 44-51, ISSN: 1449-2288.

Turjanski, A.G.; Vaqué, J.P.; Gutkind, J.S. (2007). MAP kinases and the control of nuclear events. *Oncogene*, Vol. 26, No. 22 (May 14), pp. 3240-3253, ISSN: 0950-9232.

Vayalil, P.K.; Mittal, A.; Katiyar, S.K. (2004). Proanthocyanidins from grape seeds inhibit expression of matrix metalloproteinases in human prostate carcinoma cells, which is associated with the inhibition of activation of MAPK and NF kappa B. *Carcinogenesis*, Vol. 25, No. 6 (Jun), pp. 987-995, ISSN 0143-3334.

Visconti, R.; Cerutti, J.; Battista, S.; Fedele, M.; Trapasso, F.; Zeki, K.; Miano, M.P.; de Nigris, F.; Casalino, L.; Curcio, F.; Santoro, M.; Fusco, A. (1997). Expression of the neoplastic phenotype by human thyroid carcinoma cell lines requires NF-iB p65 protein expression. *Oncogene*, Vol. 15, No. 16 (Oct 16), pp. 1987-1994, ISSN: 0950-9232.

Wajant, H. & Scheurich, P. (2001). Tumor necrosis factor receptor associated factor (TRAF)2 and its role in TNF signaling. *The International Journal of Biochemistry & Cell Biology*, Vol. 33, No. 1 (Jan), pp. 19-32, ISSN: 1357-2725.

Wang, J.; Kuiatse, I.; Lee, A.V.; Pan, J.; Giuliano, A.; Cui, X. (2010). Sustained c-Jun-NH2-kinase activity promotes epithelial-mesenchymal transition, invasion, and survival of breast cancer cells by regulating extracellular signal-regulated kinase activation. *Molecular Cancer Research*, Vol. 8, No. 2 (Feb), pp. 266-277, ISSN: 1541-7786.

Wang, H.Y.; Cheng, Z.; Malbon, C.C. (2003). Overexpression of mitogen-activated protein kinase phosphatases MKP1, MKP2 in human breast cancer. *Cancer Letters*, Vol. 191, No. 2 (Mar 10), pp.229-237, ISSN: 0304-3835.

Wang, S.; Liu, Z.; Wang, L.; Zhang, X. (2009). NF-kappaB signaling pathway, inflammation and colorectal cancer. *Cellular & Molecular Immunology*, Vol. 6, No. 5 (Oct), pp. 327-334, ISSN: 1672-7681.

Wang, X.S.; Diener, K.; Manthey, C.L.; Wang, S.; Rosenzweig, B.; Bray, J.; Delaney, J.; Cole, C.N.; Chan-Hui, P.Y.; Mantlo, N.; Lichenstein, H.S.; Zukowski, M., Yao, Z. (1997). Molecular cloning and characterization of a novel p38 mitogen-activated protein kinase. *The Journal of Biological Chemistry*, Vol. 272, No. 38 (Sep 19), pp. 23668-23674, ISSN: 0021-9258.

Wang, W.; Abbruzzese, J.L.; Evans, D.B.; Larry, L.; Cleary, K.R.; Chiao, P.J. (1999). The nuclear factor-IB transcription factor is constitutively active in human pancreatic adenocarcinoma cells. *Clinical Cancer Research*, Vol. 5, No. 1 (Jan), pp. 119-127, ISSN: 1078-0432.

Werlen, G.; Hausmann, B.; Naeher, D; Palmer, E. (2003). Signaling life and death in the thymus: timing is everything. *Science*, Vol. 299, No. 5614 (Mar 21), pp. 1859-1863, ISSN: 1095-9203.

Whyte, J.; Bergin, O.; Bianchi, A.; McNally, S.; Martin, F. (2009). Key signalling nodes in mammary gland development and cancer. Mitogen-activated protein kinase signalling in experimental models of breast cancer progression and in mammary gland development. *Breast Cancer Research*, Vol. 11, No. 5 (), pp. 209, ISSN: 1465-5411.

Wiegmann, K.; Schutze, S.; Kampen, E.; Himmler, A.; Machleidt, T.; Kronke, M. (1992). Human 55-kDa receptor for tumor necrosis factor coupled to signal transduction cascades. *The Journal of Biological Chemistry*, Vol. 267, No. 25 (Sep 5), pp. 17997-18001, ISSN: 0021-9258.

Wood, C.D., Thornton, T.M.; Sabio, G.; Davis, R.A.; Rincon, M. (2009). Nuclear localization of p38 MAPK in response to DNA damage. Int J Biol Sci; 5:428-37.

Wu, J.T. & Kral, J.G. (2005). The NF-kappaB/IkappaB signaling system: a molecular target in breast cancer therapy. *Journal of Surgical Research*, Vol. 123, No. 1 (Jan), pp. 158-169, ISSN: 0022-4804.

Zebisch, A.; Czernilofsky, A.P.; Keri, G.; Smigelskaite, J.; Sill, H.; Troppmair, J. (2007). Signaling through RAS-RAF-MEK-ERK: from basics to bedside. *Current Topics in Medicinal Chemistry*, Vol. 14, No. 5 (), pp. 601-623, ISSN: 1568-0266.

Zhang, C.; Zhu, H.; Yang, X.; Lou, J.; Zhu, D.; Lu, W.; He, Q.; Yang, B. (2010). P53 and p38 MAPK pathways are involved in MONCPT-induced cell cycle G2/M arrest in human non-small cell lung cancer A549. *Journal of Cancer Research and Clinical Oncology*, Vol. 136, No. 3 (Mar), pp. 437-445, ISSN: 0171-5216.

Zhang, Y.X. & Kong, C.Z. (2008). The role of mitogen-activated protein kinase cascades in inhibition of proliferation in human prostate carcinoma cells by raloxifene: an in vitro experiment. *Zhonghua yi xue yi chuan xue za zhi*, Jan 22;Vol. 88, No. 4 (), pp. 271-5, ISSN: 0376-2491.

Zhao, M.; New, L.; Kravchenko, V.V.; Kato, Y.; Gram, H.; di Padova, F.; Olson, E.N.; Ulevitch, R.J.; Han, J. (1999). Regulation of the MEF2 family of transcription factors by p38. *Molecular and Cellular Biology*, Vol. 19, No. 1 (Jan), pp. 21-30.

Zheng, B.; Fiumara, P.; Li, Y.V.; Georgakis, G.; Snell, V.; Younes, M.; Vauthey, J.N.; Carbone, A., Younes, A. (2003). MEK/ERK pathway is aberrantly active in Hodgkin disease: a signaling pathway shared by CD30, CD40, and RANK that regulates cell proliferation and survival. *Blood*, Vol. 102, No. 3 (Aug 1), pp. 1019-1027, ISSN: 0006-4971.

Zhou, G.; Bao, Z.Q.; Dixon, J.E. (1995). Components of a new human protein kinase signal transduction pathway. *The Journal of Biological Chemistry*, Vol. 270, No. 21 (May 26), pp. 12665-12669, ISSN: 0021-9258

Zhu, Y.; Culmsee, C.; Klumpp, S.; Krieglstein, J. (2004). Neuroprotection by transforming growth factor-beta1 involves activation of nuclear factor-kappaB through phosphatidylinositol-3-OH kinase/Akt and mitogen-activated protein kinase-extracellular-signal regulated kinase1,2 signaling pathways. *Neuroscience*, Vol. 123, No. 4, pp. 897-906, ISSN: 0306-4522.

Zubelewicz, B.; Muc-Wierzgon, M.; Wierzgon, J.; Romanowski, W.; Mazurek, U.; Wilczok, T.; Podwinska, E. (2002). Genetic disregulation of gene coding tumor necrosis factor alpha receptors (TNF alpha Rs) in follicular thyroid cancer-preliminary report. *Journal of Biological Regulators & Homeostatic Agents*, Vol.16, No. 2 (Apr-Jun), pp. 98-104, ISSN: 0393-974X.

Permissions

The contributors of this book come from diverse backgrounds, making this book a truly international effort. This book will bring forth new frontiers with its revolutionizing research information and detailed analysis of the nascent developments around the world.

We would like to thank Philippe E. Spiess, for lending his expertise to make the book truly unique. He has played a crucial role in the development of this book. Without his invaluable contribution this book wouldn't have been possible. He has made vital efforts to compile up to date information on the varied aspects of this subject to make this book a valuable addition to the collection of many professionals and students.

This book was conceptualized with the vision of imparting up-to-date information and advanced data in this field. To ensure the same, a matchless editorial board was set up. Every individual on the board went through rigorous rounds of assessment to prove their worth. After which they invested a large part of their time researching and compiling the most relevant data for our readers. Conferences and sessions were held from time to time between the editorial board and the contributing authors to present the data in the most comprehensible form. The editorial team has worked tirelessly to provide valuable and valid information to help people across the globe.

Every chapter published in this book has been scrutinized by our experts. Their significance has been extensively debated. The topics covered herein carry significant findings which will fuel the growth of the discipline. They may even be implemented as practical applications or may be referred to as a beginning point for another development. Chapters in this book were first published by InTech; hereby published with permission under the Creative Commons Attribution License or equivalent.

The editorial board has been involved in producing this book since its inception. They have spent rigorous hours researching and exploring the diverse topics which have resulted in the successful publishing of this book. They have passed on their knowledge of decades through this book. To expedite this challenging task, the publisher supported the team at every step. A small team of assistant editors was also appointed to further simplify the editing procedure and attain best results for the readers.

Our editorial team has been hand-picked from every corner of the world. Their multi-ethnicity adds dynamic inputs to the discussions which result in innovative outcomes. These outcomes are then further discussed with the researchers and contributors who give their valuable feedback and opinion regarding the same. The feedback is then collaborated with the researches and they are edited in a comprehensive manner to aid the understanding of the subject.

Apart from the editorial board, the designing team has also invested a significant amount of their time in understanding the subject and creating the most relevant covers. They scrutinized every image to scout for the most suitable representation of the subject and create an appropriate cover for the book.

The publishing team has been involved in this book since its early stages. They were actively engaged in every process, be it collecting the data, connecting with the contributors or procuring relevant information. The team has been an ardent support to the editorial, designing and production team. Their endless efforts to recruit the best for this project, has resulted in the accomplishment of this book. They are a veteran in the field of academics and their pool of knowledge is as vast as their experience in printing. Their expertise and guidance has proved useful at every step. Their uncompromising quality standards have made this book an exceptional effort. Their encouragement from time to time has been an inspiration for everyone.

The publisher and the editorial board hope that this book will prove to be a valuable piece of knowledge for researchers, students, practitioners and scholars across the globe.

List of Contributors

Paul Bradley and Philippe E. Spiess
Department of Urologic Oncology, Moffitt Cancer Center, Tampa, FL, USA

Thomas Tallberg
The Institute for Bio-Immunotherapy, Helsinki, Finland

Faik Atroshi
Pharmacology & Toxicology, ELTDK, University of Helsinki, Finland

Makoto Aoshima and Kazuyoshi Yata
Institute of Mathematics, University of Tsukuba, Ibaraki, Japan

Malin Åkerfelt, Ville Härmä and Matthias Nees
Medical Biotechnology Knowledge Centre, VTT technical Research Centre of Finland Turku, Finland

Sophia Marsella-Hatziieremia, Pamela McCall and Joanne Edwards
University of Glasgow, UK

Carmen Veríssima Ferreira, Renato Milani, Eduardo Galembeck and Hiroshi Aoyama
University of Campinas, Brazil

Willian Fernando Zambuzzi
Federal Fluminense University, Brazil

Thomas Martin Halder
TopLab GmbH, Germany

V'yacheslav Lehen'kyi and Natalia Prevarskaya
INSERM, Laboratoire de Physiologie Cellulaire, Equipe labellisée par la Ligue, contre le cancer, Villeneuve d'Ascq and Université de Lille 1, Villeneuve d'Ascq, France

Heidi Schwarzenbach
Department of Tumour Biology, Center of Experimental Medicine, University Medical, Center Hamburg-Eppendorf, Hamburg, Germany

Yao Huang and Yongchang Chang
St. Joseph's Hospital and Medical Center, Phoenix, Arizona, USA

James R. Marthick, Adele F. Holloway and Joanne L. Dickinson
Menzies Research Institute Tasmania, University of Tasmania, Australia

Xiaoying Wang, Marina V. Mikhailova and Alexei G. Basnakian
University of Arkansas for Medical Sciences and Central Arkansas Veterans Healthcare System Little Rock, Arkansas, USA

Glenn Tisman
Cancer Research Building, Whittier, CA, USA

Gonzalo Rodríguez-Berriguete, Benito Fraile, Laura Galvis, Ricardo Paniagua and Mar Royuela
Department of Cell Biology and Genetics. University of Alcalá, Madrid, Spain